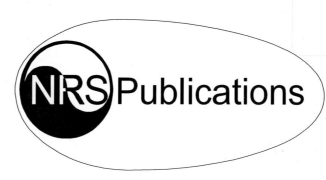

Visual Textbook of Nutritional Medicine
is a product of the
NRS Publications Education Series

Please see our website for
updates on new publications
and seminars
www.nutritionreviewservice.com.au

**Acknowledgements**

Interclinical Laboratories for the use of TMA graphs
My patients for letting me learn so much
The NRS staff for their constant support
Mr. Les Spartalis for his unswerving support
Mr. Henry Osiecki for pointing me in the right direction
Richard P Feynman for answering the Babylonian versus Greek question.
Myke Stanbridge for showing me what scientific investigation is really about.
Blake Graham for making me even more determined to simplify Nutritional Medicine
My Grandmother for giving me her right brain

ISBN  0-9756920-5-4
Title: Visual Textbook of Nutritional Medicine

# Contents

I've always had a problem with structured learning systems. Most of my teachers would attest to this fact. I've always had a problem with textbooks too. Often there would be just one gem in a chapter, and trying to find that sentence quickly would prove very frustrating. Most textbooks I have read were either too verbose or not organised well enough to allow rapid access to the information. I decided that my textbok would be unlike others in that it would allow users from a wide variety of backgrounds to access information for many purposes. In that sense it is more like a quick reference guide.

I designed this text to be used in 3 ways. The first is to outline the basic biochemistry of key nutrients such as Zinc and Vitamin C. Previously, this is something that has been poorly done. Most of the effort seems to have been about minerals with very little enzyme functions like sodium, potassium and calcium.

The second is to outline the process of nutrient flow and the points at which it may go wrong.

The third is to provide a framework for analysis of common medical problems from a molecular/atomic level.

## The 'Bottom line"

# Nutrient not there

**Nutrient Flow**
$\left\{\begin{array}{l}\text{Low in Environment}\\ \text{Low in food}\\ \text{Poor absorption}\\ \text{Pre-cellular wastage}\\ \text{Channelopathy}\end{array}\right.$

# Nutrient ineffective

**Nutrient Blockade**
$\left\{\begin{array}{l}\text{Toxic elements}\\ \text{Drugs}\end{array}\right.$

The bottom line is that there are 2 ways to generate symptoms. Either the nutrient isn't there or it is blocked by something. Traditional approaches that concentrate on deficiencies are totally out of date. They ignore the vast work of Tissue mineral science and metallotoxicology.

There would be some who would criticize such an effort because I didn't mention "such and such". At then end of the day it comes down to atoms anyway, so deeper discussions about larger compounds such as herbs and glyconutrients can only be of use if the end point of action of such compounds is fully understood.

Such writers are not in a position to criticize others who wish to be more reductionist.

Hope you enjoy it.

This book was not designed to detail all the research, but to find themes in the research and provide understanding of the mechanisms that produce health and those that create disease. That is why we use so many graphics. These graphics help us summarise processes or large amounts of research data to unify what we know and give access to information directly in order to solve clinical problems. So basically this book is about problem solving and there are several ways of using it.

The example on the next page might be one that the practitioner would use for a person with ADD/ADHD.

## 1] Clinical Charts

This would involve looking at the clinical chart for this condition. This chart has the biochemical pathway for Noradrenaline. Disruptions to this pathway could cause the syndrome. The table lists (in the rows) the nutrients required to make Noradrenaline and (in the columns) the antagonists that would block this pathway. Sometimes the blocks occur because of multiple, cumulative blocks, and not necessarily just one toxin. Also, clinically we find combinations of low nutrients *and* toxin blockade.

## 2] Nutrient Charts

If, for instance zinc was low or being blocked by another metal, then one might expect zinc deficiency symptoms systemically. The Zinc chart summarizes the types of symptoms by category (anatomical and functional). Charts like these tell us that cations can be blocked in multiple tissues at one time creating "clusters" of symptoms.

## 3] Process Charts.

Other mechanisms are described in the charts that may not be obvious from the text. They help us understand symptom complexes that are not directly related to nutrients, but to failed processes. For instance if digestion is poor then food fragments (or peptides) might embolise to tissues outside the gastrointestinal tract. This poor digestion might then cause hyperactivity, but not through interference with Noradrenaline.

## 4] Nutrient flow

The diagrams below the others refer to nutrient flow. The "scope of agriculture" diagram shows how the farming process introduces heavy metals (like Cadmium) into the food chain. The significance of the Zinc series is that Cadmium will be taken up by plants and then by humans (and their babies). It generates disturbing questions about the vigilance of monitoring by health authorities and explains why TMA's might be abnormal from birth. Those patients who are symptomatic from these toxins may have some compensatory mechanisms at fault, such as increased vulnerability to absorb such toxins (enhanced bio-availability, reduced defence) or faulty cation containment systems through genetics or poor antioxidant levels.

## 5] Final explanation

So when they are all combined, there is an understanding of both the symptom cluster and the process that generated them. This allows us to explain the symptoms and how the illness developed. It also gives us the direction of treatment.

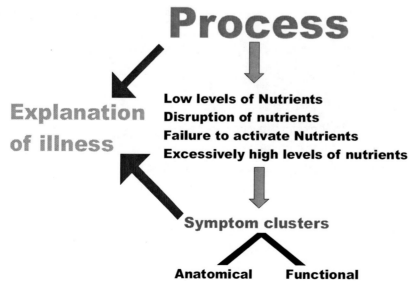

**Process**

**Explanation of illness**

**Low levels of Nutrients**
**Disruption of nutrients**
**Failure to activate Nutrients**
**Excessively high levels of nutrients**

**Symptom clusters**

**Anatomical      Functional**

## Clinical Charts

## Individual Nutrient Charts

## Chapters on Process

### Consequences of poor digestion

Foreign proteins →
- Dizziness, Tinnitus
- Fatigue, Hyperactivity, Agitation
- Pain
- Cough, Wheeze
- Urinary frequency
- Joint pain, Joint stiffness
- Itch, Rash

### Zinc Balance

NRS

**IN** / **OUT**

IN:
Milk*
Beef*
Liver*
Herring
Oysters
Sunflower seeds
Pumpkin seeds
Ginger
Whole grains
Yeast

OUT:
Sweating
Menstrual Fluid
Urine (increased by Food Colouring 102)
Pregnancy
Breast feeding
Faeces
Diuretics, ACE inhibitors
Stress & Anaesthetics
OCP & HRT
Vitamin B6 deficiency

* Zinc deficient soils create zinc deficient cows

Blocked by
Mercury
Cadmium
High Copper

### Zinc Deficiency

Plasma Zinc < 11 µmol/L or Red Cell Zinc < 200 µmol/L

Low Stomach Acid
Salicylate Intolerance

Skin: Dermatitis, Dry Skin, Eczema, Warts, Psoriasis, Pimples, Hair loss, Tinea, Thrush, Stretch Marks

Hair & Nails: Brittle nails, Hair Loss, Early Greying

Lung: Asthma, Bronchitis, Pneumonia, Chest infections

Allergy: Hay fever, Runny nose, Itchy skin

Brain: Disrupted sleep, Poor Memory, Moodiness, Depression, Poor coping with stress, Temper outbursts

Children: Hyper activity, Fidgeting, Pre-dinner tantrums

Joints: Joint pain, Joint stiffness

Sexual Function: Loss of libido, Infertility, Missed periods

Metabolic: Raised Cholesterol, Low Sugar 3 hours after meals, Alcohol Intolerance

Immune System: Frequent sore throats, Colds & Sinusitis, Ear infections, Gastroenteritis, Thrush, Boils/pimples, Delayed healing, Prolonged infections, Conjunctivitis, Low White cell count

### Nutrients important for prevention of ADD ADHD

Proteins
Zinc B1 B6 → (Tyrosine A.al)
**L-Phenylalanine**
Folate from B3 B6 Vit C (Phenylalanine Hydroxylase)
**L-Tyrosine**
Folate from B2 B6 Vit C (Tyrosine Hydroxylase)
**L-Dopa**
Zinc Magnesium B6 Vit C (Dopa Decarboxylase)
**Dopamine**
Copper Vit C (Dopamine Hydroxylase)
**Noradrenaline**

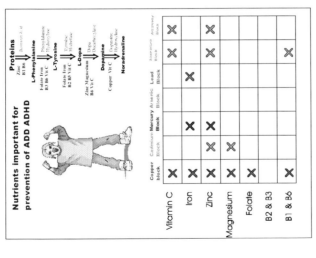

| | Copper Block | Cadmium Block | Mercury Block | Arsenic Block | Lead Block | Aluminium Block | Accessory Block |
|---|---|---|---|---|---|---|---|
| Vitamin C | X | | | | | | X |
| Iron | X | | X | | X | | |
| Zinc | X | X | X | | | | X |
| Magnesium | X | X | | | | | |
| Folate | X | | | | | | |
| B2 & B3 | | | | | | | |
| B1 & B6 | X | | | | | X | |

## Scope of Agriculture

**Raw Materials**
Oxygen
Nitrogen
Carbon
Minerals
Water

**Production**
Pest control

→

Growth accelerators

**Produce**

**Consumption**

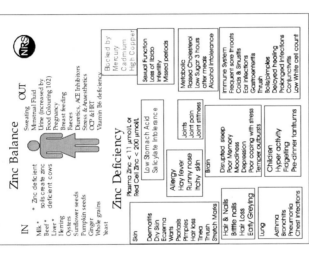

### The "zinc series" of the periodic table

| Zn | Cd | Hg |
|---|---|---|
| 30 | 48 | 80 |
| Zinc | Cadmium | Mercury |

Plants will substitute
Zinc Cadmium Mercury

Humans will substitute
Zinc, Cadmium Mercury

# A Unified Theory of Medicine?

This book is about bringing together wisdom from several scientific disciplines. Sometimes information only makes sense when parts of a puzzle are viewed concurrently by several people in separate disciplines, but for whom there is a common interest. It's like one of those trick graphics; suddenly the old lady jumps out at you, but then you can see the young woman too. Same graphic, different appreciation. By throwing ideas at my friends in different fields, I was able to use their experience to make insights into how the body works and therefore why it might not work. All the research has been done in basic sciences to allow us to bring it together. I have tried to bring together some of it in the references.

I do not wish to ignore other fields of research by focusing on cation function and metallotoxicology, but in clinical practice, problems relating to these areas occur with the greatest frequency.

The argument goes something like this. In order to achieve higher levels of evolution, it became necessary for life forms to incorporate more resources from their environment. The problem with this is that containment systems and more complex control mechanisms were required. For example, increasing anaerobic metabolism for faster movement generates free radicals and carbon dioxide. What becomes of these? How does the organism transport oxygen to the tissues and deal with the free radicals and carbon dioxide? I suggest the book "Oxygen" by Nick Lane (Oxford Press) as an excellent summary of this.

In order to deal with hydroxyl radicals, it became necessary to provide very fine control of free metals within the cells. We want some, but not too many in the wrong place. We need to "lock up the cations". The tendency to disrupt biological systems is related to electro negativity of the charged ion. The better the organism can use these metals without harming itself, the greater the biological advantage.

For instance, bulk ions like sodium and potassium create electrical charge stability in cells, but are not really used for many enzymes. Metals like copper and iron are used predominantly for enzymes and not electrical potential. Calcium and magnesium are little of both. What is interesting about magnesium is that you cannot seem to have too much of it in the cells. It is ubiquitous and the intracellular to extra cellular ratio is about 700:1. Calcium however is heavily contained within cells and not free to roam around like magnesium is. Magnesium turns up as a co-factor in many more enzymes than Calcium, because of its ability to donate electrons for biochemical reactions. We can see from the table the Copper is more electronegative than Hydrogen and yet far more teaching time is given to pH control than to copper control in medical school curricula. In order to avoid pro-oxidant states it is just as important to control Copper, as it is pH! Because of the high prevalence of water, Hydrogen ion management was a very basic step in evolution. The management systems are prevalent in very basic organisms. The point is that *all* the metals with greater electro negativity than hydrogen need to be controlled and when they are not, tissues give warning signs that something is wrong. The answer is not to give drugs to solve the problems, but to listen carefully and make biochemical correlates with the symptoms. When a tissue is having problems with intracellular magnesium, it sends a message to its owner to do something about it. These messages do not automatically mean magnesium deficiency. In order to understand where the problem is we embark on the analysis of nutrient flow.

There is not one single test that can define the problem. We need symptoms, examination, blood, tissue and sometimes urine to work it out. This is the province of Diagnostic Orthomolecular Medicine (DOM), and if this method was taught to doctors generally, we would use far fewer drugs and probably enjoy looking after patients more. For readers who want details about the theory behind this work, see the last Chapter "Some technical stuff".

Hence this is the following sequence that DOM follows.
1] Interpret the symptoms biochemically
2] What links these symptoms?
3] What is the process driving this?
4] What compensatory mechanisms have failed?
5] In what order should the treatment should be carried out?

# Ions , electronegativity and management problems

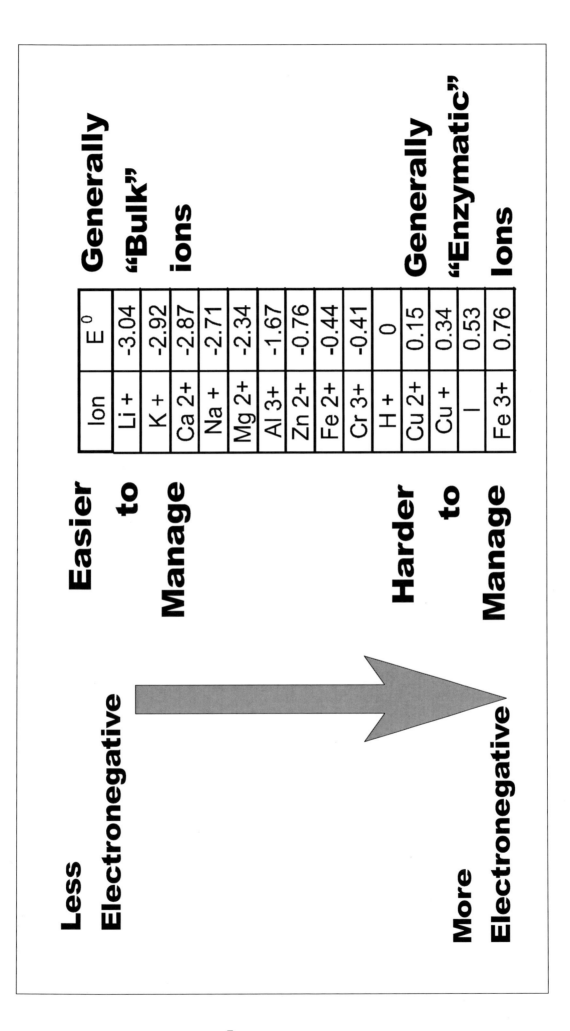

| Ion | $E^0$ |
|-----|-------|
| Li + | -3.04 |
| K + | -2.92 |
| Ca 2+ | -2.87 |
| Na + | -2.71 |
| Mg 2+ | -2.34 |
| Al 3+ | -1.67 |
| Zn 2+ | -0.76 |
| Fe 2+ | -0.44 |
| Cr 3+ | -0.41 |
| H + | 0 |
| Cu 2+ | 0.15 |
| Cu + | 0.34 |
| I | 0.53 |
| Fe 3+ | 0.76 |

**Generally "Bulk" ions**

**Generally "Enzymatic" Ions**

**Easier to Manage**

**Harder to Manage**

**Less Electronegative**

**More Electronegative**

At the end of the day all observations made on the physical world are due to photons and electrons. Because of their electron donating and accepting properties, cations allow us to observe indirectly photons and electron interactions. But *they* are easier to correlate clinically than photons or electrons. Because of the prominence of cation functions in biological systems, it is possible to distil all our observations about health down to problems with cations (bottom line: either ***not there*** or being ***blocked***). Vitamins can be created and modified but minerals are fixed in amount on this planet and not interchangeable.

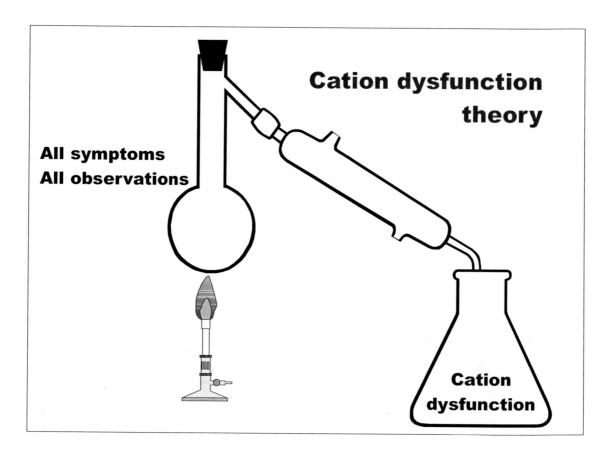

Cation levels in soils directly influence Vitamin levels in plants, which are the major source of Vitamins in our diets. Boron affects B-Vitamins in Turnip greens. Manganese affects Vitamin C in Cabbages etc. Any animal we eat has grazed on those plants and so any Vitamins we get from animals have also been affected by soil levels of cations. Digestion of such Vitamins is reliant upon stomach acid and enzymes, which are heavily reliant upon Zinc. In our bodies, all the vitamins need minerals (especially the divalent cations) to activate them. No minerals, no functioning Vitamins! So it comes down to cations as the most fundamental nutrients in the body.

Let's say that one made seven biochemical observations in patients with illness. What if these were

1] Abnormal mineral levels (cations like sodium, magnesium, copper etc)

2] Toxic Minerals like Lead, Mercury, Cadmium

3] Abnormal glucose control

4] Undermethylation

5] Over methylation

6] Presence of pyrrole's in the urine

7] Abnormalities of EFA function.

Cation dysfunction Theory could explain such findings and link the observations with some more fundamental explanation. The reader will find that the chapters in this book will be able to explain the findings. Therefore I make no apologies that dysfunction of cations is the basis for most of this book.

The term Nutritional Medicine (NM) often misleads doctors into thinking that the specialty primarily involves diets and lifestyle changes. Orthomolecular Medicine is probably a better description but it has a rather tarnished reputation. So we resort to the term Nutritional Medicine so as not to alienate our patients and colleagues.

Page one of any pathology textbook will tell you that by the time disease is detectable by microscopy there must have been a structural change. The structural change must have involved an alteration in the biochemistry which steers the cell in a direction away from the one that nature had intended. They will say look up a biochemistry book to find out what this change entails. The biochemistry books fail to link the pathobiochemistry with the clinical symptoms and everybody basically passes the buck. The truth is that nutritional medicine *links* the various specialties and as the middleman, explains of all observed phenomena.

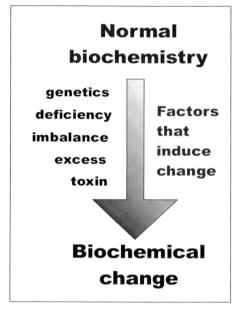
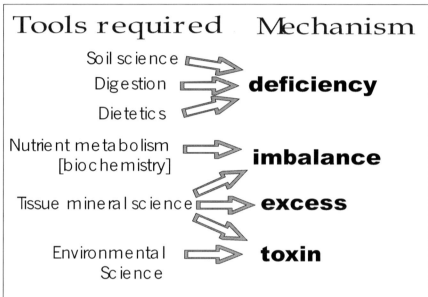

The process that drives normal biochemistry to abnormal biochemistry involves any combination of five factors. Genetics, deficiency, excess, imbalance or toxins. In order to understand these processes, there are tools required and access to the appropriate literature. Most of these tools were *never* taught to doctors and the source of the literature was never pointed out because it involved technical areas "outside of our business". So in order to solve certain problems, new areas of knowledge must be learned. These include soil science, Dietetics, tissue mineral science and Environmental science. Only after being armed with these extra tools can a full analysis be made. The problem is that many doctors do not wish to exceed the boundaries of what they were taught because their teachers in medical school or post graduate training programs threatened them if they did. Consequently potentially useful pieces of information presented to them were probably discarded.

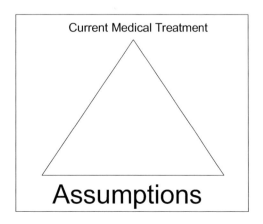

This is an example of how medicine deals with information. Let's say you got a puzzle for your birthday. You look at the box's cover quickly and say, "It's a beach scene". You start sifting through the pieces. You find an air conditioner. What is this doing here? Obviously packed in the wrong box- throw it out. Next you find a Ferrari. What is this doing here? Obviously packed in the wrong box- chuck it out. Next a 747. What is this doing here? Obviously packed in the wrong box- chuck it out. Finally, you finish the puzzle and there are pieces missing. Well, the beach scene was near the Gold Coast. The aircon was the top of a beach house. The Ferrari was a reflection in a pair of expensive sunglasses. The 747 was in the edge of the picture because the flight path comes over the beach. This how medicine deals with information outside the square. Nutritional medicine NEVER throws away a piece. Two very good examples of this are the Introns associated with DNA and Glial cells in the brain. Both of these were basically ignored in their importance before, and now we have to go back and count these "pieces" again!!

The problem is that the pieces come from a variety of scientific disciplines, each with their own nomenclature and histories. This creates a problem for linear thinkers. Everything is connected to everything! For the narrow minded brainwashed medical profession, this type of mindset is *intolerable* and unfortunately it involves *unlearning* some things. It involves questioning the objectivity of some key concepts in medicine and in fact it involves key concepts at the very bottom of the Aristotelian based knowledge pyramid, of which we are so proud. Could our hallowed teachers have been wrong? Could they have been *really* wrong? Could *their* teachers have been wrong too?

Moreover, who controls the curriculum of a medical school? Who controls not only what is included, but also what is *excluded* from such curricula? At this point, the issues become political. Unfortunately many issues in nutritional medicine *are* political, especially about toxins in the environment. Many nutritional medicine doctors harbor anti-establishment sentiment, because they see the truth behind the illness that confronts them every day. The truth ignored by the majority of the profession. People who tell the truth have never been popular in history. The world turns predominately because the majority of the affluent create a reality and stick to it by consensus. Working in Nutritional Medicine is very much like the X-files of medicine. Thousands of anecdotes adding up to a huge conspiracy. The conspiracy to perpetuate chronic illness. And behind that, the vested interests in that outcome.

One good example of this refers to the biochemistry of serotonin. The pathway is depicted below. It includes the cofactors (never emphasized in medical schools of course). We say to the patients that they have a "chemical abnormality" and that they need more chemicals to fix this. We never ask, "Why can't this patient *make* serotonin?" If the biochemistry has been worked for 20 years, then why are we encouraged to use SSRI's instead of investigating such patients?

Moreover, supplements containing tryptophan and hydroxy-tryptophan are either unavailable or Schedule 4 items. This is where the politics enter the equation

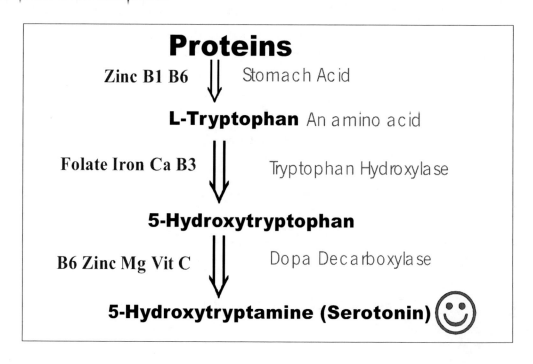

Ordinarily our bodies work transparently to us, just like using a motorcar. We turn the key, the engine starts and we never have to understand about transistors, ignition, fuel injection, pistons, exhausts etc. We only take note when something goes wrong. Bodies are the same. Symptoms are cells crying out for help. Just like babies, if we can decode the cry, we can deduce why the baby is crying. There are 4 reasons why they might cry. 1] Reduced intake. 2] Rapid loss 3] Poor tissue uptake. 4] Intracellular blockade. The key to analyzing a nutritional problem is to find out what is the process that has affected nutrient flow.

# How to analyse a problem

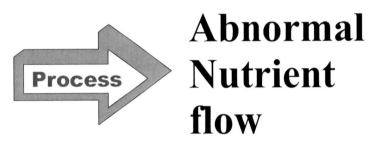

**Environmental issues**

**Nutrient function**

**Biochemical pathways**

**Failed compensatory mechanisms**

Process → **Abnormal Nutrient flow**

In general, each nutrient is carefully adjusted within a range. Low levels cause problems and there is evidence that high levels also cause problems. The diagram below demonstrates such a relationship with say immune activity. Too low a level is associated with immunodeficiency, but too high a level is associated with inmmunodepression. For many years we thought that Vitamin C was exempt from this rule, but recently this exemption has been queried.

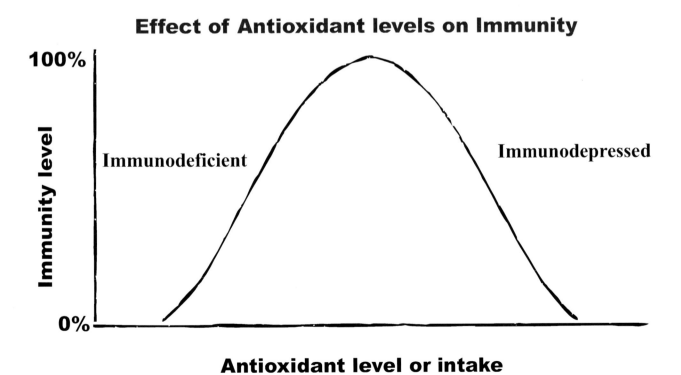

**Effect of Antioxidant levels on Immunity**

Immunity level — 100% ... 0%

Immunodeficient

Immunodepressed

**Antioxidant level or intake**

1] Reduced Intake can be caused by any problem in the food chain that connects the environment to the gut. This includes poor food choices!

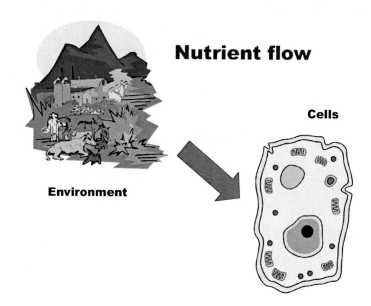

2] Poor digestive efficiency will lead to both malabsorption and lack of defence against the immunogenicity of food. Only inert molecules should traverse the intestinal wall. The very things one could give safely intravenously.

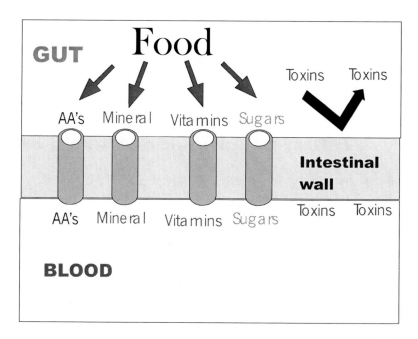

3] Rapid loss might mean enhanced liver excretion, lowered renal threshold, might mean oxidation within the blood stream, or heavy menstrual loss.

4] Intracellular blockade means that the levels of a nutrient might be normal or high, but the function is "cancelled out" by another compound. For example Mercury has a 1000 fold antagonism to zinc. This concept leads us to the idea of Nutrients and Antinutrients.

A theme which readers may have picked up from my articles relates to the concept of balance within biological systems. This is a feature of eastern medicine, which is generally not incorporated into western science, perhaps with the exception of physics. Balance can be described as "when two opposing components create equilibrium in a biological system". In other words, these can be naturally opposing components like zinc and copper or a nutrient and its counteracting *antinutrient* such as zinc and cadmium. A list below shows examples of such nutrient antinutrient combinations.

# Anti-nutrients

**Lead** blocks Iron Calcium Molybdenum
Manganese Chromium Sulphur Cobalt

**Mercury** blocks Zinc selenium iron sulphur cobalt
transmembrane ion channels

**Cadmium** blocks Zinc Magnesium Selenium Sulphur

**Arsenic** blocks Vit E selenium sulphur boron

**Aluminium** blocks Vit E Vit C Vit B1 Zinc Selenium
Sodium Potassium Phosphorus

**Antimony** blocks Zinc Selenium

In this situation, minerals are somewhat easier to understand because we could mentally imagine one mineral blocking anothers function within an enzyme. What is poorly understood is that Antinutrients can cause havoc within cells without being labelled as toxic i.e. below "toxic" levels. The definitions of toxicity are primarily defined by industry, not medicine. These industries wish to define toxicity by the least sensitive method of detection. Tissue mineral analysis is the most sensitive method of detection of heavy metals; hence industry will not use this tool. This spills over into the medical profession, who cannot understand why hair analysis is so useful for the improvement of health.

**Very important Concept**

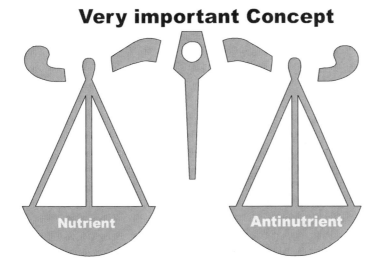

13

The point is this: you cannot understand the level of a nutrient unless you measure its *opposing* component. For instance, a normal ferritin in the presence of lead, will still give symptoms of iron deficiency. A normal red cell zinc in the presence of excess copper will still give the symptoms of zinc deficiency. A normal red cell magnesium in the presence of cadmium will still give symptoms of magnesium deficiency. Just measuring the blood levels and making assumptions about the opposing component *will not always work*. In fact it may lead to unnecessary and prolonged supplementation, with the eventual increasing of dose to control symptoms. If the copper is rising, then you need more Vitamin C over time to prevent say bleeding gums.

Balance is not just a simple set of scales; it involves three or four-dimensions. The figure below shows that copper, zinc, magnesium and molybdenum need to be in balance for correct energy cycles. Abnormalities of this tetrahedron and the main problem in chronic fatigue syndrome. Another figure shows the balance between magnesium, sodium, potassium and calcium. The balance of this tetrahedron determines nervous system function. When one combines the two, with magnesium in the centre, we see that alterations in one eventually lead to a change in the other tetrahedral balance. *These balances cannot be determined by blood test*. Only a tissue sample will provide this type of information. Biochemistry occurs in the tissues, not the blood. More importantly the solution requires understanding *why* the imbalance occurred and at which point, did disruption occur.

# Mineral balance and function

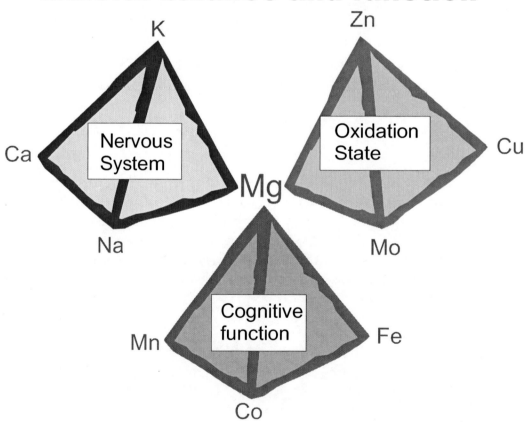

My final point is this: an analysis of why the tetrahedra gets out of balance is paramount in finding a long-term solution. Secondly, those who prescribe nutrients without an appreciation of Anti-nutrients and balance do not understand the whole process of illness.

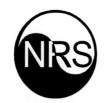

# Introduction to Nutritional Medicine

## Lecture 1
## Principles of NM

When I started in general practice I realized and I had not been taught everything and I needed to know to make my patients get better. In order to find out what was wrong with them I had to read outside the literature in which I've been indoctrinated.

What I realized was the amount of information was vast and yet it seemed to be hidden in some little repository away from the medical profession

So I started a personal journey of investigation

What you will see today and tomorrow is the culmination of five years of research

## Nutrition in the broadest terms

Visual aesthetics

Air          Food

Learning          Acoustics

Water          Love

Spirituality

To really put any scientific work into context we must be humble .

We must realize that there are more things that nurture us than we put in our mouths.

## Process

Explanation
of illness

Low levels of Nutrients
Disruption of nutrients
Failure to activate Nutrients
Excessively high levels of nutrients

Symptom clusters

Anatomical          Functional

To explain the illness to our patient involves understanding the processes that drive symptoms

These processes include low levels of nutrients, disruption of nutrients, failure to activate them, and possibly excessively high levels of nutrients

Patients who have illness for any length of time will usually have more than one symptom.

The symptoms develop as clusters and are usually a failure of divalent cations to function properly.

What's interesting is that there is a large body of research that has been done on dysfunction of these cations, but the research is scattered in many different disciplines.

Symptom clusters occur anatomically for instance in the skin, muscle, lung.

They also occur functionally. That is a disruption to blood sugar control or cognitive dysfunction.

By understanding the processes that cause disruptions to nutrients and by understanding the symptom clusters we can explain the illness to ourselves and to the patient using tangible concepts.

# Genesis of disease

Page one of any pathology textbook will tell you that by the time you can detect a structural change in an organism there must have been a change in the biochemistry.

So there is a change from normal to abnormal with the spectrum as shown on the slide. By the time pathological change occurs it is quite an obvious disease. Medicine is very good with dealing with obvious disease.

Early symptoms show up as symptom clusters and at this point the disease could be reversed.

So you can see that there is a point where the patient loses wellness. They are not really sick but they are not really well either. These symptoms are cells crying out for help. When the cry goes unheeded for long enough, then pathological change will ensue and cause disease.

**Abnormal**                              **Normal**

| Pathological change | Biochemical change | Normal biochemistry |
|---|---|---|
| Gross Symptoms | Early symptoms | No symptoms |

## Driving forces of Biochemical Change

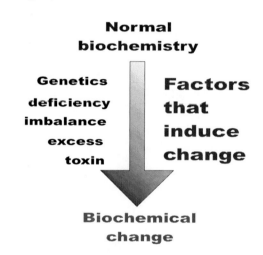

Normal biochemistry

Genetics
deficiency
imbalance
excess
toxin

**Factors that induce change**

Biochemical change

So what are the driving forces of this biochemical change? The five factors can be analyzed. They are genetics, deficiency, imbalance, excess and toxins.

The tools required to understand these mechanisms involve soil science, digestion, dietetics, nutrient metabolism tissue mineral science and environmental science.

## Tools required     Mechanism

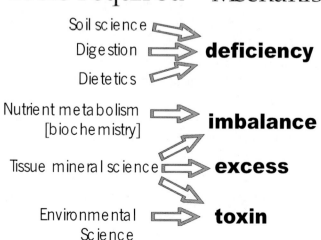

Soil science
Digestion
Dietetics

**deficiency**

Nutrient metabolism [biochemistry]

**imbalance**

Tissue mineral science

**excess**

Environmental Science

**toxin**

Most of these tools have not been taught to doctors and in general they have no idea how to access them after leaving medical school. And yet they are the basic driving forces that create the diseases of the patients they see everyday. This is a travesty. We will be using these tools during the next two days. We'll be using these tools to understand why people get sick.

## What is nutritional medicine?

1. The way medicine should be

2. Using biochemistry to heal

3. The eclectic use of all published and anecdotal data for improving health

4. Really listening to patients and using the most appropriate and least toxic method to help them.

5. The use of vitamins and minerals to prevent and heal illness

6. The restoration of health by the rebalancing of cell processes.

So what is nutritional medicine? Here are six definitions that you can ponder on. My favorite is probably number four. Why number four? Last year one and a half thousand Australians died from medication-related illnesses. There were 140,000 hospital admissions related to medications. There were 400,000 reported adverse drug reactions. Now, knowing how pressured doctors are and reluctant to criticize the system, the real adverse reaction rate must be closer to 4 million per year. That is why I like definition number four.

# Rules of Nutrition

1. There is no average person.

2. There is no average or typical cell – each cell is a specialist cell.

3. Each cell has an output that defines it.

4. Drug companies control studies and publications.

5. Doctors are threatened not to exceed the boundaries of what they were taught.

So what are the rules of nutrition? The first one is that there is no average person; each person is as unique as their fingerprints. The second rule is that there is no average or typical cell. Each cell is a specialist cell. The Third rule is that each cell has an output that defines it. An eye cell sees, and a heart cell pumps blood. The fourth rule is that drug companies control studies and publications. When your doctor leaves medical school, most of the information plonked on his desk is, glossy brochures produced by drug companies. Rule five, is that doctors are threatened not to exceed the boundaries of what they were taught. If you examine how the tertiary institutions work, you'll see that these are basically using a model called "conformational learning". That is, you don't pass until you conform. You may have the right answer, but if it is not the answer your teachers want then you don't pass. Medicine is a very good example of this.

# Sources of information

1] Basic biochemistry
2] Basic physics
3] Descriptive studies
   a) Deprivation studies
   b) Single agent trials

4] Pathological observations
5] Personal observation

**Constant updating of basic biochemistry**

Theoretically five sources of information should lead to a constant updating of basic biochemistry. These are basic biochemistry, basic physics, descriptive studies,

## "Blind spots" in Modern Medicine

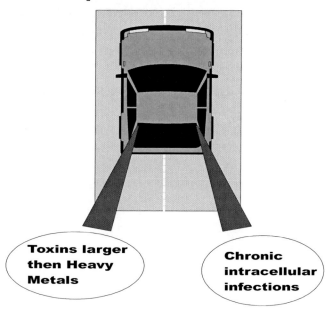

**Toxins larger then Heavy Metals**

**Chronic intracellular infections**

Another problem is that doctors are not really told the limits of their diagnostic capabilities. In fact, there are two blind spots in modern medicine. The first one is any toxin with an atomic mass larger than a heavy metal. And second is chronic intracellular infections. Judging by the number of people on this planet with these problems. You can see why complimentary health practitioners are so popular.

I heard a story (and I am not sure it if it is true) about Harvard Medical School. The story goes like this. When the medical students finally graduate, the Dean gets up and congratulates them. And he gives them one of those "good news-bad news" stories. He says, "I've got some bad news, and some really bad news. The bad news is that about one third of what we taught you is incorrect. The really bad news is that we don't know which third it is".

*"Biochemistry should understood, not just memorised. "*

**Linus Pauling**

*"Biochemistry mostly occurs in the tissues, not in the blood"*

**21st century Nutritionist**

Here are another couple of good quotes. "Biochemistry should be understood, not just memorized". This is from Linus Pauling. The second quote is "Biochemistry, mostly occurs in the tissues, not in the blood". This is from me. And as we understand more about tissue mineral analysis, you will understand why I say this.

## First axiom of nutritional medicine

You cannot assess a nutrient in isolation of its opposing component

For example an analysis of magnesium is not complete without
an analysis of copper, boron and cadmium

The first axiom of nutritional medicine is "You cannot assess a nutrient in isolation of its opposing component". For example what does a Magnesium level mean without an analysis of Copper, boron or Cadmium? Because these other minerals are in balance with magnesium and alter its function within the cell.

## Second axiom of nutritional medicine

Do not assume that because a nutrient is required in small amounts that it is not important

An analogy.
The amount of rubber used in constructing an aeroplane is very small compared to total mass.

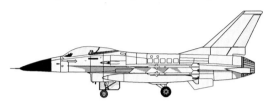

The second axiom of nutritional medicine is do not assume that because the nutrient is required in small amounts that it is not important. When you read biochemistry books you often read throwaway lines, like "Chromium is a trace element and therefore is not as important as sodium". The analogy is imagine the amount of rubber used in constructing an aeroplane. The total weight of the tyres is very small. Yet imagine trying to do without them when you land the plane?

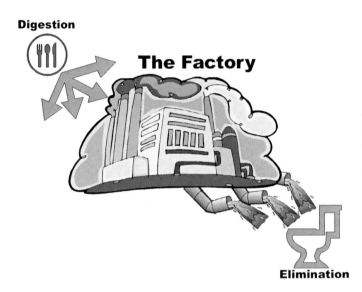

A useful analogy (and I'm glad the philosopher to Gurdjieff agrees) is to think of the human body as a three-storey factory. The input to the factory is basically digestion, and the effluent from the factory is elimination.

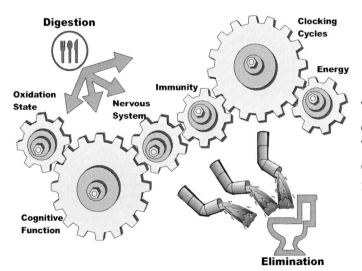

Take the roof off the factory and you see the workings of it within. And these look like cogs within a machine. Taking a closer look, we can subdivide the six cogs into oxidation state, cognitive function, the nervous system, immunity, clocking cycles, and energy.

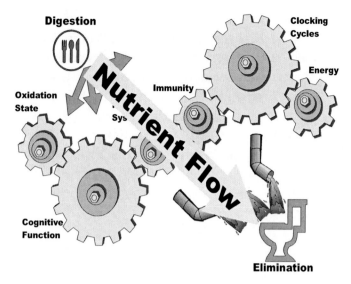

By analyzing nutrient flow through the machine, we understand the mechanism of disease states.

# Concepts of DOM

**Nutrient flow**

**Oxidation state management**

**Cation containment**

**Tissue cooperation**

**Antinutrients**

There are five concepts of Diagnostic Orthomolecular Medicine.

These are, nutrient flow, oxidation state management, cation containment, tissue cooperation, and antinutrients. As the lectures progress, you will see these concepts, turn up quite frequently.

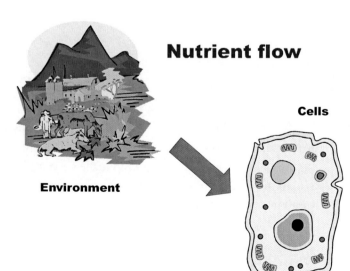

Let's take the first example of nutrient flow. A nutrient has to come from the environment (that is the exterior) and traverse many hurdles to get into the cells.

## Nutrient utilisation

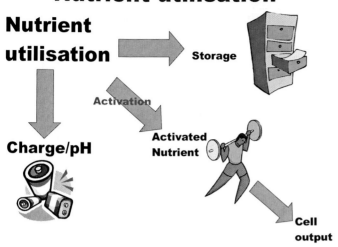

Once it gets to the cells, three things can happen to it. It can be stored, it can be activated, or it can play a part in the charge or pH of the cell.

## Scope of Agriculture

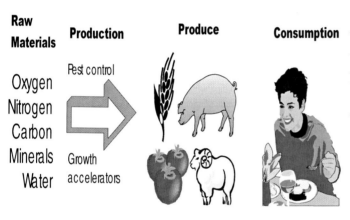

The step from the environment into the organism involves the scope of agriculture. Agriculture takes raw materials, processes them through a production method to create what we eat. The production method involves pest control and growth acceleration. This tampering is where toxins are introduced to the organism.

# Generation of symptoms

1] Lack of nutrient (malabsorption)

2] Poor tissue uptake (Channelopathy)

3] Enhanced loss (Tissue bypass)

4] Nutrient blockade (Intracellular antagonism)

So what causes symptoms? First of all, the lack of a nutrient. This is called malabsorption, but it may involve poor dietary choices or be related to the scope of agriculture. The second is poor tissue uptake or Channelopathy. The third reason is enhanced loss or tissue bypass. And the last is nutrient blockade or intracellular antagonism.

## 1] Lack of nutrient (malabsorption)

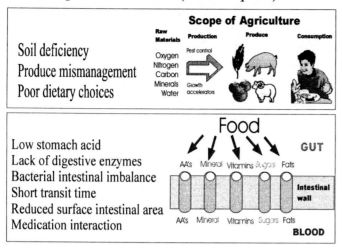

Soil deficiency
Produce mismanagement
Poor dietary choices

Low stomach acid
Lack of digestive enzymes
Bacterial intestinal imbalance
Short transit time
Reduced surface intestinal area
Medication interaction

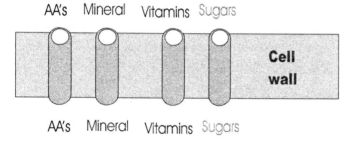

In the case of lack of nutrient, soil deficiency and produce mismanagement contribute to low levels of nutrients in the food we eat. Equally, another problem is poor dietary choices. When magnesium deficient patients see a list of foods that contain magnesium, they will often say, "I don't eat *any* of those things". After you ingest the produce it's the gastrointestinal tract, and a number of other factors that produce malabsorption. Low stomach acid, a lack of digestive enzymes, imbalance of the intestinal flora, reduced time for absorption (intestinal hurry), and interaction with medications are all factors, which reduce the transfer of nutrients from the gut to the bloodstream.

## 2] Poor tissue uptake (Channelopathy)

**BLOOD**

AA's    Mineral    Vitamins    Sugars

Cell wall

AA's    Mineral    Vitamins    Sugars

**Cells**

The second reason is poor tissue uptake or Channelopathy. What this means is that the passage of nutrients across cell membranes from the blood to the cells is blocked.

# Effect of Mercury

OUTSIDE **Membrane Channels**

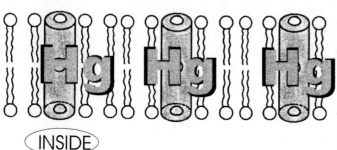

INSIDE

One example of this is Mercury. Mercury causes significant Channelopathies. The hallmark of this problem is a longing. The cells are "starving in a sea of plenty". A very good example of this is diabetes. Imagine not being able to transport glucose, across cell membranes, and then it would build up in the blood. What this means is that there may be the focal areas of Channelopathy in a person, which give rise to symptoms in these areas. Imagine a calf muscle, not being able to import magnesium. The blood level may be normal, the tissue mineral analysis level may be normal, but the patient responds to magnesium. According to the Nobel prizewinners for physiology and medicine in 1991, Channelopathy, may be the commonest cause of chronic illness.

## 3] Enhanced loss (tissue bypass)

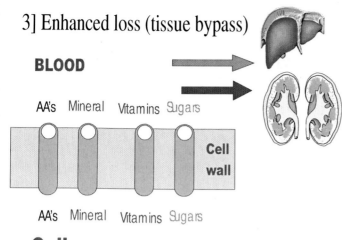

**BLOOD**

AA's  Mineral  Vitamins  Sugars

Cell wall

AA's  Mineral  Vitamins  Sugars

**Cells**

The third problem is enhanced loss or tissue bypass. One example is in the trace elements. After absorption from the small intestine, trace elements like Iron or Manganese all go to the liver via the portal vein. The liver may then decide to immediately excrete that mineral into the bile.

## Anti-nutrients

| | |
|---|---|
| **Lead** | blocks Iron Calcium Molybdenum Manganese Chromium Sulphur Cobalt |
| **Mercury** | blocks Zinc selenium iron sulphur cobalt transmembrane ion channels |
| **Cadmium** | blocks Zinc Magnesium Selenium Sulphur |
| **Arsenic** | blocks Vit E selenium sulphur boron |
| **Aluminium** | blocks Vit E Vit C Vit B1 Zinc Selenium Sodium Potassium Phosphorus |
| **Antimony** | blocks Zinc Selenium |

The fourth reason, that causes symptoms is nutrient blockade, or intracellular antagonism. This means that adequate levels of a nutrient in a cell may be ineffectual, because of another compound. For example, lead, the heavy metal will block Iron, Calcium, Molybdenum, Manganese, Chromium, Sulphur and Cobalt. Which means a patient may appear Iron deficient clinically, but have a normal level of Iron, by any method you care to measure it. When the lead opposes Iron, the Iron cancels out behaving as if it was not there. This is the concept of anti -nutrients.

## 4] Nutrient blockade (Intracellular antagonism)

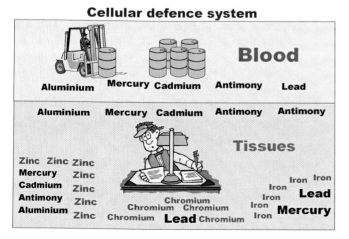

**Cellular defence system**

There are specific methods to deal with toxins like lead. Tissue mineral analysis may show these methods being utilized without showing the lead. Here's another quote "Toxins exert their effect at a distance". Sometimes the only clue is a raised Chromium level on a tissue mineral analysis (TMA). As the patient goes through a catharsis, we see the lead being excreted at a later date.

# Genes dictate _where_ toxins go

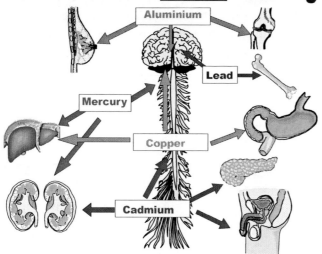

Genes actually dictate where the toxins go. There are genes that may send Cadmium or aluminum to the central nervous system. If you have one of these genes and you have the exposure and the oxidative stress, then you will develop some neurodegenerative disorder like multiple sclerosis or amyotrophic lateral sclerosis.

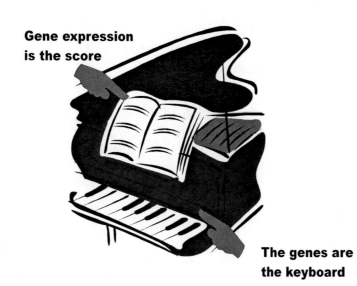

**Gene expression is the score**

**The genes are the keyboard**

The subject of genetics has come under some review recently. There is a new science called Epigenetics. It turns out that a lot of the genetic material in the nucleus was thought of as junk. We thought that only the nice double Helix could possibly store information. That even within the double Helix only transcription units could possibly store information. Transcription units are those that code for a protein. And over 50 years we have ignored non-transcription units and the other proteins associated with DNA. This is a major blunder. The genetics books being rewritten as we speak. The upshot of this is that we now think of genes rather differently. The genes are like the piano keyboard and gene expression is the score. If you have a slightly out of tune F sharp, but you never play that key you will never know about this problem. And if you did press this key it could be drowned out by the noise of the other keys. And gene expression is the volume control. It is not an all or none phenomenon

There are various factors that determine the volume of gene expression, one of the most important of these is S-adenosyl-methionine or SAMe.

## Driving forces of Biochemical Change

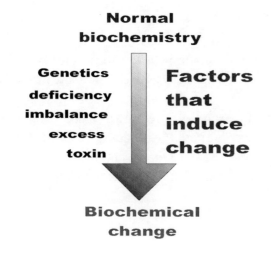

**Normal biochemistry**

**Genetics deficiency imbalance excess toxin**

**Factors that induce change**

**Biochemical change**

So when it comes to genetics already taught to doctors, this maybe part of the one third of the incorrect information, just like the Dean of Harvard Medical School said. But it also means that we need not be defeatist about the influence of genetics in disease, because genes can be turned on and off by environment and Lifestyle, which are changeable.

## Soil & environmental Science Basics

1. Humans thrive in areas where they were _meant_ to survive

2. To bend nature, humans have to use chemicals

3. Australian soils are low in zinc, molybdenum, manganese and selenium

4. Pesticides were widely used in metro areas as well as farms and forrests

6. Many metro areas were originally maket gardens or small farms

7. Clay liners were NOT always used in refuse pits

8. In the mandatory recording of pesticide use , Farming has previously been exempt from the National Register

## Charged ions

| "Bulk" ions low Mol Wt | | |
|---|---|---|
| Sodium<br>Potassium<br>Calcium | Strong<br>containment<br>systems | VERY few<br>enzymes<br>use these<br>as cofactors !!!!!! |

| Microminerals | | |
|---|---|---|
| Magnesium<br>Zinc<br>Iron<br>Copper<br>Manganese<br>Molybdenum<br>Selenium<br>Chromium<br>Cobalt | Mostly cations (two plus charge)<br>Electron donors<br>Containment systems _except_ Mg | Hundreds<br>of enzymes<br>use these<br>as cofactors!!!!!! |

So here is the bad news about Soil and environmental science basics. Humans live in areas where they were meant to survive. To bend nature we have to use chemicals. Australian soils are low in Zinc, Molybdenum, Manganese and Selenium. Pesticides were widely used in metropolitan areas as well as farms and forests. Many Metro areas were originally market gardens or small farms. When they were sold for residential housing, they still contained the residues of the pesticides. Clay liners were not always used in refuse pits. Which means the lead acid batteries leaking the lead; the car tyres are leaking Cadmium into the groundwater. In the mandatory recording of chemical use pesticides used for farming have been previously exempt from the National register. We have no idea how much pesticides were used on our farms. We do, however, know something about the usage in Tasmania. The reason is that as it is an island all imports were described on manifests on ships or planes. If Tasmania is in anyway indicative, then we are in big trouble.

The next slide is about charged atoms in cells. I have split these into bulk ions and micro minerals. Most of medical school teaching focuses on the low molecular weight bulk ions like sodium, potassium and Calcium. Very few enzymes used these cofactors and yet the bulk of biochemistry is about enzymes. The enzymes of the body use mostly the micro minerals (especially divalent cations) like magnesium, Zinc, Iron & Manganese. So why did they spend so much time telling us about sodium and potassium and Calcium? It begs the question about who controls the curriculum in medical schools? What is the motivation behind the curriculum? And why did our teachers, stop reading the research after the seventies? Why wasn't the biochemistry being updated?

# "The single most successful strategy to prevent hydroxyl radicals was the ability to hide intracellular metals

**Professor Bilinski**

It seems Professor Bilinski believes that cation containment was a huge evolutionary step. What this means is that we need our metals in the cell, but not too much of them at any one time.

# "Lock up your cations !"

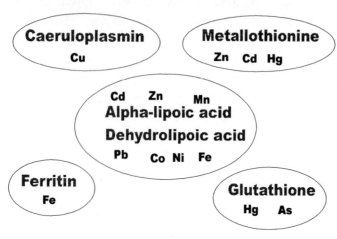

So we created cation cages. I call this "lock up your cations". And these systems, which include caeruloplasmin, ferritin, metallothionine, glutathione and Lipoic acid are all important for the containment of good metals and bad ones.

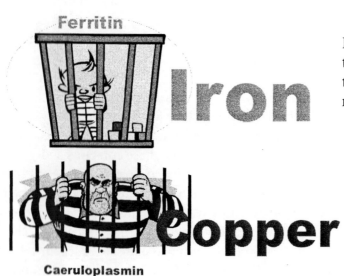

For instance, ferritin and caeruloplasmin mechanisms to control Iron and Copper. Why do we need to control Iron and Copper? Because they are very electro negative, more so than hydrogen ion.

## Metallothionine Structure

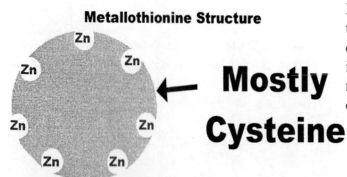

Mostly Cysteine

Metallothionine is a method that uses Zinc and cysteine to control Copper and heavy metals, like Mercury in various tissues, like the skin, the stomach, the intestine the liver and the brain. Abnormalities of metallothionine help us understand the clinical picture of autism.

# 3] Nutrient blockade (Intracellular antagonism)

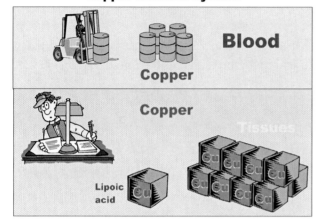

**Copper defence system**

Lipoic acid is one of the methods of controlling Copper. If the cell accumulates Copper, then Lipoic acid may be used to contain it.

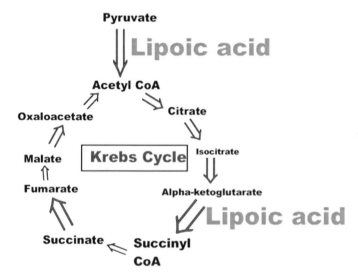

That is, if you can spare enough from the Krebs cycle.

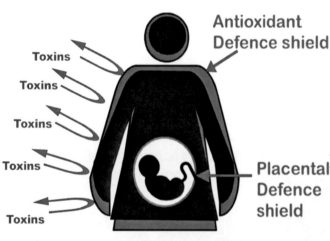

All in all, the antioxidant defence shield protects us from toxins trying to invade us and our babies.

# Antioxidants

| Metals | Vitamins | Bioflavonoids |
|---|---|---|
| Zinc | Vitamin A | Beta carotene |
| Copper | Vitamin C | grapeseed extract |
| Manganese | Vitamin E | pine bark extract |
| Selenium | Vitamin K | lycopene |
| Molybdenum | | quercetin |
| | | rutin |
| | | hesperidin |

These antioxidants might be categorized into three types metals, vitamin C and bioflavonoids.

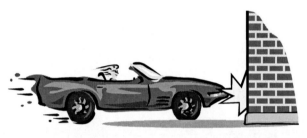

**Antioxidant air-bag**

At the end of the day, they are like the airbag in the car that protects you from getting injured when you crash.

## Defence shield down

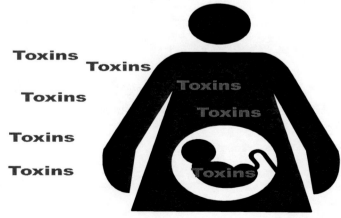

Toxins

Toxins

Toxins

Toxins

Toxins

Toxins

Another problem is that when the defence shield is down toxins can invade you and your unborn child. We see this more commonly today than ever before.

# Toxin infiltration

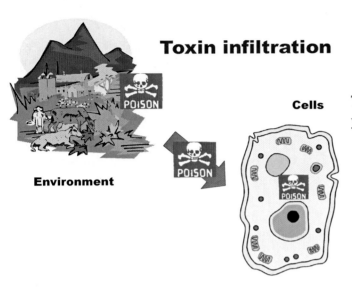

**Environment**

**Cells**

Toxins can "hitch a ride" with the nutrients to get into your cells.

# Toxin infiltration

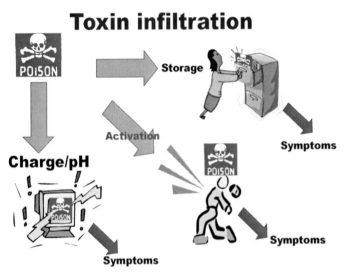

**Storage**

**Activation**

**Charge/pH**

**Symptoms**

**Symptoms**

**Symptoms**

Once a toxin infiltrates you, it can do damage in three ways. You may store it with your nutrients, and this will give rise to symptoms. The toxin may affect the activation of nutrients. This will also give symptoms. And finally the toxin may affect the charge or the pH of the cell. This may give rise to electrical instability or excessive, acidity or alkalinity.

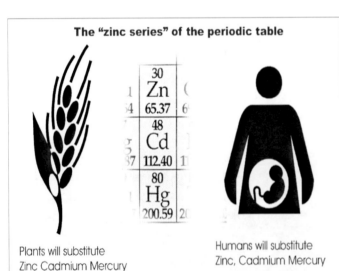

The "zinc series" of the periodic table

| | 30 | |
|---|---|---|
| 1 | Zn | ( |
| 4 | 65.37 | 6 |
| | 48 | |
| r | Cd | |
| 7 | 112.40 | 1 |
| | 80 | |
| | Hg | |
| | 200.59 | 2( |

Plants will substitute
Zinc Cadmium Mercury

Humans will substitute
Zinc, Cadmium Mercury

A very good example of this is the passage of Cadmium and Mercury into the cells, when they hitch a ride with Zinc in the food chain. The Zinc series of the periodic table shows that Zinc, Cadmium and Mercury have similar atomic structures. Unfortunately, in biological systems, there'll be confusion between the three minerals. That means that if a plant is presented with Zinc, Cadmium or Mercury, then it will not distinguish between them. That means that Cadmium and also Mercury will "hitch a ride with Zinc" into the plant. Then the humans who eat the plant eat the Cadmium and the Mercury.

# Cadmium infiltration

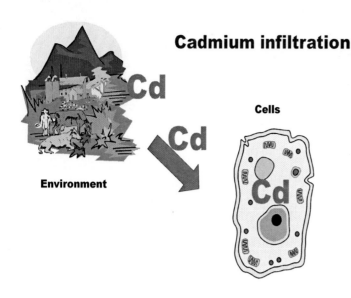

Take for instance Cadmium, which is plentiful in our superphosphate fertilizers. How does Cadmium getting to fertiliser you may ask? Well Cadmium is found in the earth's crust and accumulates in rock phosphate. When we convert rock phosphate to superphosphate, we increase the bioavailability of Cadmium. We make it more digestible. In this way, superphosphate is may contain up to 20 mg per kilo of Cadmium. We fertilise wheat, with superphosphate we harvest the wheat, we eat the bread, we get the Cadmium. An adult will accumulate about 20 to 30 g of Cadmium in a lifespan.

# Defence systems

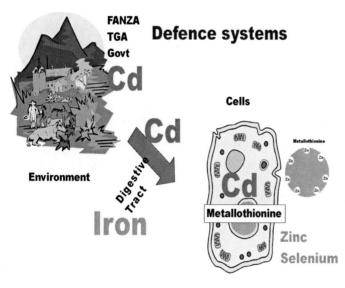

The best protection against Cadmium ingestion is Iron. The more Iron you have the less Cadmium you absorb. Iron deficiency effects about 12% of the global population. Most of these people are women and children. If Cadmium does get into the cell the next protective mechanism called metallothionine. Metallothionine needs Zinc (lots of Zinc) and the Sulphurous amino acid cysteine.

# Anti-nutrients

| | |
|---|---|
| **Lead** | blocks Iron Calcium Molybdenum Manganese Chromium Sulphur Cobalt |
| **Mercury** | blocks Zinc selenium iron sulphur cobalt transmembrane ion channels |
| **Cadmium** | blocks Zinc Magnesium Selenium Sulphur |
| **Arsenic** | blocks Vit E selenium sulphur boron |
| **Aluminium** | blocks Vit E Vit C Vit B1 Zinc Selenium Sodium Potassium Phosphorus |
| **Antimony** | blocks Zinc Selenium |

The problem with Cadmium and its ilk, is that this toxic element will block nutrients in the cells. Lead for instance, will block Iron, Calcium, Molybdenum, Manganese, Chromium, Sulphur and Cobalt. This will not show up a blood test. "Biochemistry occurs in the cells, not the blood". Only a tissue sample will show this. And even the tissue sample may not give a true picture of the total amount of this toxic element.

# Nutrients and Anti-nutrients

| | Copper block | Cadmium Block | Mercury Block | Arsenic Block | Lead Block | Aluminium Block | Antimony Block |
|---|---|---|---|---|---|---|---|
| Sodium | | | | | | ✗ | |
| Potassium | | | | | | ✗ | |
| Magnesium | ✗ | ✗ | | | | | |
| Calcium | | | | | ✗ | | |
| Iron | ✗ | | ✗ | | ✗ | | |
| Zinc | ✗ | ✗ | ✗ | | | ✗ | ✗ |
| Chromium | | | | | ✗ | | |
| Selenium | | ✗ | ✗ | ✗ | | ✗ | ✗ |
| Molybdenum | ✗ | | | | ✗ | | |
| Manganese | ✗ | | | | ✗ | | |
| Phosphorus | | | | | | ✗ | |
| Vitamin B1 | ✗ | | | | | ✗ | |
| Vitamin C | ✗ | | | | | ✗ | |
| Vitamin E | ✗ | | | ✗ | | ✗ | |
| Folate | ✗ | | | | | | |
| Boron | ✗ | | | ✗ | | | |

Here is the table showing the effect of these anti-nutrients. What you should note from this table is the effect of Copper overload. Too much Copper is very disruptive to intracellular nutrients. One of the reasons is that Copper is very electro-negative. That means that we must have very good control systems to keep it caged up. "Lock up your cations" otherwise they will attack you.

## Very important Concept

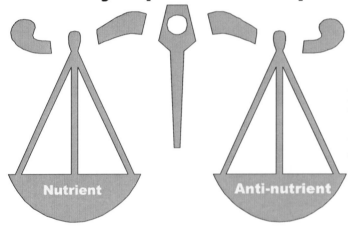

Because toxins get stored with nutrients, they find a balance in the cell. Disrupting toxins will cause problems, if it is not done gently. Sometimes this means improving organ drainage first, like improving liver function before detoxifying the patient.

Biology

Commerce

Politics

My final comment is that industry defines toxicity; industry inserts toxins into our bodies. Governments monitor industries, governments monitor toxicities. Therefore in medical practice, we see the result of biology taking a back seat to commerce and politics. To control a population, it is better to keep them slightly sick, so you can keep an eye on them. If they are too healthy, they will rise up against you.

## Biochemical interpretation of symptoms and the relationship to nutrient flow.

By using the questionnaire, we can determine the amount of cellular dysfunction. Symptoms are just tissues crying out for attention, like a baby does. If we can decode the cry, we can work out what is wrong. Moreover we can determine *why* it is wrong.

This involves the concept of nutrient flow. From the environment to the final utilisation of the nutrient, Nutrient flow is vulnerable at any or indeed *all* points of this flow.

Nutrients come from our environment and their flow can be monitored and their functions characterised. The end result is that they perform a function, which is normally taken for granted by the organism.

# Nutrient flow

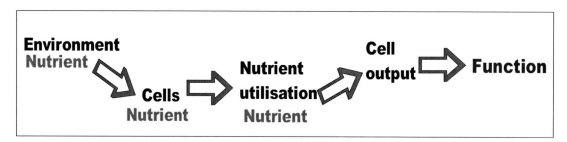

In the case of malabsorption as below, we can see the effect "down stream" of the flow, which generates symptoms. An analysis of the abnormal flow identifies where the block is and shows us how to rectify the problem by dealing with both the *process* that caused it and the *compensatory* mechanism that failed to prevent it.

**The patient would score highly for these questionnaire symptoms of digestive dysfunction.**

# Nutrient flow

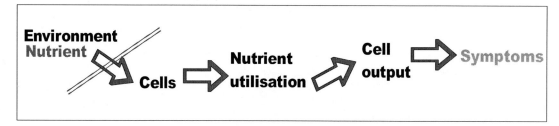

**These symptoms are often due to Zinc, Vitamin C or Iron deficiency/blockade.**

| *Topic* **Digestion** | Have you had…… | never | In the past | Recently | frequently |
|---|---|---|---|---|---|
| | Heartburn or reflux | | | | |
| | Bloating after meals | | | | |
| | Constipation | | **Zinc and/or Helicobacter** | | |
| | Burping, Farting or wind | | | | |
| | diarrhoea or loose stools | | | | |
| | Nausea (feeling like vomiting) | | | | |
| | Stomach ulcers or Stomach pain | | | | |

**This group is generally zinc deficiency /blockade.**

| Immune system | | | | | |
|---|---|---|---|---|---|
| Tonsillitis | | | | | |
| Cold sores | | | | | |
| Conjunctivitis | | | | | |
| Sore throat | | Zinc, iron or | | | |
| Mouth ulcers | | Vitamin C | | | |
| Ear infection | | | | | |
| Sinus infection | | | | | |
| Boils or pimples | | | | | |
| Thrush | | | | | |
| Genital infection | | | | | |
| Urinary infection | | | | | |

These are symptoms of the infamous Estrogen Dominance syndrome and often accompany high TMA copper levels.

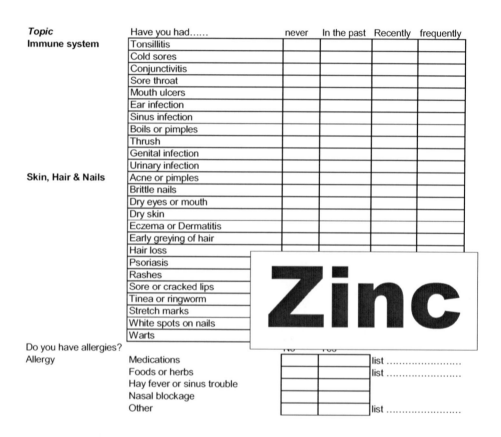

| Topic | Have you had...... | never | In the past | Recently | frequently |
|---|---|---|---|---|---|
| **Immune system** | Tonsillitis | | | | |
| | Cold sores | | | | |
| | Conjunctivitis | | | | |
| | Sore throat | | | | |
| | Mouth ulcers | | | | |
| | Ear infection | | | | |
| | Sinus infection | | | | |
| | Boils or pimples | | | | |
| | Thrush | | | | |
| | Genital infection | | | | |
| | Urinary infection | | | | |
| **Skin, Hair & Nails** | Acne or pimples | | | | |
| | Brittle nails | | | | |
| | Dry eyes or mouth | | | | |
| | Dry skin | | | | |
| | Eczema or Dermatitis | | | | |
| | Early greying of hair | | | | |
| | Hair loss | | | | |
| | Psoriasis | | | | |
| | Rashes | | Zinc | | |
| | Sore or cracked lips | | | | |
| | Tinea or ringworm | | | | |
| | Stretch marks | | | | |
| | White spots on nails | | | | |
| | Warts | | | | |

Do you have allergies?

| Allergy | | No | Yes | |
|---|---|---|---|---|
| | Medications | | | list ....................... |
| | Foods or herbs | | | list ....................... |
| | Hay fever or sinus trouble | | | |
| | Nasal blockage | | | |
| | Other | | | list ....................... |

The next symptoms are associated with low molybdenum levels on TMA.

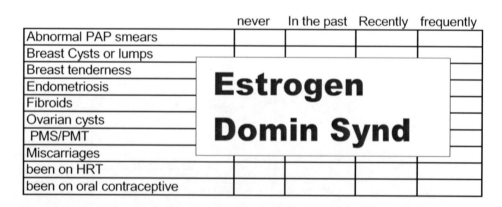

| Gynaecological | never | In the past | Recently | frequently |
|---|---|---|---|---|
| Abnormal PAP smears | | | | |
| Breast Cysts or lumps | | | | |
| Breast tenderness | | | | |
| Endometriosis | | Estrogen | | |
| Fibroids | | Domin Synd | | |
| Ovarian cysts | | | | |
| PMS/PMT | | | | |
| Miscarriages | | | | |
| been on HRT | | | | |
| been on oral contraceptive | | | | |

| | | never | In the past | Recently | frequently |
|---|---|---|---|---|---|
| **Lung** | Asthma or Emphysema | | | | |
| **Skin, Hair & Nails** | Tinea or ringworm | | | | |
| | Thrush | | | | |
| **Heart** | Angina or Chest pain | | | | |
| | Palpitations or Irregular heart rate | | | | |
| | Have you had...... | never | In the past | Recently | frequently |
| **Nervous system** | Agitation or Anxiety | | | | |
| **Muscle system** | Irritability | | | | |
| | Migraine or other headache | | | | |
| | Poor night vision | | | | |
| | Gout | | | | |

**Mo**

| | | | | |
|---|---|---|---|---|
| **Blood disorders** | Iron deficiency | | | |
| **Have you ever suffered from.....** | | | | |
| | Osteo Arthritis | | | |
| | Gout | | | |
| **Have you had cancer?** | | No | Yes | Year |
| **Cancer** | Breast | | | |
| | Stomach or Colon | | | |
| | | No | Yes | Year |
| **Have you ever had** | Candida | | | |

This group are associated with abnormalities of magnesium.

| | | never | In the past | Recently | frequently |
|---|---|---|---|---|---|
| Heart | Angina or Chest pain | | | | |
| | cold hands & feet | | | | |
| | Fluid retention | | | | |
| | Heart Attack | | | | |
| | Heart failure | | | | |
| | Heart murmur | | | | |
| | High blood pressure | | | | |
| | Palpitations or Irregular heart rate | | | | |
| | | never | In the past | Recently | frequently |
| Sleep | disrupted sleep | | | | |
| | insomnia | | | | |
| | snoring | | | | |
| | daytime tiredness | | | | |
| | unrefreshed sleep | | | | |

**Mg**

| | | | | | |
|---|---|---|---|---|---|
| | Have you had...... | | | | |
| **Nervous system** | Agitation or Anxiety | | | | |
| **Muscle system** | Irritability | | | | |
| | Migraine or other headache | | | | |
| | Poor night vision | | | | |
| | Gout | | | | |
| | Dizziness or Vertigo | | | | |
| | Facial twitching | | | | |
| | fidgeting or Restless legs | | | | |
| | Fits or seizures | | | | |
| | Blurred vision | | | | |
| | Leg/foot or hand cramps | | | | |
| | carpal tunnel syndrome | | | | |
| | Depression | | | | |
| | Memory loss | | | | |
| | Chronic pain | | | | |
| | Mood swings or Irritability | | | | |
| | Muscle pain or ache | | | | |
| | Muscle weakness/heaviness | | | | |
| | Pins & needles / Numbness | | | | |
| | Poor concentration | | | | |
| | Poor balance | | | | |
| | Tinnitus (ringing in the ears) | | | | |
| | Tremor of the hands | | | | |
| | Weakness of a limb | | | | |

These symptoms are commonly associated with high copper on TMA.

| Topic | Please tick the appropriate column<br>Have you had…… | never | In the past | Recently | frequently |
|---|---|---|---|---|---|
| Digestion | Nausea (feeling like vomiting) | | | | |
| | Constipation | | | | |
| | Gall bladder problems | | | | |
| Skin, Hair Nails | Stomach ulcers or Stomach pain | | | | |
| | Early greying of hair | | | | |
| | Rashes | | | | |

| | Do you have allergies? | No | Yes | | |
|---|---|---|---|---|---|
| Allergy | Hay fever or sinus trouble | | | list …………………… | |
| | Nasal blockage | | | list …………………… | |

| Topic | | never | In the past | Recently | frequently |
|---|---|---|---|---|---|
| Gynaecological | Abnormal PAP smears | | | | |
| | Breast Cysts or lumps | | | | |
| | Breast tenderness | | | | |
| | Endometriosis | | | | |
| | Fibroids | | | | |
| | Ovarian cysts | | | | |
| | PMS/PMT | | | | |
| | Miscarriages | | | | |
| | been on HRT | | | | |
| | been on oral contraceptive | | | | |

**Copper overload**

| | | No | Yes | Year |
|---|---|---|---|---|
| Any Liver problems? | Abnormal liver function tests | | | |
| | Liver damage or Fatty liver | | | |

| Topic | | never | In the past | Recently | frequently |
|---|---|---|---|---|---|
| Sleep | disrupted sleep | | | | |
| | insomnia | | | | |

| Topic | Have you had…… | never | In the past | Recently | frequently |
|---|---|---|---|---|---|
| Nervous system | Agitation or Anxiety | | | | |
| Muscle system | Irritability | | | | |
| | Migraine or other headache | | | | |
| | Depression | | | | |
| | Memory loss | | | | |

| | | No | Yes | Year |
|---|---|---|---|---|
| Blood disorders | Iron deficiency | | | |
| | Easy bruising | | | |
| Have you had cancer? | | No | Yes | Year |
| Cancer | Breast | | | |
| | Ovary or uterus | | | |
| Do you have any of these? | | No | Yes | |
| Hormone | Thyroid problems | | | |

## Nutrient flow

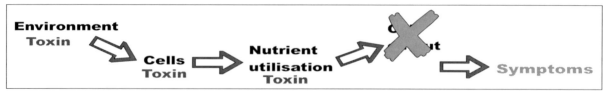

Sometimes toxins "hitch a ride" with the nutrients

Another common scenario is the introduction of toxins into a biological system. This may lead to symptoms also by the effect on cellular utilisation of nutrients (see section on B-Vitamins) . With this concept we can identify two major areas of concern. The first is the effect on modern agriculture on the food chain. The second is the transfer of nutrients from the exterior to the final destination (intracellular binding sites).

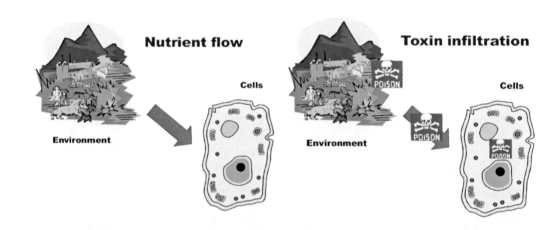

There are several defence systems that deal with toxins. Firstly the gut should either repel or destroy them (see Zinc section). Secondly, the liver should destroy or sequester them. And thirdly, the cell has methods of dealing with toxins that stray into the tissues.

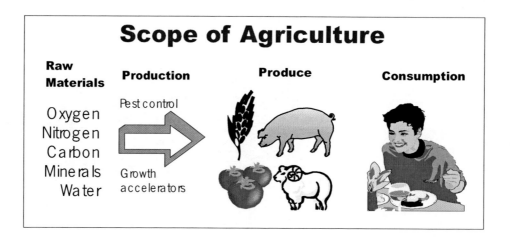

Furthermore disease states will modify the nutrient flow, particularly of minerals. The notable examples which lead to excess are iron, copper and manganese.
The effect of toxins can be summarised by the table below.

And finally we arrive at the guidelines for Diagnostic Orthomolecular Medicine as practised at the NRS (Nutrition Review Service).

**Guidelines for Clinical Nutritional Medicine**

1] What is the *main* complaint?

2] Interpret the symptoms biochemically

3] What are the links between the symptoms?

4] Is digestion involved?

5] Is hormone imbalance involved?

6] Could it be a channelopathy?

7] What tests will be needed to confirm the abnormal biochemistry/pathology?

8] What is the process driving this abnormal biochemistry?

9] What normal compensatory mechanisms have been compromised?

10] What are the aims of treatment? Channel repair, Restock , Detox, Repair, Restore defence or aid digestion?

10] In what order should these be carried out?

# Nutrients and antinutrients

| | Copper block | Cadmium Block | Mercury Block | Arsenic Block | Lead Block | Aluminium Block | Antimony Block |
|---|---|---|---|---|---|---|---|
| Sodium | | | | | | X | |
| Potassium | | | | | | X | |
| Magnesium | X | X | | | | | |
| Calcium | | | | | X | | |
| Iron | X | | X | | X | | |
| Zinc | X | X | X | | | X | X |
| Chromium | | | | | X | | |
| Selenium | | X | X | X | | X | X |
| Molybdenum | X | | | | X | | |
| Manganese | X | | | | | | |
| Phosphorus | | | | | | X | |
| Vitamin B1 | X | | | | | X | |
| Vitamin C | X | | | | | X | |
| Vitamin E | X | | | X | | X | |
| Folate | X | | | | | | |
| | | | | | | | |

Topologically, the human body is like a torus. That is the "inside" of us (digestive tract) is actually the outside. This poses the problem of security against things that may hurt us. In the years of past it wase just bacteria, viruses and fungi, and luckily our stomach acid and the immune system did the trick. These days we have preservatives, food colourings, heavy metals and other nasties to deal with. So what's the problem? With a physiology basically thousands of years old, we are struggling to cope with the ingested dangers of the 21st Century. So we need to promote the natural defence system that includes the stomach and the liver. The consequences of poor digestion are shown in the diagram and are due to incompletely digested proteins (peptides) lodging (embolising) in various tissues and causing them to malfunction.

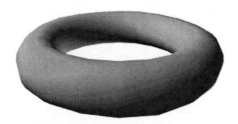

# A torus

So many people have symptoms such as reflux, heartburn, bloating after meals and they do not realise that these are the symptoms of a failing defence system. These are the symptoms of reduced stomach acid and they are the start of many impending disasters about to befall the people who have them. Just reducing stomach acid will impair the ability to absorb Iron, Calcium and Magnesium. Bad enough you may say, but these people also will have trouble with the digestion of the salicylates (natural aspirins). These foods include citrus, tomatoes, pineapple, kiwi fruit, strawberries, stone fruit, capsicum, chilli, mushrooms and onions. These plants accumulate natural aspirins as a defence mechanism to avoid being eaten before ripening. The only species who take them off the tree fully laden with salicylates are humans; and they do this for money and to take short cuts with nutrition. Salicylate intolerance was a rare thing 50 years ago, but now it is almost as common as helicobacter.

Which brings us the next piece of our digestive puzzle. Helicobacter was discovered when investigators were trying to find out why some people got ulcers when on anti-inflammatory drugs. It turns out that helicobacter made them more likely to get an ulcer in the stomach. Well guess what relatives the anti-inflammatory drugs have? Aspirins (salicylates). So, those people with salicylate intolerance may well have Helicobacter brewing in their stomachs.

---

### Why Helicobacter causes Mineral Deficiencies

Helicobacter (H. Pylori) causes inflammation of the stomach
The function of the stomach is to produce acid for meals.
Any organ that's inflamed **does not function properly**

Encephalitis (inflammation of the brain) causes impaired thinking.
Retinitis (inflammation of the eye) causes reduced vision
Otitis media (inflammation of the middle ear) causes hearing impairment.
Myocarditis (inflammation of the heart) causes heart failure.           **examples**
Bronchitis causes shortness of breath.
Hepatitis (inflammation of the liver) causes liver impairment.
Nephritis (inflammation of the kidney) causes impaired kidney function.
Pancreatitis (inflammation of the pancreas) causes impaired insulin production.
Synovitis (inflammation of the joint lining) causes joints that can't bend.

For some reason, the Gastroenterologists feel that the stomach should be the *only* exception.
So actually, an inflamed stomach lining will not produce *enough* acid when food is eaten.
You need acid to absorb iron, calcium and magnesium.

Helicobacter is a chronic stomach infection of worldwide epidemic proportions. It gained notoriety when it was discovered that it could cause stomach ulcers. When this information came out, everyone said "But nothing can live in the stomach; it's too acidic". Well, the truth of the matter is that we were all told that the stomach killed anything nasty as part our defence system, and so hearing the Helicobacter was the exception was rather odd. We were told that this bug is so perverse that it loves acid, and that is why we must suppress acid. The obvious (and completely overlooked) corollary hypothesis is that helicobacter could only survive if the *acid was low* and the commonest reason for this would be zinc deficiency. What happens if your zinc is chronically low? You get low stomach acid and reduced defence against infections! You might say that this would suggest that zinc could be useful in the treatment of Helicobacter infections, and yes, there are some studies, which have used zinc for Helicobacter eradication.

This is not the only anomaly. Helicobacter supposedly causes gastritis. Most tissues when inflamed do not function properly, and yet the gastroenterologists claim that stomach acid must be high. Of all the medical examples above, you can see that indeed gastritis is a *special condition* according to the medical specialists in this field of digestion. Really? There is one more anomaly. Helicobacter is supposed to cause ulcers. Apparently, forty percent of Australians have helicobacter. Quite clearly then, *most people* with helicobacter *do not develop ulcers*. What factors predispose those to getting the ulcers? Probably low zinc.

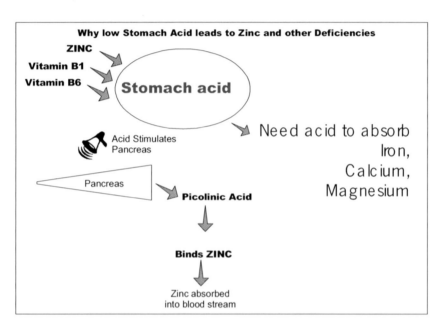

Now, many of my patients turn up with the diagnosis of "Candida". The two commonest reasons for this overgrowth of this yeast is low stomach acid and lack of acidophilus in the intestine. Try this experiment. Put some pieces of melon in the fridge for a couple of weeks. What you will find is a heavy growth of a white fungus. This is Candida albicans. Stomach acid is supposed to kill fungi, right? Then these fungi should be killed if there is adequate digestive power in the stomach. So the best treatment is not just a low Candida diet, not just antifungals, but put back the defence system! Give them Zinc, Vitamin B1, Vitamin B6 or digestive enzymes supplements or just plain Betaine hydrochloride (which converts to stomach acid) As for the acidophilus. The name says it all. Philos means to love, for example paedophile. These bacteria need an acid environment to survive, so low stomach acid creates an environment hostile to these organisms in the intestine. They also like molybdenum and zinc, and you know how much of these we get in our diet! A good intestinal environment will protect from food poisoning, travellers diarrhoea, and antibiotic induced thrush and probably from bowel cancer. One of the functions of molybdenum is to detoxify sulphites and carcinogens such as nitrosamines in the diet. Hence, the association of gastric tract cancers with low molybdenum. This was demonstrated in China about 20 years ago.

The widespread problems with digestion are causing major illness but in indirect ways. The reduction of the topical defence system, the impaired absorption of important nutrients like Zinc and Selenium and the increased incidence of food intolerances (as opposed to food allergies) are powerful driving forces towards ill health. Fix the gut and the rest falls into place.

Just to reinforce why stomach acid is so important in the chain of digestion, the diagram below depicts the connection between the production of gastric acid and the absorption of Zinc and other minerals. The take home message is this. If you don't make acid, you don't absorb zinc, and if you don't absorb zinc, you don't make stomach acid.

List of foods with a very high content of salicylates:-

Fruit: Sultanas (dried), prunes, raisins (dried), currants (dried), raspberry, redcurrant, grape, loganberry, blackcurrant, youngberry, cherry, orange, blueberry, plum, pineapple, boysenberry, guava, apricot, blackberry, cranberry, date, strawberry, rock melon, tomatoes and tomato products (pastes, sauce, puree).

Vegetables: gherkin, endive, champignon, radish, olives, capsicum, zucchini, chicory, hot pepper, chili, snow peas/unshelled peas.

Nuts: Almonds, water chestnuts.

Spices & Sauces: Cumin, chicory, cayenne, sage, vinegar (cider), aniseed, mace, curry, paprika, thyme, Worcester Sauce, dill, turmeric, Vegemite, Marmite, rosemary, oregano, garam marsala, mixed herbs, mint, cumin canella, tarragon, mustard, Five Spice, pickles.

Drinks: Tea - all brands, alfalfa, peppermint. Cereal coffee -Nature's Cuppa, any with chicory content Alcohol - liqueurs, port, wine, rum, and cider

Other - MSG, Chinese food, Parmesan cheese, aspirin, tartrazine (food colouring 102), benzoates (food additives 210-211), Licorice, peppermints, honey, mints/Minties

**Helicobacter and hypochlorhydria**

Cater, R. E. 2nd. Helicobacter (aka Campylobacter) pylori as the major causal factor in chronic hypochlorhydria. Med Hypotheses. 39:367-374, 1992.

Cave, D. R., et al. Effect of a Campylobacter pylori protein on acid secretion by parietal cells. Lancet. 2:187-189, 1989.

El-Omar,.E. M., et al. Divergent effects of H. pylori on acid secretion. Gut. 37(Supplement 2):A6, 1995.

Gaby, A. R. Helicobacter pylori eradication: are there alternatives to antibiotics? Alternative Medicine Review. 6(4):355-366, 2001.

Graham, D. Y., et al. Iatrogenic Campylobacter pylori infection is a cause of epidemic achlorhydria. Am J Gastroenterol . 83:974-980, 1988.

Halter, F., et al. Long-term effects of Helicobacter pylori infection on acid and pepsin secretion. Yale J Biol Med. 69:99-104, 1996.

# Consequences of poor digestion

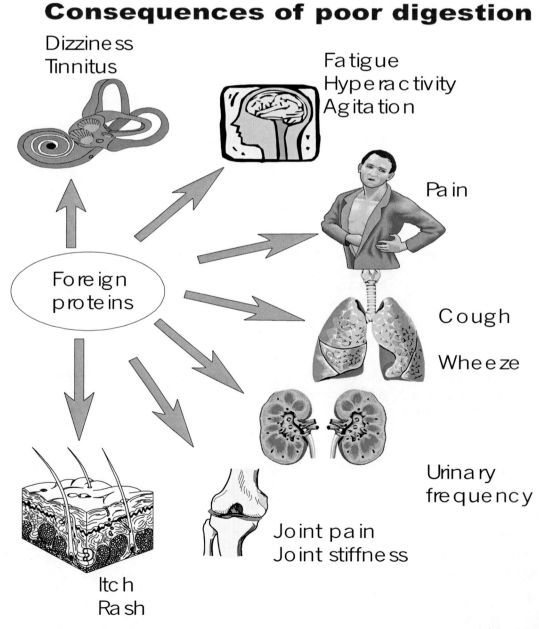

Dizziness
Tinnitus

Fatigue
Hyperactivity
Agitation

Pain

Foreign proteins

Cough

Wheeze

Urinary frequency

Joint pain
Joint stiffness

Itch
Rash

Some interesting research from the chronic fatigue syndrome literature has revealed a set of conditions called Channelopathies. The name refers to the ion channels that allow metallic ions in and out of the cell, but could be applied more broadly to the passage of Nutrients into the cell and the release of Toxins out of the cell. The best-known example of Channelopathy is Cystic Fibrosis due to an abnormality of chromosome 7. This involves the "chloride" channel.

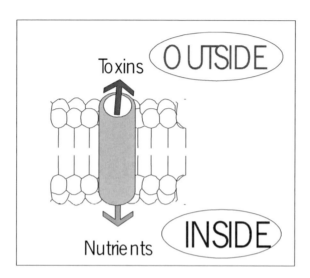

Some specific examples would include well-known one-way channels such as inflowing potassium and the anti-port (counter pump) system of Sodium and Potassium. Of note is that Magnesium is required for one of these Potassium channels and Vitamin B6 is needed for the Na/K Anti-port pump.

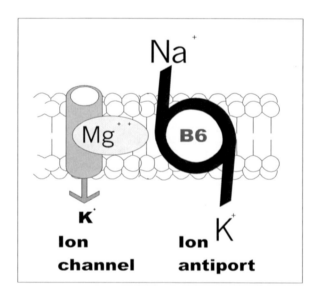

If we take a look at the passage from the gut to the cells, we see 2 important hurdles that need to be traversed. The Intestinal wall, and the target cell wall and in the case of the brain, the glial cells.

It is well known that glutamine is helpful for the intestinal wall passage while taurine is useful for the target cell wall passage. In general Amino Acids may play important roles in ion "delivery" systems, and this explains why some patients do better on Amino Acid Chelate supplements.

A common channelopathy is the disruption to the Na/K pump due to organophosphate pesticides. Organochlorines probably affect Cu/K or Cu/Mo pumps. This explains why such pesticides cause copper retention disorders.

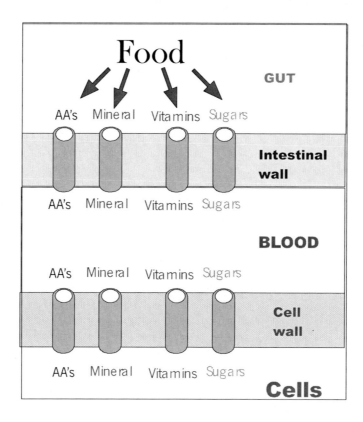

Interestingly, these channels sit in "vats" of oil including the essential fatty acids (EFA's). The oils vary with blood group. When we test a person's blood group we subject the surface of the cell to a biochemical reaction and depending on the reaction we determine the blood group. This means that the cell wall is different for each blood group and this difference is actually coded for on Chromosome 9. The table below summarises the different Omega 3, 6 & 9 requirements according to blood group. AB group's need the same as B, which are Flax seed oil capsules. These oils have been used in many conditions and may be diagnosistic in some Channelopathies at 6 to 9 grams per day.

| Essential Fatty Acids (EFA's) | | |
|---|---|---|
| **A** | $\Omega$ 3 | Fish oil |
| **O** | $\Omega$ 3 & 6 | Evening Primrose oil Borage or Starflower |
| **B** | $\Omega$ 3, 6 & 9 | Flaxseed oil |
| Channelopathy is a problem with channels | | |

Blood Group

Many patients are diagnosed with hyperglycaemia. Most are started on empirical treatments without any investigation as to why this happened. There is much already in the literature to help define more accurately what type of diabetes the patients might have, but nobody bothers to check. My point is this: why not check if there is a cause that is amenable to nutritional management at the time of diagnosis?

Please refer to the figure schematic below.

There are two sources of glucose. Firstly, from starches and sugars in the diet and from the liver during fasting, especially overnight. Dietary glucose requires digestive enzymes to correctly digest carbohydrates. Carbohydrates release sugars as differing rates. This rate has been referred to as the glycaemic index. The higher the index, the faster the sugar rises. The maximum is pure glucose at 100.

The liver makes glucose to prop up the blood sugar level, rather like a treasury props up a country's currency. The important nutrients are zinc, magnesium and Vitamin B6.

The next phase is the productions and storage of insulin. Zinc, manganese and sulphur are important nutrients for this. Next comes insulin release and this is dependent upon magnesium. Think of magnesium as a valve that allows the correct and appropriate release of insulin. Glucose stimulates as release of insulin from the pancreas.

Once insulin is in the blood stream, it acts as the front door to let glucose into the cells, where it used for fuel. But to get into the cell the glucose needs an entry ticket. This is the Glucose tolerance factor. It contains chromium, vanadium and Vitamin B3. In addition, Chromium and vanadium need to be in balance. Alternatively, there is a side door entry, which can utilise Vitamin C, Vitamin E, selenium, arginine (an amino acid) or taurine (also an amino acid).

The problem we have is that zinc and selenium are low in the soil and magnesium levels have fallen in our diets since broad acre farming. Refining carbohydrates destroys chromium and vanadium. Overall we have increased the glycaemia index of our diets. High glycaemic index diets waste chromium. Add these up, and you have a significant problem.

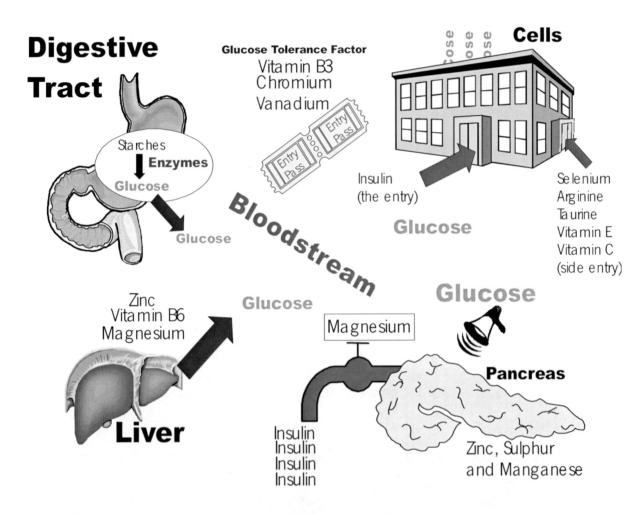

# References

1] Abraham A. S., et al. The effects of chromium supplementation on serum glucose and lipids in patients with and without non-insulin dependent diabetes. Metabolism. 41:768-771, 1992

2] Anderson R., et al. Beneficial effects of chromium for people with Type II Diabetes. Diabetes. 45(Suppl. 2):124A/454, 1996

3] Anderson R.A., Roussel A-M, Zouari N., et al. Potential antioxidant effects of zinc and chromium supplement in people with type II diabetes mellitus. J Am Coll Nutr. 20(3):212-218, 2001

4] Anderson R. A., et al. Chromium supplementation of human subjects: Effects on glucose, insulin, and lipid variables. Metabolism. 32:894-899, 1983

5] Anderson R. A., et al. Supplemental chromium effects on glucose, insulin, glucagon, and urinary chromium losses in subjects consuming low-chromium diets. American Journal of Clinical Nutrition. 54:909-916, 1991

6] Anderson R. A., et al. Elevated intakes of supplemental chromium improve glucose and insulin variables in individuals with type 2 diabetes. Diabetes. 46:1786-1791, 1997

7] Anderson R. A. Nutritional factors influencing the glucose/insulin system: chromium. J Am Coll Nutr. 16(5):404-410, 1997

8] Baly D., et al. Effect of manganese deficiency on insulin binding, glucose transport & metabolism in rat adipocytes. J Nutr. 120:1075-1079, 1990

9] Boden G., et al. Effects of vanadyl sulfate on carbohydrate and lipid metabolism in patients with non-insulin-dependent diabetes mellitus. Metabolism. 45:1130-1135, 1996

10] Boyd S. G., et al. Combined dietary chromium picolinate supplementation and an exercise program leads to a reduction of serum cholesterol and insulin in college-aged subjects. J Nutr Biochem. 9:471-475, 1998

11] Cam M. C., et al. Distinct glucose lowering and beta cell protective effects of vanadium and food restriction in streptozotocin-diabetes. Eur J Endocrinol. 141(5):546-554, 1999

12] Chan et al. The role of copper, molybdenum selenium and zinc in nutrtion and health. Clin Lab Med. 18(4): 673-85, 1998

13] Chauser A. Zinc, Insulin and Diabetes. J of American College of Nutrition 17(2): 109-115, 1998

14] Cohen N., et al. Oral vanadyl sulfate improves hepatic and peripheral insulin sensitivity in patients with non-insulin-dependent diabetes mellitus. Journal of Clinical Investigations. 95(6):2501-2509, 1995

15] Combs G.F. and Combs S.B. The Role of Selenium in Nutrition. Academic Press, Inc., Orlando, USA, 1986

16] Corica F., Allegra A., Di Benedetto A., et al. Effects of oral magnesium supplementation on plasma lipid concentrations of patients with non-insulin-dependent diabetes mellitus. Magnes Res. 7:43-47, 1994

17] Davies S., et al. Age-related decreases in chromium levels in 51,665 hair, sweat, and serum samples from 40,872 patients - implications for the prevention of cardiovascular disease and type II diabetes mellitus. Metabolism. 46(5):469-473, 1997

18] Evans G. W. The effect of chromium picolinate on insulin controlled parameters in humans. Int J Biosocial Medical Research. 11:163-180, 1989

19] Evans G. W., et al. Chromium picolinate increases membrane fluidity and rate of insulin internalization. J Inorg Biochem. 46(4):243-250, 1992

20] Fugii S., Takemura T., Wada M., et al. Magnesium levels in plasma, erythrocyte, and urine in patients with diabetes mellitus. Horm Metab Res. 14:161-162, 1982

21] Haglund et al. Evidence of a relationship between childhood onset type 1 diabetes and low groundwater concentration of zinc. Diabetes Care Aug. 19:8 873-5, 1996

22] Jing M.A., Folsom A.R., Melnick S.L., et al. Associations of serum and dietary magnesium with cardiovascular disease, hypertension, diabetes, insulin, and carotid arterial wall thickness: the ARIC study. J Clin Epidemiol. 48:927-940, 1995

23] Kelly G. S. Insulin resistance: lifestyle and nutritional interventions. Alternative Medicine Review. 5(2):109-132, 2000

24] Leach R.M.,Jr. Metabolism & Function of Manganese. Trace elements in Human Health & Disease. Vol.III.

25] Lee N. A., et al. Beneficial effect of chromium supplementation on serum triglyceride levels in NIDDM. Diabetes Care. 17(12):1449-1452, 1994

26] Mather H. M., et al. Hypomagnesemia in diabetes. Clin Chem Acta. 95:235-242, 1979

27] McNeill J. Enhanced in vivo sensitivity of vanadyl-treated diabetic rats to insulin. Canadian Journal of Physiology and Pharmacology. 68(4):486-491, 1996

28] Mechegiani E., et al. Zinc-dependent low thymic hormone level in type I diabetes. Diabetes. 12:932-937, 1989

29] Mertz W., et al. Present knowledge of the role of chromium. Federation Proceedings. 33:2275-2280, 1974

30] Nakamura T., et al. Kinetics of zinc status in children with IDDM. Diabetes Care. 14:553-557, 1991

31] Niewoener C. B., et al. Role of zinc supplementation in type II diabetes mellitus. Am J Med. 63-68, 1988

32] Paolisso G., et al. Improved insulin response and action by chronic magnesium administration in aged NIDDM subjects. Diabetes Care. 12(4):265-269, 1989

33] Paolisso et al. Hypertension, diabetes and insulin resistance: the role of intracellular magnesium. Am J Hypertens. 10:3 346-55, 1997

34] Pepato M. T., et al. Effect of oral vanadyl sulfate treatment on serum enzymes and lipids of streptozotocin-diabetic young rats. Mol Cell Biochem. 198(1-2):157-161, 1999

35] Pidduck H.G., et al. Hyperzincuria of diabetes mellitus and possible genetic implications of this observation. Diabetes. 19:240-247, 1970

36] Preuss H.G., et al. Chromium update: examining recent literature 1997-1998. Curr Opin Clin Nutr Metab Care. 1:509-512, 1998

37] Poucheret P., et al. Vanadium and diabetes. Mol Cell Biochem. 188(1-2):73-80, 1998

38] Prout T.E., et al. Zinc Metabolism in Patients with Diabetes Mellitus. Metabolism. 9:109-17, 1960

39] Pryor K. Nutritional approaches to optimal blood glucose and insulin levels: key factors in longevity and resistance to diabetes and other degenerative diseases. Vitamin Research News. April 2000

40] Rabinowitz M. B., et al. Effects of chromium and yeast supplements on carbohydrate and lipid metabolism in diabetic men. Diabetes Care. 6(4):319-327, 1983

43] Rao K.V.R., et al. Effect of zinc sulfate therapy on control and lipids in type I diabetes. JAPI. 35:52, 1987

44] Rayman M.P. The importance of selenium to human health. Lancet. 356(9225): 233-241, 2000

45] Reaven G. Role of insulin resistance in human disease. Diabetes. 37:1595-1607, 1998

46] Resnick L. Magnesium in the pathophysiology and treatment of hypertension and diabetes mellitus: where are we in 1997? Am J Hypertension. 10:368-370, 1997

47] Rubinstein A.H. Manganese-induced hypoglycemia. The Lancet. 2:1348-1351, 1962

48] Rubenstein A.H., et al. Hypoglycemia induced by manganese. Nature. 194:188-9, 1962

49] Sakurai H., et al. Insulin-like effect of vanadyl ion on streptozotocin-induced diabetic rats. J Endocrinol. 126(3):451-459, 1990

50] Seelig M.S.,et al. Low Magnesium: A Common Denominator in Pathologic Process in Diabetes Mellitus, Cardiovascular Disease and Eclampsia. Journal of the American College of Nutrition, October; 11(5): 608/Abstr 39, 1992

51] Sjogren A., et al. Oral administration of magnesium hydroxide to subjects with insulin dependent diabetes mellitus. Magnesium. 121:16-20, 1988

52] Sjogren A. et al. Magnesium, potassium and zinc deficiency in subjects with type II diabetes mellitus. Acta Med Scand. 224(5):461-466, 1988

53] Singh R.B., et al. Current zinc intake and risk of diabetes and coronary artery disease and factors associated with insulin resistance in rural and urban populations of North India. J Am Coll Nutr. 17:564-570, 1998

54] Stapleton S.R. Selenium: an insulin-mimetic. Cell Mol Life Sci. 57(13-14): 1874-1879, 2000

55] Striffler J. S., et al. Chromium improves insulin response to glucose in rats. Metabolism. 44:1314-1320, 1995

56] Striffler J. S., et al. Dietary chromium decreases insulin resistance in rats fed a high-fat, mineral-imbalanced diet. Metabolism. 47:396-400, 1998

57] Striffler J. S., et al. Overproduction of insulin in the chromium-deficient rat. Metabolism. 48:1063-1068, 1999

58] Toplack H., et al. Addition of chromium picolinate to a very low calorie diet improves the insulin-glucose ratio after weight reduction. International Journal of Obesity. 19(2):s057, 1995

59] Uehara S., et al. Clinical significance of selenium level in chronic pancreatitis. J Clin Biochem Nutr. 5:201-207, 1988

60] Wallace E. C. Diabetic epidemic. Energy Times. 9(4):24-28 1999

61] Watts D.L. The nutritional relationships of manganese. J. Orthomol. Med. 5(4):219-22, 1990

An important aspect of Nutritional Medicine relates to the metallic containment systems that have evolved especially relating to charged ions. Bulk ions get lots of airplay in medical schools, but infact play *very little* part in enzyme functions. Microminerals however carry out most of the enzymatic reactions, but get extremely little mention in medical school curricula. Perhaps their teachers stopped reading after 1960?

# Charged ions

## "Bulk" ions low Mol Wt

| | | |
|---|---|---|
| Sodium<br>Potassium<br>Calcium | Strong<br>containment<br>systems | VERY few<br>enzymes<br>use these<br>as cofactors !!!!!! |

## Microminerals

| | | |
|---|---|---|
| Magnesium<br>Zinc<br>Iron<br>Copper<br>Manganese<br>Molybdenum<br>Selenium<br>Chromium<br>Cobalt | Mostly cations (two plus charge)<br>Electron donors<br>Containment systems <u>except</u> Mg | Hundreds<br>of enzymes<br>use these<br>as cofactors!!!!!! |

The importance of these containment systems was aptly summarized by Professor Bilinski. What we need then is *some* of these minerals, but not *too many* of them in the wrong place. Despite what vitamin supplement companies push, it is clear that more is *not* better!

In order to deal with them (divalent cations) we have a system that can store them and release them when necessary. A bit like letting out your hounds when you want to chase a fox.

# "Lock up your cations !"

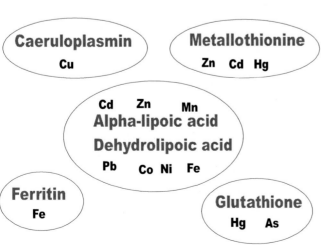

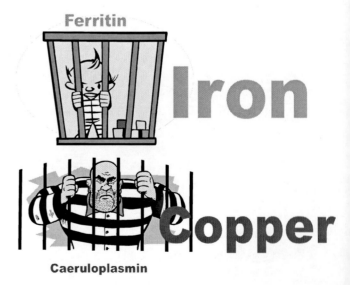

## Metallothionine Structure

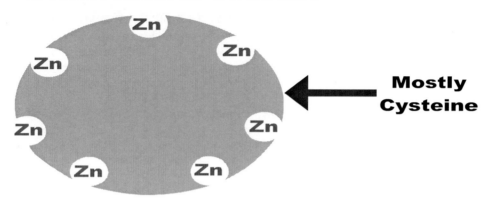

Better-known examples are ferritin and caeruloplasmin for containing copper and iron. Copper and iron have high electro negativities and pose real problems to cell in order to use them safely.

Another metalloprotein is Metallothionine, which is predominantly the sulfurous amino acid cysteine with seven zinc atoms. This compound forms part of defence system against heavy metals and too much copper. It is distributed in the gastrointestinal tract, skin, liver and brain. Disorders of it cause symptoms ranging from dairy intolerance to autism. See the chapter on zinc for more on this.

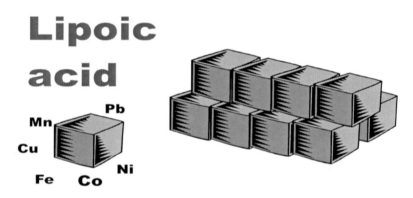

Another containment system is Alpha Lipoic Acid (ALA). ALA can complex with most divalent cations (2 plus positive ionic charge atoms). It is a valuable method of metal control within cells.

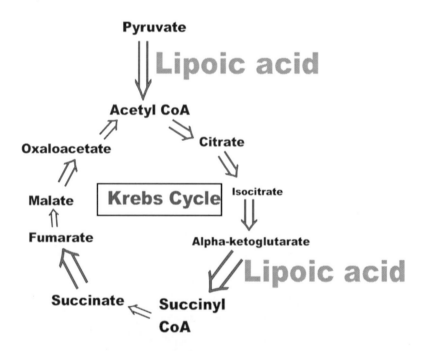

That is, if you can *spare* some of it from the Krebs cycle. This means that there may be a resource management problem for cells facing both oxidative stress and toxic metals. This could lead to neuro-degenerative conditions like Alzheimer's and Multiple Sclerosis.

Cells utilize nutrients in 3 ways; Storage/ Structure, Enzyme functions and charge/pH management. Activated nutrients utilization often defines the output of the cell. It is integral to what it does.

There are various mechanisms of intracellular antagonism and the offending atoms are listed with the nutrients they block or destroy. This is why one must know the level of **both** molecules in order to know how symptoms are being generated. The most potent blockade is by Mercury, then Cadmium.

As toxins arrive, they are stored in various parts of the cell, often inadvertently with a nutrient. This may "tie up" nutrients which get involved with this misuse. It may mean that higher levels are needed to function because normal levels "cancel out" in the presence of toxins. The analogy is like needing to use more accelerator if you have the parking brake stuck on. Antagonism of Zinc by mercury is said to be 1000:1 and Cadmium 100:1.

# Cellular defence system

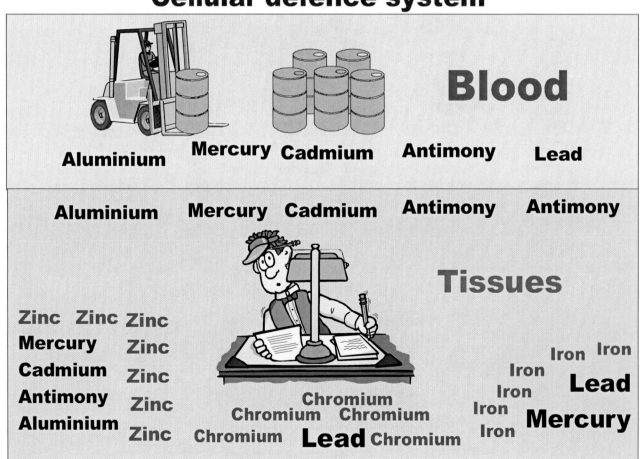

This section will examine the importance of Zinc, Molybdenum, Magnesium and Copper in the creation of a normal oxidation state within the cell. The final balance of free radicals and antioxidants affects many functions including energy production and the prevention of cancers. These minerals are involved (not to the exclusion of others of course) and imbalances within the tetrahedron will impact on the oxidation state and on other tetrahedra such as the nervous system and cognitive function.

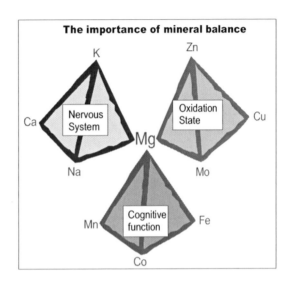

Let's look at Copper and Magnesium's contribution to the balance. The final common pathway for the production of ATP (the energy currency of most cells in the body) requires a series of electron transfers through a series of structures within the wall of the mitochondria (energy producers). The final pathway is depicted below. Although iron turns up in many of these cytochromes, the last 2 are significantly affected by copper and magnesium. An imbalance in these will affect the efficiency of electron transport and pH (acidity) levels in these powerhouses.

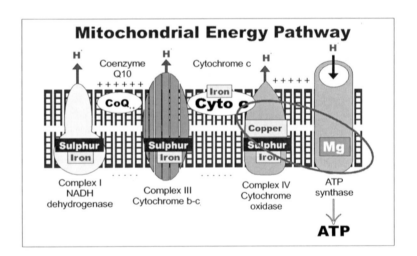

The next relationship to examine the Copper: Zinc ratio. The enzyme Superoxide dismutase is important for controlling free radical generation and disposal. However its character will change depending upon the balance of these 2 minerals. When copper is abundant the enzyme exhibits a pro-oxidation characteristic, and when zinc is in abundance it displays antioxidant features.

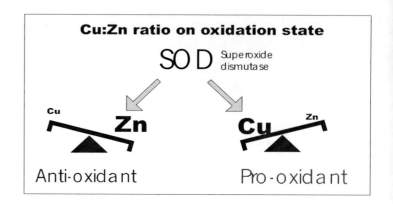

The next in the tetrahedron is Copper and Molybdenum. These 2 minerals strongly affect pH (acidity) levels in the tissues. Many enzymes do not like to be out of range for pH and mitochondria are very sensitive to pH levels as the generation of protons (ionised hydrogen atoms) affects ATP levels. The system is usually very nicely balanced (as long as Copper and Molybdenum are too).

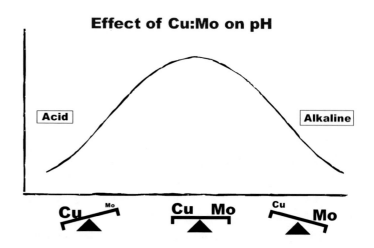

The last relationship to examine is the Zinc:Magnesium ratio. The best example of this the Cori cycle. When lactate is produced by muscle, it should be recycled to glucose by the liver. Adequate levels of magnesium and zinc are required by muscle to convert glucose to lactate. At the other end, the liver needs adequate levels of zinc and magnesium to convert the lactate back to glucose. Zinc is required for lactate Dehydrogenase.

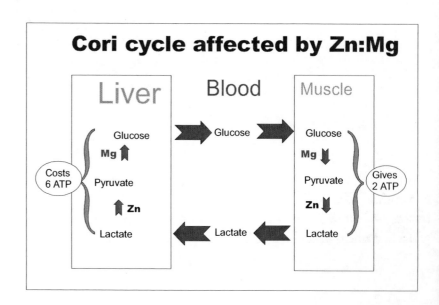

This section will look at how we arrive at the tetrahedron relating to nervous system function. The balance of these important charged ions determines the majority of nerve behaviour and understanding the reasons behind this can lead to rebalancing of nerve circuits and substantial reduction of symptoms.

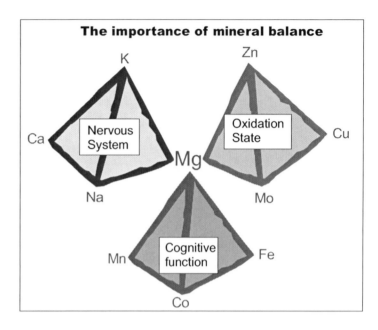

We start with nerve transmission. The propagation of the action potential is through the flux of sodium and potassium along the path of the nerve cell. Ordinarily sodium is excluded from the cell while potassium is accumulated. The electrical impulse is created when sodium flows into the cell and potassium out of the cell. This continues until the nerve impulse hits the terminal neuron. At this point the impulse will trigger the flow of calcium into the nerve cell (voltage gated calcium channel). It is the sudden rise of calcium that causes the neurotransmitter to be released into the synaptic cleft and stimulate the next nerve. As soon as calcium rushes into the cell, it is transported back out in order for the nerve (and mitochondria) to recover. So the release is short and sharp to give maximum effect, but not to linger on.

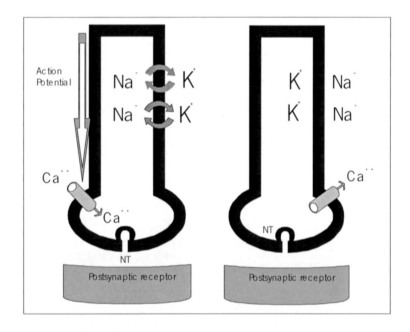

Most textbooks will depict this process as in the above diagram. However, we know that the mitochondria are in abundance in the terminal neurone and that these organelles make the neurotransmitters using ATP, which has to be generated by glucose utilisation. If we analyse the steps involved in making ATP, we see that magnesium is needed for 12 out of the 22 steps. Hence magnesium must be in abundance in the terminal neuron. So let's add the background magnesium into the equation. It turns out then, that the resting state is when magnesium is in abundance and the neuron transmitter release state is when calcium is in abundance.

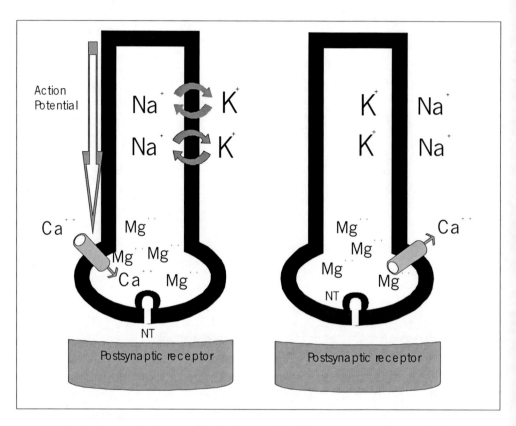

So to summarise, the nerve transmission is dependent upon the balance of sodium to potassium, while the neurotransmitter release is dependent upon the balance of calcium and magnesium. The whole system then needs all four minerals in balance, which is best depicted by a tetrahedron (four sided 3-D shape). It also transpires that ATP is a neurotransmitter that allows glial cells to "eavesdrop" on neurones.

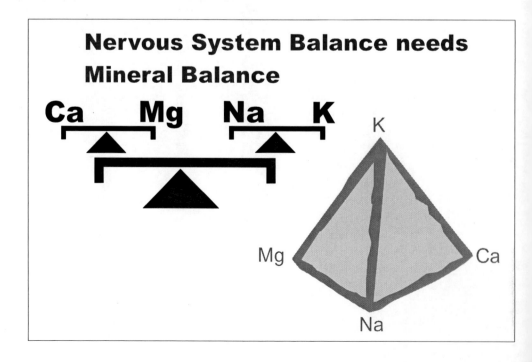

# Hormone system interactions

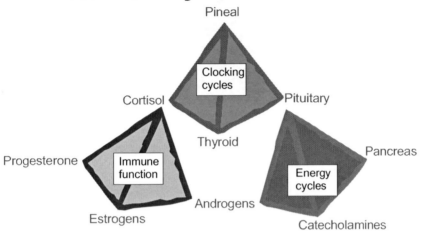

This section will attempt to show how important clocking cycles are to human health. Disruption to these cycles is common and frequently misunderstood. One example is circadian dysrhythmia.

The first link will be the best known of these, which is the menstrual cycle. The pituitary and female hormones interact as shown.
The pituitary sends messages to the ovary (FSH & LH) to ovulate and the ovary sends messages (estrogens) back to confirm. Between the two glands they create a 28-day cycle (in most women).

# Pituitary- Ovarian interaction

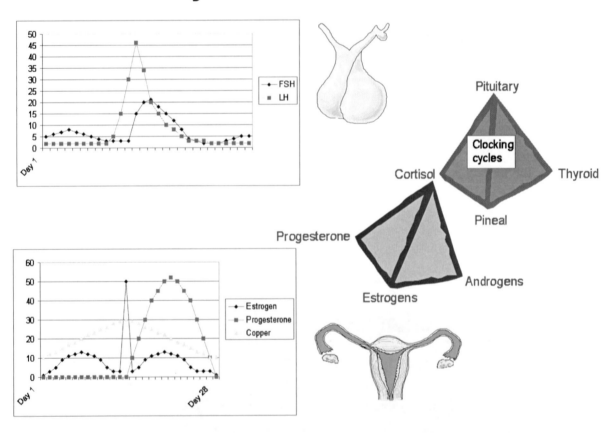

The next interaction is between the pituitary, ovary and thyroid. The conversion of T4 to T3 requires progesterone and selenium (see section on Selenium). Any rise in T3 is associated with a rise in core temperature. After ovulation, the corpus luteum makes progesterone; therefore more T3 is made which makes the core temp rise after ovulation.

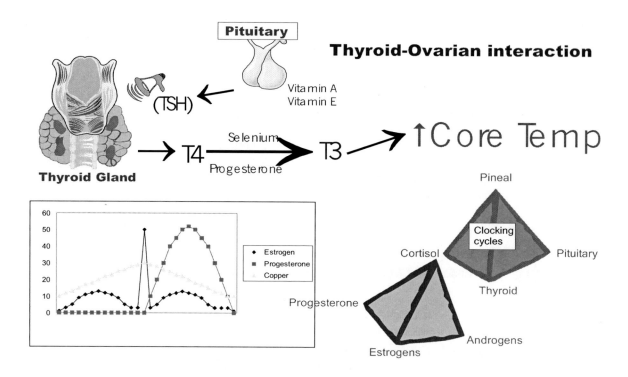

The next link is the production of DHEA modulated by melatonin. It explains the relationship between sleep times and longevity.

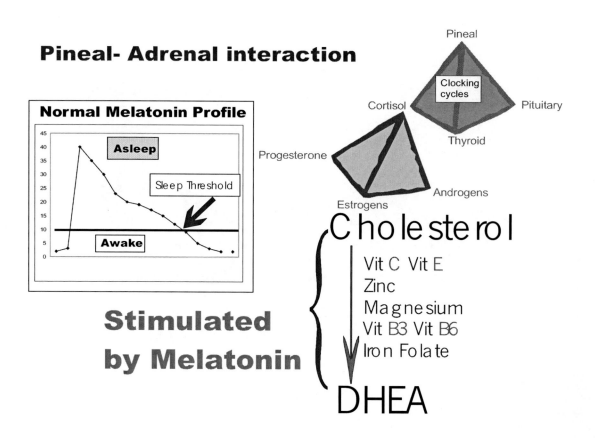

Abnormalities of this Tetrahedron are common, the best known being Syndrome X.

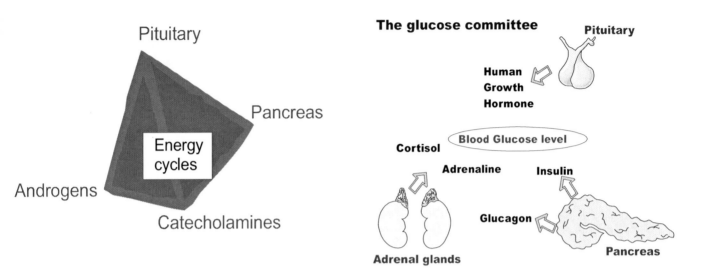

Another way of looking at this problem is by examining the "glucose committee". If these endocrine organs stop communicating correctly then obesity and blood sugar problems arise.

Which brings us to the importance of the pancreas. This organ is special in that it is an endocrine and exocrine gland. It is the interface between the inside and outside. In order for it to work, it needs a combination of trace elements and amino acids. In all, 17 different amino acids are needed for insulin. Tryptophan (which is not needed to make insulin) is required by the liver and kidney to make picolinate which bonds zinc and the other trace elements. The system relies upon a good and varied protein diet and god stomach acid production in order to get the 18 amino acids to make this part of the glucose committee run properly. Failure of any of these lead to pancreatic malfunction and hence disturbances of glucose metabolism and then adrenal and pituitary function.

# Pancreas

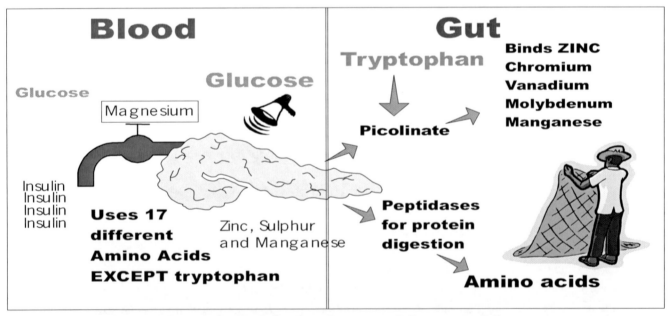

## In total 18 out of 20 Amino acids used by pancreas

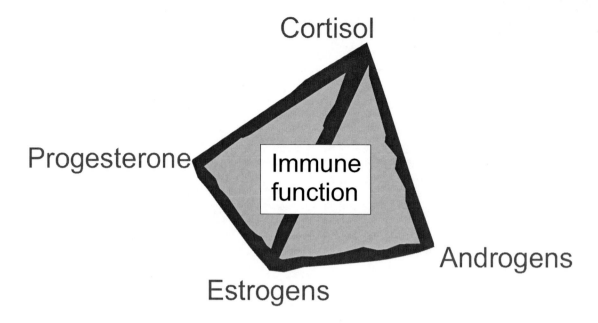

The balance of hormones affects immunity. The immune tetrahedron depicts this. The following explains how this conclusion is made.

The family of white cells includes the granulocytes and lymphocytes and as further work is carried out each subset is further delineated and their functions are mapped out.

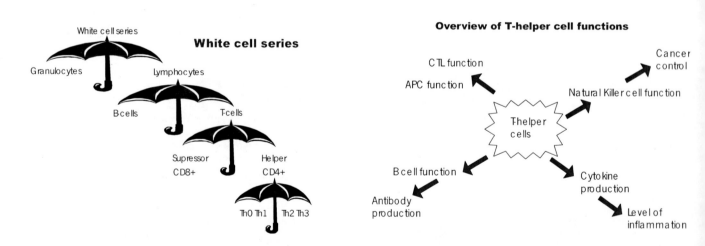

T-helper cell function determines a significant amount of immune activity both within the lymphocyte subsets and outside these subsets.

Helper cell balance affects antibody production as well as cytokine release and natural killer cell function also. Keeping Th-1 and Th-2 subsets responsibly balanced will keep an immune system from over-reacting to its own tissues, but vigilant against infections and cancers.

Certain factors can cause a Th-2 predominant system. These are listed on the next page. High Estrogen or low Progesterone and/or a low DHEA can do this. This explains why some autoimmune disorders are more common in females and may vary in the pregnant state. Extreme variations in DHEA/Cortisol balance will also affect immunity. The best examples are the immune defects in *both* Addison's disease and Cushing's.

The balance between the hormone groups, Estrogens, Progesterone, Cortisol and Androgens, will affect the balance of the T-Helper cell subsets and one aspect of this might be antibody production, another inflammation, rates of allergy and infections.

## Spectrum of Th1 Th2 imbalance

| Th1 Excess | Th2 Excess |
|---|---|
| Hashimoto's | Allergies |
| Multiple Sclerosis | Hayfever & Rhinitis |
| DM type 1 | Asthma |
| Ulcerative Colitis | Urticaria |
| Crohn's disease | SLE |
| Coeliac disease | Haemolytic anaemia |
| Rheumatoid arthritis | Thrombocytopenia |
| Sjogren's syndrome | Scleroderma |
| alopecia totalis | IBS |
| Vitiligo | CFS |
| Psoriasis | Fibromyalgia |
| Sunburn | Grave's disease |
| Alzheimer's disease | Cancer |
| Parkinson's disease | Eczema |
| Sarcoidosis | Polymyalgia rheumatica |
| Acute Allograft rejection | Buerger's syndrome |
|  | Endometriosis |

## Factors pushing Th2 up

Estrogen: progesterone balance
Low DHEA
Low Zinc
High Copper: Zinc Ratio
Low B Vitamins
Low Vitamin C
Low Vitamin A
Low selenium

# Th2

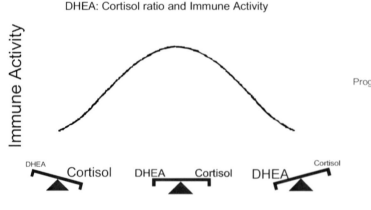

DHEA: Cortisol ratio and Immune Activity

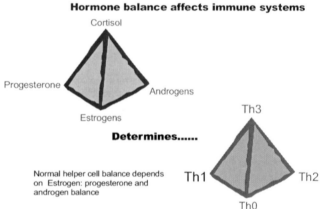

Hormone balance affects immune systems

Normal helper cell balance depends on Estrogen: progesterone and androgen balance

57

Studies on Coenzyme Q10 date back 30 years. The range of investigation includes not only studies showing that lower levels are found in a variety of diseases, but also that therapy with Coenzyme Q10 was beneficial in a variety of diseases. An interesting story about Coenzyme Q10 was about Karl Folkers the first person to synthesise it. At the time he worked for the pharmaceutical company Merck. Instead of being praised for this discovery, he was told to dump everything because Merck was about to launch a diuretic for heart failure and hypertension. The very conditions that Coenzyme Q10 could have been used for! The patent for Coenzyme Q10 was sold to a Japanese company and the rest is history.

## Factors reducing Coenzyme Q10 production

1. Cholesterol Lowering agents (Pravachol, Zocor etc)

2. Beta blockers (Atenolol, Metoprolol)

3. Phenothiazines (Stelazine, Chlorpromazine)

4. Tricyclic Antidepressants (Tofranil, Trytptanol etc)

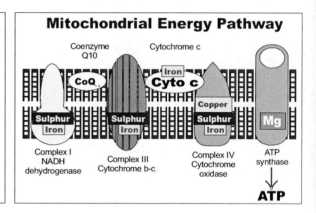

**Mitochondrial Energy Pathway**

Coenzyme Q10    Cytochrome c

CoQ    Iron    Cyto c    Copper

Sulphur Iron    Sulphur Iron    Sulphur Iron    Mg

Complex I NADH dehydrogenase    Complex III Cytochrome b-c    Complex IV Cytochrome oxidase    ATP synthase

**ATP**

Interestingly, there are many studies showing that certain commonly used medications lower the levels of this cofactor. What's more important however, is that this information should be present in the prescribing information of these drugs. What if patients taking prescription medication were given this supplement to counteract the side effects of their drugs? Then this would mean that doctors would have to be told what Coenzyme Q10 actually was. If they knew what it was, then they would realise that this supplement could be used successfully for the very medical conditions they were being told to treat with drugs! They might be tempted to try the supplement first, which would rob the drug companies and the "specialists" of income and kudos.

## Sources of coenzyme Q10
1] Meat (only if digestion good)

2] Intestinal flora

3] Endogenous production

## Nutrients needed for Coenzyme Q10 production
Magnesium
Vitamin B2, B3, B5, B6, B12
Folic Acid
Vitamin C
Selenium

The final energy chain that drives most of the cells in the body (all except the red blood cells) needs Coenzyme Q10 as the second step. This is the energy cycle that drives the entire heart!
The other steps involve iron. How many people could avoid a bypass if their iron levels were optimised?
What are the sources of Coenzyme Q10? Dietary (especially red meat), gut bacterial production (certain strains of E. Coli) and endogenous production (see diagram showing biochemical pathways).

Coenzyme Q10 looks a bit like a short snake with a big head. The head is the "Q" and the tail is the "10". A Coenzyme is a cofactor, which enhances the effectiveness of an enzyme, but isn't protein based. The "Q" comes from quinate and the "10" comes from the fact that the "tail" of Coenzyme Q10 has 10 carbon atoms. So this means that Coenzyme Q10 is made in two bits. The quinate comes from Tyrosine and is bent into a ring form like a benzene molecule. (left side of the pathway). The "10" part comes from joining a 2-carbon part with a 3-carbon part to make a 5–carbon part and then joining the two 5-carbon parts to make the "10". Finally you join the head to the tail.

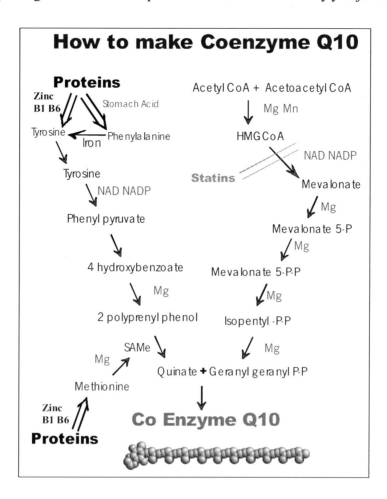

There are several interesting features of the biochemical pathways. Firstly, magnesium is heavily involved. This puts it at risk of blockade by copper. Secondly a cofactor called SAMe is also required. Lastly is where the cholesterol lowering agents block the pathway to make Coenzyme Q10. They block HMGCoA reductase, which is an important

## Coenzyme Q10 studies

Cancer prevention and treatment
Ischaemic Heart disease prevention and treatment
Heart failure prevention and treatment
Diabetes prevention and treatment
High blood pressure prevention and treatment
Stroke prevention and treatment
Glaucoma prevention and treatment
Chronic fatigue syndrome prevention and treatment
Alzheimers disease prevention and treatment

step in the synthesis of Coenzyme Q10. How long has medicine known this? 20 years!

The range of conditions that may respond to Coenzyme Q10 are listed. They are part of the modern "unexplained" epidemic of diseases, mostly fatal. Isn't it time the medical profession woke up from their coma and start looking at the evidence in their own literature?

**Negative effects of drugs on Coenzyme Q10 starting from 1975**

1] Aberg F., Appelkvist E.L. & Broijersen A., et al. Gemfibrozil-induced decrease in Serum Ubiquinone and Alpha- and Gamma-Tocopherol levels in men with Combined Hyperlipidaemia. Eur J Clin Invest. 28(3):235-42, 1998

2] Appelkvist E.L., Edlund C. & Low P., et al. Effects of Inhibitors of Hydroxymethylglutaryl Coenzyme A Reductase on Coenzyme Q and Dolichol Biosynthesis. Clin Investig. 71(8 Suppl):S97-102, 1993

3] Bargossi A.M. Grossi G. & Fiorella P.L., et al. Exogenous CoQ10 Supplementation Prevents Plasma Ubiquinone Reduction Induced by HMG-CoA Reductase Inhibitors. Mol Aspects Med. 15(suppl):187-93, 1994

4] Belichard P., Pruneau D. & Zhiri A. Effect of a Long-Term treatment with Lovastatin or Fenofibrate on Hepatic and Cardiac Ubiquinone levels in Cardiomyopathic Hamster. Biochem Biophys Acta. 1169(1):98-102, 1993

5] De Pinieux G., Chariot P. & Ammi-Said M., et al. Lipid-Lowering Drugs and Mitochondrial Function: Effects of HMG-CoA Reductase Inhibitors on Serum Ubiquinone and Blood Lactate/Pyruvate Ratio. Br J Clin Pharmacol. 42(3):333-7, 1996

6] Folkers K., Langsjoen P. & Willis R., et al. Lovastatin decreases Coenzyme Q levels in humans. Proc Natl Acad Sci U S A. 87(22):8931-4, 1990

7] Ghirlanda G., Oradei A. & Manto A., et al. Evidence of Plasma CoQ10-Lowering Effect by HMG-CoA Reductase Inhibitors: A Double-Blind, Placebo-Controlled Study. J Clin Pharmacol. 33(3):226-9, 1993

8] Mortensen S.A., Leth A. & Agner E., et al. Dose-Related decrease of Serum Coenzyme Q10 during treatment with HMG-CoA Reductase Inhibitors. Mol Aspects Med. 18(suppl):S137-44, 1997

9] Watts G.F., Castelluccio C. & Rice-Evans C., et al. Plasma Coenzyme Q (Ubiquinone) Concentrations in patients treated with Simvastatin. J Clin Pathol. 46(11):1055-7, 1993

10] Willis R.A., Folkers K. & Tucker J.L., et al. Lovastatin decreases Coenzyme Q levels in rats. Proc Natl Acad Sci U S A. 87(22):8928-30, 1990

**Some studies dating back to 1970**

Brude, I. R., et al. Peroxidation of LDL from combined-hyperlipidemic male smokers supplied with omega-3 fatty acids and antioxidants. Arterioscler Thromb Vasc Biol. 17(11):2576-2588, 1997.

Digiesi, V., et al. Mechanism of the action of coenzyme Q10 in essential hypertension. Curr Ther Res. 51:668-672, 1992.

Digiesi, V., et al. Coenzyme Q10 in essential hypertension. Mol Aspects Med. 15(Supplement):257-263, 1994.

Folkers, K., et al. Evidence for a deficiency of coenzyme Q10 in human heart disease. Int J Vit Res. 40:380, 1970.

Folkers, K., et al. Biochemical rationale and myocardial tissue data on the effective therapy of cardiomyopathy with coenzyme Q10. Proceedings of the National Academy of Sciences. 82:901, 1985.

Folkers, K., et al. Survival of cancer patients on therapy with coenzyme Q10. Biochemical and Biophysical Research Communications. 192(1):241-245, 1993.

Gaby, A. R. The role of coenzyme Q10 in clinical medicine. Part II. Cardiovascular disease, hypertension, diabetes mellitus and infertility. Alt Med Rev. 1(3):168-175, 1996.

Greenberg, A., et al. Coenzyme Q10: A new drug for cardiovascular disease. Journal of Clinical Pharmacology. 30: 596-608, 1990.

Hanaki, Y., et al. Coenzyme Q10 and coronary artery disease. Clin Investig. 71:S112-S115, 1993.

Langsjoen, P. H., et al. Response of patients in classes III and IV of cardiomyopathy to therapy in a blind and crossover trial with coenzyme Q10. Proceedings of the National Academy of Sciences, USA. 82(12):4240-4244, 1985.

Langsjoen, P. H., et al. Effective and safe therapy with coenzyme Q10 for cardiomyopathy. Klinische Wochenschrift . 66(13):583-590, 1988.

Langsjoen, P. H, et al. A six-year clinical study of therapy of cardiomyopathy with coenzyme Q10. Int Journal of Tissue Reactions. 12(3):169-171; 1990.

Langsjoen, P.H., et al. Pronounced increase in survival of patients with cardiomyopathy when treated with coenzyme Q10 and conventional therapy. International Journal of Tissue Reactions. 12(3):163-168, 1990.

Langsjoen, P., et al. Treatment of essential hypertension with coenzyme Q10. Mol Aspects Med. 15(Supplement):S265-S272, 1994.

Langsjoen, H., et al. Usefulness of coenzyme Q10 in clinical cardiology: a long-term study. Mol Aspects Med. 15(Supp):S165-S175, 1994.

Littaru, G. P., et al. Deficiency of coenzyme Q10 in human heart disease, part II. Int J Vit Nutr Res. 42:413, 1972.

Lockwood, K., et al. Apparent partial remission of breast cancer in 'high risk' patients supplemented with nutritional anitoxidants, essential fatty acids and coenzyme Q10. Molecular Aspects of Medicine. 15(Supplement):S231-S240, 1994.

Lockwood K., et al. Partial and complete regression of breast cancer in patients in relation to dosage of coenzyme Q10. Biochemical and Biophysical Research Communications. 199(3):1504-8, 1994.

Lockwood, K., et al. Progress on therapy of breast cancer with vitamin Q10 and the regression of metastases. Biochemical and Biophysical Research Communications. 212(1):172-177, 1995.

Mellstedt, H., et al. A deficiency of coenzyme Q10 (CoQ10) in cancer patients in Sweden. In: Eighth International Symposium on Biomedical and Clinical Aspects of Coenzyme Q. The Molecular Aspects of Medicine. 1994.

Mortensen, S. A. Perspectives on therapy of cardiovascular diseases with coenzyme Q10 (ubiquinone). Clinical Investigator. 71:S116-S123, 1993

Mortensen, S. A., et al. Coenzyme Q10: Clinical benefits with biochemical correlates suggesting a scientific breakthrough in the management of chronic heart failure. Int J Tissue React. 12(3):155-162, 1990.

Neuzil, J., et al. Alpha-tocopherol hydroquinone is an efficient multifunctional inhibitor of radical-initiated oxidation of low density lipoprotein lipids. Proc Natl Acad Sci USA. 94:7885-7890, 1997.

Portakal, O., et al. Coenzyme Q10 concentrations and antioxidant status in tissues of breast cancer patients. Clin Biochem. 33:279-284, 2000.

Sinatra, S.  Coenzyme Q10 and cancer.  Sixth International Congress on Anti-Aging and Bio-Med Techn Conf Las Vegas 11-13 Dec 1998.

Singh, R. B., et al.  Randomized, double-blind placebo-controlled trial of coenzyme Q10 in patients with acute myocardial infarction.  Cardiovascular Drugs Ther.  12(4):347-353, 1998.

Singh, R. B., et al.  Serum concentration of lipoprotein(a) decreases on treatment with hydrosoluble coenzyme Q10 in patients with coronary artery disease: discovery of a new role.  Int J Cardiol.  68(1):23-29, 1999.

Yamagami, T., et al.  Bioenergetics in clinical medicine.  Studies on coenzyme Q10 and essential hypertension.  Research Communications in Chemical Pathology and Pharmacology.  11(2):273-278, 1975.

Yamagami, T., et al.  Bioenergetics in clinical medicine.  VIII.  Administration of coenzyme Q10 to patients with essential hypertension.  Research Communications in Chemical Pathology and Pharmacology.  14(4):721-727, 1976.

Yamagami, T., et al.  Effect on Q10 on essential hypertension, a double blind controlled study.  Biomed and Clin Aspects of CoQ10.  5:337-344, 1986.

Yu, C. A., et al.  Studies on the ubiquinone-protein interaction in electron transfer complexes.  Biomed and Clin aspects of CoQ10.  4:57-68, 1984.

**My first point is to explain that the data about nutrition and cancer has been collated for over a century. In case you have any doubts about how ignorant Doctors are about this information, I have provided a short list at the end of this chapter. "My case rests your honour".....**

Copper excess and Cancer.

The university of Michigan published a paper, which showed that molybdenum supplements could alter the outcomes of cancer patients. It was called "Treatment of metastatic cancer with tetrathiomolybdate (ed molybdenum salt), an anti-copper, anti-angiogenic agent: Phase I study". It showed that starving tumours of copper could arrest their growth. Other studies have shown that molybdenum will affect a variety of cancers either orally or topically in humans and animal models. It begs the question of copper's involvement in the cause of cancer.

Certainly copper excess is related in part to Xenoestrogen exposure. This class of compound (especially the Organochlorines) are progressively being labelled as carcinogens. Hence the cause of the copper overload is also the carcinogen.

Secondly high coppers are always associated with deficiency of molybdenum, which is copper's most effective controller. This explains the mounting number of studies linking molybdenum deficiency to cancer of oesophagus, breast, stomach and colon.

Thirdly, copper has a Jekyll and Hyde personality. At normal levels it behaves itself but at high levels it blocks zinc, iron and magnesium and destroys by oxidation Vitamin C, Folic Acid and Vitamin E and Vitamin B1 (thiamine). Vitamin C and Folic Acid deficiency are associated with cancers like Larynx, Prostate, Breast, Cervix, Uterus, Melanoma, Bladder, Stomach and Pancreas.

Immunorestoration.

This involves the identification of the biochemical mechanisms that caused the cancer and its spread. Studies since early last century have accumulated about the reasons cancer occurs. Even "Nutritional" doctors do generally not attempt using the studies in a clinical setting. The importance of restoring the immune system to normal involves analysing why it failed. Whatever the chosen mode of clearance be it surgery, radiotherapy or chemotherapy, the conditions that caused the cancer are *still present* in the body. This is why recurrences occur. A cancer progresses in the following steps.

1] The process begins with a carcinogen. There are 3 groups, chemicals, metals and radiation. These compounds cause DNA mutation. The cell auditors, zinc and magnesium normally check this process.

2] The next step involves abnormal cell replication. Every cell in our body has a "self-destruct button" called Apoptosis. This button should always be pushed if the cell becomes abnormal. The requirements for an intact mechanism include balance between a) Estrogen and Progesterone, b) good energy cycles, c) a balance between iron and copper and d) a balance between copper and the longevity hormone DHEA (dehydroepiandrosterone). The balance of Estrogen and progesterone affects two important genes. P53 is an apoptosis gene. Its expression is dependent on progesterone levels. BCL-2 is a cancer gene and its expression is affected by Estrogen levels (ALL estrogens, endogenous and foreign eg xenoestrogens). One of the mechanisms of apoptosis is brought about by the passage of Cytochrome C leaving the mitochondria and triggering the apoptosis "button". The availability of free cytochrome C is dependent upon iron copper balance. The more copper, the less cytochrome C, the less apoptosis occurs. The level of free radicals to antioxidants also affect apoptosis. Since DHEA reduces copper's oxidizing power, Copper: DHEA ratio affects apoptosis. We make DHEA from Cholesterol and the rate of production is affected by Melatonin. The production of melatonin is complex and requires many steps and cofactors.

3] Any cells that attempt to migrate are controlled by a security patrol of lymphocytes. This security patrol needs zinc, iron, and selenium, Vitamin C, Vitamin D and Vitamin E.

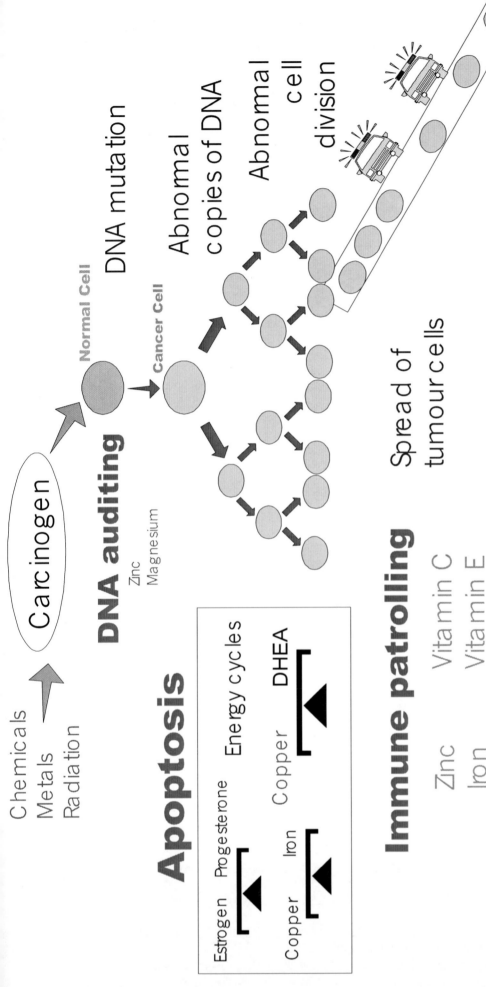

Chemicals
Metals
Radiation

Carcinogen

Normal Cell

DNA mutation

**DNA auditing**

Zinc
Magnesium

Cancer Cell

Abnormal
copies of DNA

Abnormal
cell
division

**Apoptosis**

Estrogen   Progesterone   Energy cycles

Copper        Copper      DHEA

Iron

Spread of
tumour cells

**Immune patrolling**

Zinc       Vitamin C
Iron        Vitamin E
Selenium Vitamin D

Encouragement
of new blood supply

**Angiogenesis**

**Copper**

4] Even if the tumour cells lodge in a new environment (metastasize), they cannot survive without developing a new blood supply. This is called Angiogenesis (*angio* meaning blood vessel and *genesis* meaning new). This process is dependent upon the amount of copper in the tissues and the requirement for copper by the tumour.

So all in all, it is extremely difficult to induce a cancer in a human. Many systems have to fail. Analysing the failed systems involves blood tests and hair analysis. When all this information is collated, the mechanism of the cancer becomes clear and the mode of repair can be planned. This may involve oral supplements such as tablets, capsules and powders or intravenous supplements.

Cancer References relating to Nutrional Medicine: For a larger list see www.nutritionreviewservice.com.au look on references in the left frame.

1] Amer B.N. & Gold L.S. Natural chemicals, synthetic chemicals, risk assessment and caner. Princess Takamatsu Symp. 21:303-314, 1990

2] Bain C., et al. Diet and melanoma. An exploratory case-control study. Ann Epidemiol. 3(3):235-8, 1993

3] Barch D.H. Esophageal cancer and microelements. J Am Coll Nutr. 8(2):99-107, 1989

4] Block G., et al. Fruit, vegetables, and cancer prevention: a review of the epidemiological evidence. Nutr Cancer. 18:1-20, 1992

5] Blondell J.M. The anticarcinogenic effect of magnesium. Med Hypotheses. 6:863-71, 1980

6] Blutt .E. & Weigel N.L. Vitamin D and prostate cancer. Proc Soc Exp Biol Med. 221(2):89-98, Jun, 1999

7] Böing H., et al. Regional nutritional pattern and cancer mortality in the Federal Republic of Germany. Nutr Cancer. 7(3):121-30, 1985

8] Böing H., et al. Dietary carcinogens and the risk for glioma and meningioma in Germany. Int J Cancer 53:561-5, 1993

9] Booyens J., et al. Dietary fats and cancer. Med Hypotheses 17:351-62, 1985

10] Bostick R.M., et al. Sugar, meat, and fat intake, and non-dietary risk factors for colon cancer incidence in Iowa women (United States). Cancer Causes Control. 5:38-52, 1994

11] Bounous D.G., et al. Whey proteins in cancer prevention. Can Lett. 57:91-4, 1991

12] Broghamer W.L., et al. Relationship between serum selenium levels and patients with carcinoma. Cancer. 37:1384, 1976

13] Bruemmer B., et al. Nutrition intake in relation to bladder cancer among middle-aged men and women. Am J Epidemiol 144(5):485-95, 1996

14] Bueno-de-Mesquita HB., Gonzalez CA. Main hypotheses on diet and cancer investigated in the EPIC study. Eur J Canc Prev. 6:1-7-17, 1997

15] Burnley P.G.J., et al. Serologic precursors of cancer: Serum micronutrients and the subsequent risk of pancreatic cancer. American Journal of Clinical Nutrition. 49:895-900, 1989

16] Butterworth C.E. Jr. Effect of folate on cervical cancer. Synergism among risk factors. Ann N Y Acad Sci. 669:293-9, 1992

17] Butterworth C.E., et al. Folate status, women's health, pregnancy outcome and cancer. J Am Coll Nutr. 12(4):438-41. Review. Aug, 1993

18] Byers, R., et al. Epidemiologic evidence for vitamin C and vitamin E in cancer prevention. Am J Clin Nutr. 62(Supplement):1385S-1392S, 1995.

19] Cao G.H., et al. A study of the relationship between trace element Mo and gastric cancer. World J Gastroenterol Feb. 4(1): 55-56, 1998

20] Carroll K.K. Dietary factors in hormone-dependent cancers, in M Winick, Ed. Current Concepts in Nutrition, Volume 6: Nutrition and Cancer. New York, John Wiley & Sons, 25-40, 1977

21] Carroll K.K. Dietary fats and cancer. Am J Clin Nutr. 53:1064S-7S, 1991

22] Cheng K.K., et al. Stopping drinking and risk of oesophageal cancer. Br Med J. 310:1094-7, 1995

23] Cheng K.K., et al. Nutrition and oesophageal cancer. Cancer Causes and Control. 7:33-40, 1996

24] Chiu B C-H., et al. Diet and risk of non-Hodgkin lymphoma in older women. JAMA 275(17):1315-31, 1996

25] Chlebowski R.T., et al. New directions in the nutritional management of the cancer patient. Nutr Res. 13:3-21, 1993

26] Clark L. The epidemiology of selenium and cancer. Federation Proceedings. 44:2584-2589, 1985

27] Clark L.C., et al. Plasma selenium and skin neoplasms: A case control study. Nutr Cancer. 6:13, 1985

28] Clark L.C., et al. Effects of selenium supplementation for cancer prevention in patients with carcinoma of the skin. JAMA. 276(24):1957-63, 1996

29] Clark L.C., et al. Decreased incidence of prostate cancer with selenium supplementation: results of double-blind cancer prevention trial. Br J Urol. 81:730-734, 1998

30] Colditz G.A., et al. Increased green and yellow vegetable intake and lowered cancer deaths in an elderly population. Am J Clin Nutr 41(1):32-6, 1985

31] Coldsitz G.A. Selenium and cancer prevention: promising results indicate further trials required. The Journal of the American Medical Association. 276(24):1984, 1996

32] Colston K.W., et al. Possible role for vitamin D in controlling breast cancer proliferation. Lancet i:188-91, 1989

33] Combs G.F., et al. Can dietary selenium modify cancer risk? Nutr. Rev. 43:325-331, 1985

34] Combs G.F. Jr., et al. Reduction of cancer mortality and incidence by selenium supplementation. Med Klin. 92(Supplement 3):42-

45, 1997

35] Comee J., et al. A Case-control study of gastric cancer and nutrutuinal factors in Marseille, France. Eur J Epidemiol. 11:55-65, 1995

36] Copeland E.M. 3rd et al. Nutrition and cancer. Int Adv Surg Oncol. 4:1-13, 1981

37] Cox C et al The role of copper suppression as an antiangiogenic strategy in head and neck squamous cell carcinoma Laryngoscope apr 111 (4 pt 1) : 696-701 2001

38] Daou D.L. Natural anticarcinogens, carcinogens and changing patterns in cancer: some speculations. Enviro Res. 50(2):322-40, 1989

39] D'Avanzo B., et al. Alcohol consumption and the risk of gastric cancer. Nutr Cancer. 22:57-64, 1994

40] Davis D.L., Bradlow H.L., Wolff M., Woodruff T., Hoel D.G. and Anton-Culver H. Medical Hypothesis: Xenohormones as Preventable Causes of Breast Cancer. Env Health Persoectuves. 101:372-377, 1993

41] Delmore G. Assessment of nutritional status in cancer patients: widely neglected? Support Care Cancer. 5(5):376-80, 1997

42] Dich J., et al. Pesticides and cancer. Cancer cayses control. 8(3):420-443, 1997

43] Durlach J., Bara M. Magnesium and its relationship to oncology, in H. Sigel, A. Sigel, Eds. Metal Ions in Biological Systems. Vol. 26: Compendium on magnesium and its role in biology. New York-Basel, Marcek Dekker, 1990

44] Eichhlozer M., et al. Prediction of male cancer mortality by plasma levels of interacting vitamins: 17 year follow-up of the prospective Basal study. Int J Cancer. 66:145-50, 1996

45] Enig M.G., et al. Dietary fat and cancer trends – A critique. Fed Proc. 37:2215-20, 1978

46] Eskin B.A. Iodine and breast cancer. A 1982 update. Biol Trace Elem Res. 5:399-412, 1983

47] Esteve J., et al. Diet and cancers of the larynx and hypopharynx: the IARC multi-center study in southwestern Europe. Cancer causes Control. 7:240-52, 1996

48] Fearson K.C. Nutritional pharmacology in the treatment of neoplastic disease. Bailieres Clin Gastroenterol. 2(4):941-9, Oct, 1988

49] Fenech M. & Ferguson L.R. Vitamins/minerals and genomic stability in humans. Mutat Res. 475(1-2):1-6, Apr 18, 2001

50] Ferraroni M., et al. Selected micronutrient intake and the risk of colorectal cancer. Br J cancer. 70(6):1150-5, 1994

51] Ferrigno D., Buccheri G., Camilla T. Serum copper and zinc content in non-small cell lung cancer: abnormalities and clinical correlates. Monaldi Arch Chest Dis (Italy), Jun. 54(3) p204-8, 1999

52] Feustel A. & Wennrich R. Zinc and cadmium in cell fractions of prostatic cancer tissues of different histological grading in comparison to BPH and normal prostate. Urol Res. 12(2):147-50, 1984

53] Flaten T.P. Chlorination of drinking water and cancer incidence in Norway. Int J Epidemiol. 21(1):6-15. 1992

54] Folkers K., et al. Survival of cancer patients on therapy with coenzyme Q10. Biochem Biophys Res Commun. 192(1):241-5, 1993

55] Franceschi S., et al. Dietary factors and non-Hodgkin's lymphoma: a case-control study in the north-eastern part of Italy. Nurt Cancer. 12:333-41, 1989

56] Franceschi S. I., et al. Food groups and risk of colorectal cancer in Italy. Int J Cancer. 72:56-61, 1997

57] Frentzel-Beyme R. & Chang-Claude J. Vegetarian diets and colon cancer: the German Experience. Am J Clin Nutr. 59(suppl):1143S-52S,1994

58] Freudenheim J.L., et al. Diet, smoking and alcohol in cancer of the larynx: a case-control study. Nutr Cancer. 17:33-45, 1992

59] Fuch C.S., et al. Dietary fiber and the risk of colorectal cancer and adenoma in women. N Engl J Med. 230(3):169-76, 1999

60] Gao Y.T., et al. Risk factors for esophageal cancer in Shanghai, China. II. Role of diet and nutrients. Int J Cancer. 58(2):197-202, 1994

62] Garland C., et al. Dietary vitamin D and calcium and risk of colorectal cancer: A 19-year prospective study in men. Lancet i:307-9, 1985

63] Garland C.F., et al. Serum 25-hydroxyvitamin D and colon cancer. Eight-year prospective study. Lancet i:176-8, 1989

64] Garland M., et al. Prospective study of toenail selenium levels and cancer among women. J Natl Cancer Inst. 87(7):497-505, 1995

65] Ghadirian P., et al. International comparisons of nutrition and mortality from pancreatic cancer. Cancer Detect Prev. 15(5):357-62, 1991

66] Ghadirian P., et al. Nutritional factors and colon carcinoma: a case-control study involving French canadians in Montreal, Quebec, Canada. Cancer. 80:858-64, 1997

67] Giovannucci E., et al. A prospective study of dietary fat and risk of prostate cancer. J Natl Cancer Inst. 85(19):1571-9, 1993

68] González C.A., et al. Nutritional factors and gastric cancer in Spain. Am J Epidemiol. 139:466-73, 1994

69] Goodman M.T., et al. Diet, body size, physical activity and the risk of endometrial cancer. Cancer Res. 57:077-85, 1997a

70] Goodman M.T., et al. Association of soy and fiber consumption with the risk of endometrial cancer. Am J Epidemiol. 146(4):294-306, 1997b

71] Graf E & Eaton J. Suppression of colon cancer by dietary phytic acid. Nutr Cancer. 19(1):11-19, 1993

72] Graham S., et al. Dietary factors in the epidemiology of cancer of the larynx. Am J Epidemiol. 113(6):675-80, 1981

73] Gridley G., et al. Vitamin supplement use and reduced risk of oral and pharyngeal cancer. Am J Epidemiol. 135(10):1083-92, 1992

74] Guo How-Ran et al. Arsenic in drinking water and incidence of urinary cancers. Epidemiology. 8(5):545-50, 1997

75] Hartwig A. Role of magnesium in genomic stability. Mutat Res. 475(1-2):113-21. Review. Apr 18, 2001

76] Head K. Ascorbic acid in the prevention and treatment of cancer. Altern Med Rev. 3(3):174-186, 1998

77] Hertog M.G.L., et al. Dietary flavonoids and cancer risk in the Zutphen Elderly Study. Nutr Cancer. 22:175-84, 1994

78] Hill M. Epidemiology of meat and colorectal cancer – historical aspects. Eur Cancer Prevent News. 31:8-10, 1997

79] Hinds M.W., et al. Dietary cholesterol and lung cancer among men in Hawaii. Am J Clin Nutr. 37:192-3, 1983

80] Howe G., et al. Dietary factors and risk of pancreatic cancer: Results of a Canadian population-based case-control study. Int J Cancer. 45:604-8, 1990

81] Hrushesky W.J.M. Breast Cancer, Timing of Surgery, and the Menstrual Cycle: Call for Prospective Trial. J Women's Health. 5:555-566, 1996

82] Hrushesky W.J. Menstrual Cycle Timing of Breast Cancer Resection: Prospective Study is Overdue. J Natl Cancer Inst. 87(2):143-4, 1995

83] Hursting S., et al. Types of dietary fat and the incidence of cancer at five sites. Prev Med. 19:242-53, 1990

84] Ingram D., et al. Case-control study of phyto-oestrogens and breast cancer. Lancet. 350:990-4, 1997

85] Jacobs D.R. Jr., et al. Whole grain intake and cancer: a review of the literature. Nutr Cancer. 24(3):221-9, 1995

86] Jaga K. & Duvvi H. Risk reduction for DDT toxicity and carcinogenesis through dietary modification. J R Soc Health. 121(2):107-13. Review. Jun, 2001

87] John A.P. Dysfunctional mitochondria, not oxygen insufficiency, cause cancer to produce inordinate amounts of lactic acid: the impact of this on the treatment of cancer. Med Hypotheses. 57(4):429-431, 2001

88] Kandouz M., Siromachkova M., Jacob D., Marquet B.C., et al. Antagonism between Estradiol and Progestin on Bcl-2 Expression in Breast Cancer Cells. Int J Cancer. 68:120-125, 1996

89] Kaplan S., et al. Nutritional factors in the etiology of brain tumors. Am J Epidemiol. 146(10):832-41, 1997

90] Kaul L., et al. The role of diet in prostate cancer. Nutr Cancer. 9:123-8, 1987

91] Kirschner M.A. The Role of Hormones in the Etiology of Human Breast Cancer. Cancer. 39(6):2716-2726, 1977

92] Knekt P., et al. Serum selenium and subsequent risk of cancer among Finnish men and women. J National Cancer Institute. 82:864-868, 1990

93] Knekt P., et al. Body iron stores and risk of cancer. Int J Cancer. 56(3):379-82, 1994

94] Kolonel L.N., et al. Nutrient intakes in relation to cancer incidence in Hawaii. Br J Cancer. 44(3);332-9, 1981

95] Komada K., et al. Effects of dietary molybdenum on esophageal carcinogenesis in rats induced by N-methyl-N-benzylnitrosamine. Cancer Res. 50:2418-2422, 1990

96] La Vecchia C., et al. Intake of selected micronutrients and risk of colorectal cancer. Int J Cancer. 73:525-30, 1997

97] Lee J.R. Fluoridation and bone cancer. Editorial. Fluoride. 26(2):79-82, 1993

98] Lemon H.M. & Rodriguez-Sierra J.F. Timing of breast cancer surgery during the luteal menstrual phase may improve prognosis. Nebr Med J. 81(4):110-5, Apr, 1996

99] Levi F., et al. Dietary factors and the risk of endometrial cancer. Cancer. 71:3575-81, 1993

100] Liehr J.G. Genotoxic Effects of Estrogens. Mutat Res. 238(3):269-276, 1990

101] Lockwood K., et al. Partial and complete regression of breast cancer in patients in relation to dosage of coenzyme Q10. Biochem Biophys Res Commun. 199(3):1504-8, 1994a

102] Lockwood K., et al. Apparent partial remission of breast cancer in 'high risk' patients supplemented with nutritional antioxidants, essential fatty acids and coenzyme Q10. Molec Aspects Med. 15(suppl):S231-S240, 1994b

103] Lockwood K., et al. Progress in therapy of breast cancer with vitamin Q10 and the regression of metastases. Biochem Biophys Res Commun. 212(1):172-7, 1995

104] Luo X.M., et al. Molybdenum and oesophageal cancer in China. Federation Proceedings. Federation of the American Society for Experimental Biology. 46:928, 1981

105] Malvy D.J.M., et al. Assessment of serum antioxidant micronutrients and biochemical indicators of nutritional status in children with cancer in search of prognostic factors. Int J Vitam Nutr Res. 67:267-71, 1997

106] Martinez M.E. & Willett W.C. Calcium, vitamin D and colorectal cancer: a review of the epidemioligic evidence. Cancer Epidemiol Biomarkers Prev. 7(2):163-8, 1998

107] Mayne S.T. Nutrition intake and risk of subtypes of esophageal and gastric cancer. Cancer Epidemiol Biomarkers Prev. 10(10):1055-62, Oct, 2001

108] McCarthy M. Selenium linked to lower prostate cancer risk [letter]. Lancet. 352:713, 1998

109] McConnell K.P., et al. The relationship between dietary selenium and breast cancer. Journal of Surgical Oncology. 15(1):67-70, 1980

110] Meguid M., et al. Plasma carotenoid profiles in normals and patients with cancer. J Parenter Enteral Nutr. 12(2):147-51, 1988

111] Menkes M.S., et al. Serum beta-carotene, vitamins A and E, selenium and the risk of lung cancer. NEJM. 315:1250, 1986

112] Messina M.J., et al. Soy intake and cancer risks: a review of the in vitro and in vivo data. Nutr Cancer. 21:113:31, 1994

113] Mettlin C.J., et al. Patterns of milk consumption and risk of cancer. Nutr Cancer. 12:89-99, 1990

114] Milde et al. Serum levels of selenium, manganese, copper and iron in colorectal patients. Biol Trace Elem Res (USA) .79 (2) 107-14, 2001

115] Milner J.A. A historical perspective on garlic and cancer. J Nutr. 131(3s):1027S-31S, Mar, 2001

116] Mohr P.E., Wang D.Y., Gregory W.M., Richards M.A. and Fentiman I.S. Serum Progesterone and Prognosis in Operable Breast cancer. Br J Can. 73:1552-1555, 1996

117] Moon T.E., et al. Retinoids in prevention of skin cancer. Can Let 114:203-5, 1997

118] Nakadaira H., et al. Distribution of selenium and molybdenum and cancer mortality in Niigata, Japan. Arch Envir Health Sep. 50:5 374-80, 1995

119] Nakakoshi T. Copper and hepatocellular carcinoma. Radiology (United States), Jan. 214(1) p304-6, 2000

120] Nanba H., Hamaguchi A. & Kuroda H. The chemical structure of an antitumor polysaccharide in fruit bodies of Grifola frondosa (maitake). Chem Pharm Bull. 35:1162-1168, 1987

121] Nanba H. Antitumor activity of orally administered "D-Fraction" from maitake mushroom (Grifola frondosa). J Naturopathic Med. 1:10-15, 1993

122] Negri I., et al. Intake of selected micronutrients and the risk of breast cancer. Int J Cancer. 65:140-4, 1996

123] Nelson R.L. Is the changing pattern of colorectal cancer caused by selenium deficiency? Dis Colon Rectum. 459-461, 1984

124] Nelson R.L., et al. Serum selenium and colonic neoplastic risk. Diseases of the Colon and Rectum. 38:1306-1310, 1995

125] Newmark H.L., et al. Colon cancer and dietary fat, phosphate and calcium: A hypothesis. J Natl Cancer Inst. 72(6):1323-5, 1984

126] Newmark H.K. Vitamin D adequacy. A possible relationship to breast cancer. Adv Exp Med Biol. 364:109-114, 1994

127] Norie I.H. & Foster H.D. Water quality and cancer of the digestive tract: The Canadian experience. J Orthomol Med. 4(2):59-69, 1989

128] Orr J.W. Jr., et al. Nutritional status of patients with untreated cervical cancer. II. Vitamin assessment. Am J Obstet Gynecol. 151(5):632-5, 1985

129] Osborne M.P., et al. Upregulation of Estradiol C16-alpha-hydroxylation in HumanBreast Tissue: A Potential Biomarker of Breast Cancer Risk. J Nat Cancer Inst. 85(23):1917-1993, 1993

130] O'Toole P. & Lombard M. Vitamin C and gastric cancer: Supplements for some or fruit for all? Gut. 39:345-7, 1996

131] Parazzini F., et al. Alcohol and endometrial cancer risk: findings from an Italian case-controlled study. Nutr Cancer. 23(1):55-61, 1995

132] Peters J.M., Preston-Martin S. & London S.J., et al. Processed meats and risk of childhood leukemia. Cancer Causes Control. 5(2):195-202, 1994

133] Pearce M.L. & Dayton S. Incidence of cancer in men on a diet high in polyunsaturated fats. Lancet I:464-7, 1971

134] Pokotny J. Natural toxic substances in food. Cas Lek Cesk. 136(9):267-270, 1997

135] Porcelli B., et al. Levels of folic acid in plasma and red blood cells of colorectal cancer patients. Biomed Pharmacother. 50(6-7):303-5, 1996

136] Pozniak P.C. The carcinogenicity of caffeine and cancer: A review. J Am Diet Assoc. 85(9):1127-33, 1985

137] Prasad K.N. Modulation of the effects of tumor therapeutic agents by vitamin C. Life Sci. 27(4):275-80, 1980a

138] Prasad K.N. & Edwards-Prasad J. Vitamin E and cancer prevention: recent advances and future potentials. J Am Coll Nutr. 11(5):487-500, 1992

139] Prinz-Lingenohl R., Fohr I. & Pictrzik K. Beneficial role for folate in the prevention of colorectal and breast cancer. Nutr 40(3):98-105, Jun, 2001

140] Pritchard G.A., et al. Lipids in breast carcinogenesis. Br J Surg. 76(10):1069-73, 1989

141] Pujol P., Hilsenbeck S.G., Chamness G.C. and Elledge R.M. Rising Levels of Estrogen Receptor in Breast Cancer over 2 Decades. Cancer. 74:1601-1606, 1994

652] Rato A.G. & Pedrero J.G., et al. Melatonin blocks the activation of estrogen receptor for DNA binding. FAS EB J. 13(8):857-68, May, 1999

142] Riordan N.H., et al. Intravenous ascorbate as a tumor cytotoxic chemotherapeutic agent. Med Hypotheses. 44:207-13, 1995

143] Risch H.A., et al. Dietary fat intake and risk of epithelial ovarian cancer. J Natl Cancer Inst. 86(18):1409-15, 1994

144] Rivadeneira D.E., et al. Nutritional support of the cancer patient. CA Cancer J Clin. 48(2):69-80, 1998

145] Rodriquez C., Calle E.E., Coates R.J., Miracle-McMahill H.L., Thun M.J. and Heath C.W. Estrogen Replacement Therapy and Fatal Ovarian Cancer. Am J Epidemiol. 141:828-834, 1995

146] Rose D.P. & Hatala M.A. Dietary fatty acids and breast cancer invasion and metastasis. Nutr Cancer. 21:103-11, 1994

147] Rose D.P. & Connolly J.M. Omega-3 fatty acids as cancer chemopreventive agents. Pharmacol Ther. 83(3):217-44. Review. Sep, 1999

148] Sandler R.S., et al. Diet and risk of colorectal adenomas: macronutrients, cholesterol and fiber. J Natl Cancer Inst. 85(11):846-8, 1993

149] Sankaranarayanan R. & Mathew B. Retinoids as cancer-preventive agents. IARC Sci Publ. 139:47-5, 1996

150] Santamaria L. & Bianchi-Santamaria A. Carotenoids in cancer chemoprevention and therapeutic interventions. J Nutr Sci Vitaminol (Tokyo)Spec No:321-6, 1992

151] Salonen J.T., et al. Association between serum selenium and the risk of cancer. American Journal of Epidemiology. 120:342, 1984

152] Salonen J.T., et al. Risk of cancer in relation to serum concentrations of selenium and vitamins A and E: matched case control analysis of prospective data. British Medical Journal. 290:417-420, 1985

153] Schrauzer G.N. Selenium and cancer: A review. Bioinorganic Chemistry. 5:275-281, 1976

154] Schrauzer G.N. Anticarcinogenic effects of selenium. Cell Mol Life Sci. 57(13-14):1864-73, Dec, 20000

155] Schwartz G.G. & Hulka B.S. Is vitamin D deficiency a risk factor for prostate cancer? Anticancer Res. 10(5A):1307-11, 1990

156] Seely S. & Horrobin D.F. Diet and breast cancer: The possible connection with sugar consumption. Med Hypotheses. 11(3):319-27, 1983

157] Seelig M.S. Magnesium and other nutritional clinical deficiencies in immunologic abnormalities including allergies and neoplasms. Abstract. J Am Coll Nutr. 12:579, 1993

158] Senie R.T. & Tenser S.M. The timing of breast cancer surgery during the menstrual cycle. Oncology (Huntingt). 11(10):1509-17, Oct, 1997

159] Shering S.G., et al. Thyroid Disorders and Breast Cancer. Eur J Cancer Prev. 5(6):504-506, 1996

160] Shklar G. Mechanisms of cancer inhibition by anti-oxidant nutrients. Oral Oncol. 34:24-9, Jan, 1998

161] Siguel E.N. Cancerostatic effect of vegetarian diets. Nutr Cancer. 4(4):285-91, 1983

162] Smyth P.P. The Thyroid and Breast Cancer: A Significant Association? Ann Med. 29(3):189-191, 1997

163] Snowdon D.A. Diet and ovarian cancer. Letter to the Editor. JAMA. 254(3):356-57, 1985

164] Srivastava M., et al. Nutritional risk factors in carcinoma of the esophagus. Nutr Res. 15(2):177-85, 1995

165] Steinmetz K.A. & Potter J.D. Vegetables, fruit and cancer prevention: a review. J Am Diet Assoc. 96:1027-9, 1996

166] Stoll B.A. Can supplementary dietary fiber suppress breast cancer growth? Br J Cancer. 73:557-9, 1996

167] Stoll B.A. Eating to beat breast cancer: potential role for soy supplements. Ann Oncol. 8:223-5, 1997

168] Stoll B.A. Alcohol intake and late-stage promotion of breast cancer. Eur J Cancer. 35(12):1653-8. Review. Nov, 1999

169] Stoll B.A. Adiposity as a Risk Determinant for Postmenopausal Breast Cancer. Int J Obes Relat Metab Disord. 24(5): 527-533, 2000

170] Tisch M. & Lohmeier A., et al. Genotoxic effect of the insecticides pentachlorophenol and lindane on human nasal mucosal epithelium. Dtsch Med Wochenschr. 126(30):840-4, Jul 27, 2001

171] Toke G.B.& Dhamne B.K. A study of serum copper, serum zinc and Cu/Zn ratio as diagnostic and prognostic index in cases of head, neck and face tumors. Indian J Pathol Microbiol Apr. 33(2):171-4, 1990

172] Vanchieri C. Cutting copper curbs angiogenesis, studies show. J Natl Cancer Inst. 92(15):1202-3, Aug 2, 2000

173] Verreault R., et al. A case-control study of diet and invasive cervical cancer. Int J Cancer. 43:1050-4, 1989

174] Vlajinac H.D., et al. Diet and prostate cancer: a case-control study. Eur J Cancer. 33(1):101-7, 1997

175] Wargovich M.J. Calcium and colon cancer. J Am Coll Nutr. 7(4):295-300, 1988

176] WCRF Panel. Diet, Nutrition and the Prevention of Cancer. A Global Perspective. Washington, DC, World Cancer Research Fund/American Institute for Cancer Research, 1997

177] Whelen P., et al. Zinc, vitamin A and prostatic cancer. Br J Urol. 55(5):525-8, 1983

178] Willett W.C. & MacMahon B. Diet and cancer: An overview. N Engl J Med. 310(11):697-703, 1984

179] Witte J.S., et al. Diet and premenopausal bilateral breast cancer: a case-control study. Breast Cancer Res Treat. 42:243-51, 1997

180] Yoshizawa K., et.al. Study of prediagnostic selenium level in toenails and the risk of advanced prostate cancer. J Natl Can Inst. 90:1219-24, 1998

181] Zaichick Vye et al. Zinc in the human prostate gland: normal, hyperplastic and cancerous. Int Urol Nephrol. 29(5):565-74, 1997

182] Zhang D. & Holmes W.F., et al. Retinoids and ovarian cancer. J Cell Physiol. 185(1):1-20. Review. Oct, 2000

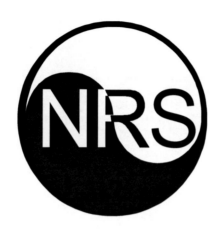

# Important Nutrients

# The B-Vitamins.

The B-Vitamin Complex has been studied extensively and there are many good texts I would refer readers to for further details. (Reavley, Groff et al, Marks & Marks and Werbach) The sources and clinical complexes are summarized in the Nutrient Charts section. What I would like to explain to the reader is the problems with nutrient flow for this group especially intracellular metabolism and the effect of antinutrients.

With respect to the levels of B-vitamins in foods, these will vary considerably with mean temperatures, time of picking and trace element levels especially manganese and boron.

Dysbiosis can affect the absorption of these vitamins, as can chronic inflammatory bowel disease. In the case of pernicious anaemia (PA), there is more evidence that the modern day PA is due to chronic helicobacter infection. There is also mounting evidence that helicobacter should not be able to survive in a stomach that makes plentiful amounts of acid. There are two possibilities; either chronic infection will lead to hypochlorhydria or the pre-existing hypochlorhydria will create an environment that helicobacter can thrive in. Long-term acid suppression is already backfiring on our species in terms of health problems such as hypertension, depression, arthritis, diabetes and chronic fatigue syndrome.

Readers may be surprised to know that the majority of B-vitamin supplements are useless unless intracellular activation can take place. The reality of the situation is that all the B-Vitamins need a mineral or another B-Vitamin to activate them. Failure to perform the activation steps will lead to symptoms being generated from tissues in the presence of *normal or even high* levels in the blood. Remember the adage "Biochemistry predominantly occurs in the tissues, not the blood".

The table below shows the examples of common B-group vitamins and their activated forms. Actually the situation is similar to Vitamin C, where dehydroascorbate in transported into cells like the adrenal glands and neutrophils and then activated by glutathione to ascorbic acid. Excess B-vitamins will also wind up in the toilet bowl like Vitamin C. Perhaps the analogy of a pistol with the safety catch would help. Imagine the B-Vitamins and Dehydroascorbate like loaded pistols. In the blood they have the safety catch on, so that they do not activate blood constituents like the clotting cascade or the Red Blood cell enzymes. They are imported into the cells and then the safety catch is switched to red (on) for live firing. Toxic elements (Such as Lead & Mercury) interfere with the activation, effectively locking the safety catch on permanently. This means that blood levels are misleading as a measure of B-Vitamin function.

## B & C Vitamin Activation
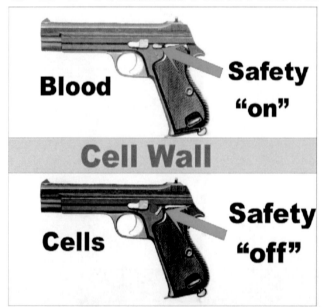

## Toxic Metal effect
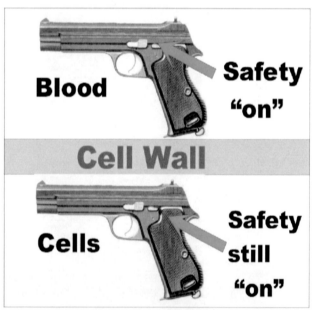

**Suggested Reading List**.

Groff et al Advanced Nutrition and Human Metabolism West Publishing Co

Mark & Marks Basic Medical Biochemistry Williams & Wilkins

Reavley Nicola The New Encyclopaedia of Vitamins, Mineral Supplements and Herbs Bookman Press.

# B-vitamin Activation

Require Mg Zn Mo Mn & other B-vitamins

| | | |
|---|---|---|
| **B1** | Thiamine | Thiamine pyrophosphate |
| **B2** | Riboflavin | Riboflavin-5-phosphate  FAD FMN |
| **B3** | Niacin | NAD Niacinamide |
| **B5** | Pantothenic acid | Co Enzyme A |
| **B6** | Pyridoxal | Pyridoxal-5-phosphate |
| **B7** | Biotin | Biocytin |
| **B 9** | Folic acid | Folinic acid D-H-F T-H-F |
| **B12** | Cyanocobalamin | Methylcobalamin Adenosylcobalamin |

# Cobalt and Vitamin B12: A marriage of Vitamin and Mineral

Vitamin B12 is a much-misunderstood vitamin. It has an unusual structure in that it contains a cobalt atom at its centre. This makes the mineral cobalt unusual too. When evaluating tissue mineral analysis (TMA), the cobalt level reveals much about the metabolism of Vitamin B12 within the cells. Other minerals come as salts. That is we can ingest calcium crystals, magnesium crystals, sodium crystals etc, but cobalt only enters the body buried inside the Vitamin B12 structure.

The following diagram explains the route of B12 and its activation. The process is vulnerable in several ways. Vegetarians have fewer foods with B12 in them. Those with helicobacter infection may develop low levels of "intrinsic factor" which is made in the stomach for the express purpose of B12 absorption. There are those with other forms of malabsorption due to low stomach acid such as pernicious anaemia and there are those patients who take drugs that suppress stomach acid. Some people are born with the lack of intrinsic factor (familial pernicious anaemia) and

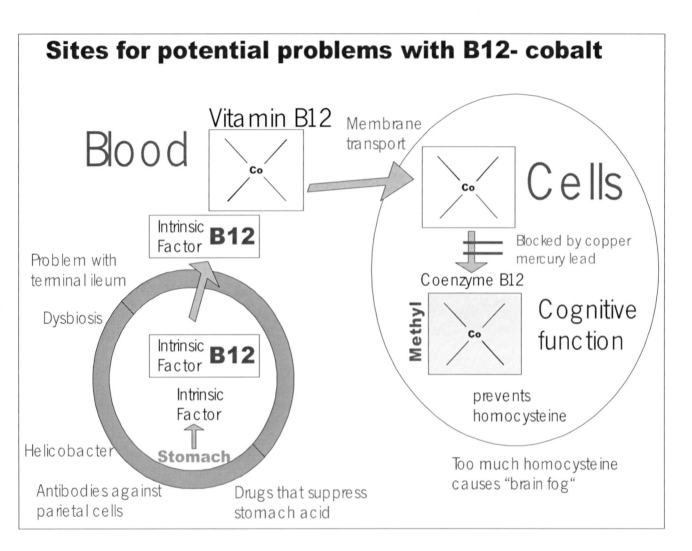

some patients (later in life) develop antibodies to the cells that make intrinsic factor (antiparietal cell antibodies). Helicobacter infection has been linked to the later onset pernicious anaemia. Either way B12 absorption falls.

The importation of Vitamin B12 from the blood into the cell requires an active transport system. This means that only a **low** level of B12 or a **high** level really mean anything. In addition to blood level, intracellular cobalt must be performed in order to truly understand the B12-cobalt cycle.

Most B-vitamins need to be converted to their active form before they will function. Mostly, minerals such as magnesium or zinc do this. For instance Zinc and B2 are required for the activation of B6. Magnesium is required for the activation of B1. In the case of Vitamin B12, its conversion to Methylcobalamin (Coenzyme B12) can be blocked by copper, lead or mercury.

The consequences of low levels of methylcobalamin are a rise in brain homocysteine. This causes a condition called "brain fog". The symptoms include "woolly thinking", noun substitution in sentences, transient memory loss, episodes of confusion, and even dementia. It has been shown that intramuscular Vitamin B12 can improve dementia patients even if they have *normal* blood levels of Vitamin B12. The reason is that by supersaturating the blood, more B12 might diffuse into the cells, which are starving for this vitamin. Of course the medical profession will always believe the blood test rather than the patient!

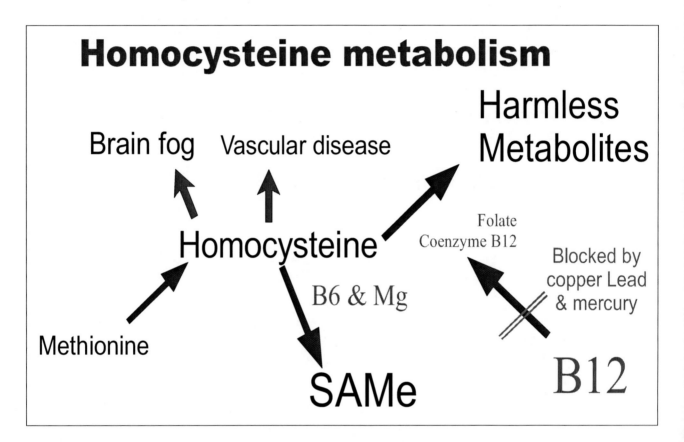

Contrary to what your doctor was taught, the strongest predictor of vascular disease is not cholesterol, but the level of homocysteine. This information was suppressed by the pharmaceutical industry for years because giving B6, B12 and folic acid could rectify the problem. When methionine is metabolised, the intermediate step is homocysteine, which causes vascular damage. Homocysteine is a "hot potato". You don't want to hang on to it for too long. In order to metabolise it quickly there are two paths one can take. The top pathway involves folate and B12 and the bottom pathway needs B6 and magnesium. In the periphery, high homocysteine causes blood vessel damage; in the brain it causes dementia or brain fog.

The table below outlines the nine possible combinations of serum B12 levels and TMA cobalt levels. The symbols indicate the possible reasons.

So to really deal with cobalt –B12 biochemistry, you need to know the levels of both. The treatment will involve the correct B12 supplement and treating the reason for the abnormality.

## Serum B12

| Tissue cobalt | LOW | Normal | HIGH |
|---|---|---|---|
| **LOW** | Malabsorption ◆ | Membrane transport problem ✷ | Membrane transport problem ✷ |
| **Normal** | Malabsorption ◆ | Normal | Membrane transport problem ✷ |
| **HIGH** | Malabsorption ◆ / Intracellular Blockade ✓ | Intracellular Blockade ✓ | Intracellular Blockade ✓ |

◆ Check for low stomach acid & helicobacter

✷ Are Ca, Mg, Na or K out too?

✓ Copper high or are lead or mercury present?

74

# C- I told you so!

The first time I ever heard of intravenous vitamin C injections I had visions of some kind of witchcraft being performed. After reviewing the extensive literature on it I understood why so many conditions might improve with such therapies, even if the therapists themselves couldn't explain why it worked.

Every retired chemist, doctor, naturopath, next-door neighbour, friend of your second cousin etc, is an armchair expert on Vitamin C, so I'll try not to bore those people. I'll try to mention information that you might not have read about in Womens Weekly or Omni.

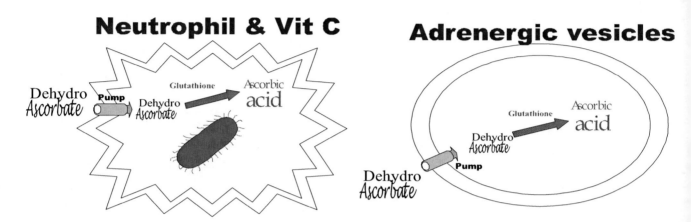

The most surprising facts about vitamin C aren't in the studies on cancer or the immune system, but the biochemistry of how the body uses it. Apart from its function in the defence against cancer, bacterial infections, fungal infections and viral infections, Vitamin C is important in asthma, sinusitis and mental illnesses.

The highest Vitamin C concentration in any tissue is found in the adrenal gland. Why would the adrenal gland store so much of it? It turns out that you need Vitamin C to make cortisol and adrenalin. Surprise surprise, that means you need more Vitamin C when you are under stress. That means that the recommended daily allowance of 60mg might not be flexible enough for people with different environmental stresses. Now isn't that interesting that something so logical might cast doubt about the appropriateness of such tables? That means that a serum Vitamin C level might underestimate the storage of the adrenal gland and the ability to make these hormones under pressure. This means that you could have symptoms of Vitamin C deficiency such as tiredness, low blood pressure or fainting well before you got scurvy.

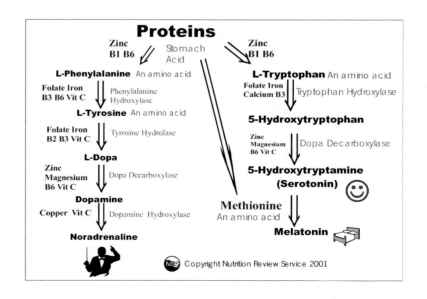

75

The next interesting fact is that the tissue second highest in Vitamin C concentration is the brain. Now what would the brain need all that Vitamin C for? Wear and tear, collagen repair? No, to make dopamine and serotonin and melatonin. Some studies suggest that it may bind to the same sites as the antipsychotics such as stelazine and chlorpromazine and act as a natural antipsychotic. Vitamin C keeps your sanity intact and your collagen intact too. So low levels of vitamin C could lead to insomnia, depression and lethargy. These studies suggest that low brain Vitamin C levels are associated with schizophrenia.

Wow, this sounds like a wonder drug, what about its function to chelate heavy metals and remove them? What about the fact that immune cells need it for killing bacteria?

Another important use of vitamin C is to make carnitine. Start with lysine (the amino Acid) and add iron and vitamin C to make carnitine. Why is this so important? All our skeletal muscles run on fatty acids to fuel them. Carnitine acts like a shovel to get these fatty acids in to the mitochondria (powerhouses in the cells). No vitamin C, and muscles don't work properly. They become weak and painful.

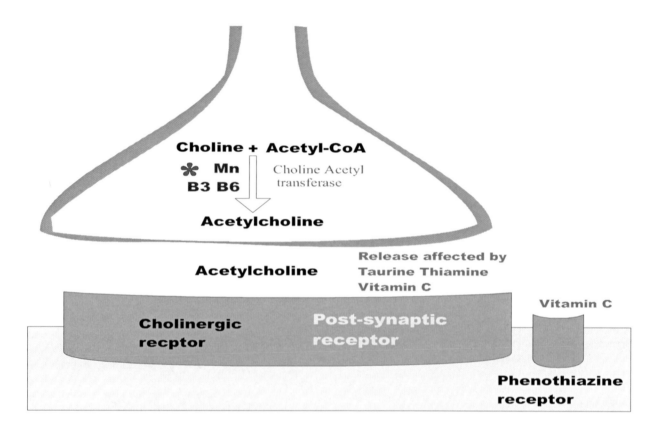

This is all very interesting you might say, but in Australia 2004, vitamin C deficiency must be a rare thing and not worthwhile checking for. We all eat heaps of Vitamin C containing foods everyday. Do we really? Lets take oranges. How much Vitamin C would there be in an orange? Well, here comes the bad news. Independent surveys of Vitamin C levels often find no vitamin C (not a molecule) in local oranges. How could such a thing happen? Well, why does the orange contain the vitamin C? It's an antioxidant. It's there to protect the seeds from oxidation long after the flesh has fallen away. When does this happen? During the last three days of ripening the salicylates (natural aspirins) leave the fruit while the antioxidants increase. The fruit ripens and falls off the tree in a natural, caring, free-range kind of way. Then, the fruit is quickly eaten by a passer-by, who gets all of the goodness.

Is this how all oranges are farmed today? You might have guessed that this is *not* what happens in the real world of commerce. So maybe our sacred sources might not be so good after all? "Oh but that's nonsense - I eat lots of broccoli". There's 58 mg in half a cup of boiled broccoli; 174 mg in 1 cup of red capsicum; 48 mg in a half cup of boiled brussel sprouts. Even a fully loaded orange has only 68mg. Does anyone really believe that in today's world, 60mg is the recommended daily allowance for Vitamin C? It should be more like 600mg! Do we believe that modern day farming techniques concentrate and preserve all the antioxidants in the fruit or vegetables?

Are we exposed to more stress than our ancestors? Are we exposed to more viruses in our lifetimes than our ancestors were? Are we exposed to more chemicals than our ancestors were? Are we getting more antioxidants in our food than our ancestors did (zinc, selenium, Vitamin C)? ***Could there be some really major problem here***? Could this contribute to the epidemics of cancer, heart disease?

Does the Health Department really care? Do the Pharmaceutical companies really care? Does the Health Insurance Commission want doctors to measure things like zinc, selenium and Vitamin C? Does it want the public to know the full truth about the real number of deficiencies such as Vitamin C? You be the judge.

So, for the ubiquitous "I never heard of it, so it can't be true" medico, there are only 87 references today. Sorry, probably not enough for you.

**PS** - Sources include: Acerola cherry, guava, capsicum, blackcurrants, kale leaves, parsley, collard leaves, kale, orange peel, turnip greens, dock, broccoli, brussel sprouts, mustard greens, watercress, cauliflower, jujube, strawberry, lemon, orange, spinach, lychee, currants, lime, grapefruit, kumquat, turnip, cantaloupe, asparagus, radish, tangerine, fennel, granadilla, okra, fresh beans, peas, melon, loganberry, tomato, blackberry, sweet potato, mung bean sprouts, lettuce, pineapple, leek, parsnip, quince, garlic, avocado, jujube.

# Enemies of Vitamin C

1. Modern farming

2. Copper excess

3. Alumimium

4. Stress

*"Don't boil your brocolli in a copper pot"*

5. Recurrent infections

6. Smoking & passive smoking

# References:

**Vitamin C, Asthma, Bronchitis and Sinusitis**

1] Anderson, R., et al. <u>Ascorbic acid in bronchial asthma</u>. South African Medical Journal. 63:649-652, 1983.

2] Bielory, L., et al. <u>Asthma and Vitamin C</u>. Annals Allergy. 73:89-96, 1994.

3] Brown, L. A., et al. <u>Ascorbate deficiency and oxidative stress in the alveolar type II cell</u>. American Journal of Physiology. 273(4 Part 1):L782-L788, 1997.

4] Haas, Elson M. <u>Staying Healthy with Nutrition</u>. Celestial Arts, Berkeley, California, USA. 1992:144.

5] Hatch, G. E. <u>Decreased preference for foods containing vitamin C and decreased concentrations of vitamin C in blood plasma are also associated with asthma</u>. American Journal of Clinical Nutrition. 61:625S-630S, 1995.

6] Sridhar, M. K. <u>Nutrition and lung health</u>. British Medical Journal. 310:75-76, 1995.

7] Mohnsenin, V., et al. <u>Ascorbic acid exerts its effect on asthmatics through prostaglandin metabolism</u>. American Thoracic Society 125, 1982.

8] Mohnsenin, V., et al. <u>Effect of ascorbic acid on response to methylcholine challenge in asthmatic subjects</u>. American Review of Respiratory Disease. 127:143-147, 1983.

ancestors? Are we exposed to more heavy metals than our ancestors (except perhaps the Romans who used lead 9] Olusi, S. O., et al. <u>Plasma and white blood cell ascorbic acid concentrations in patients with bronchial asthma</u>. Clinica Chemica Acta. 92:161-166, 1979.

10] Wolfson, D. <u>Solving sinusitis</u>. Nutrition Science News. April 2000.


**Vitamin C and Psychiatry**

11] Beauclair, L., et al., <u>An adjunctive role for ascorbic acid in the treatment of schizophrenia</u>. Clin. Psych Pharmacol. 7:282-3; 1987.

12] Cheraskin, Emanuel, MD, et al., <u>The Vitamin C Connection</u>. Harper & Row, NY, 1983.

13] Gold, Mark S., MD, et al., <u>The Good News About Depression</u>. Villard Books, NY, 1987.

14] Kanofsky, I.D., et al., <u>Ascorbate: An adjunctive treatment for schizophrenia</u>. J. Am. Coll. Nutr, 8(5):425,1989.

15] Milner G., <u>Ascorbic acid in chronic psychiatric patients: A controlled trial</u>. Br. J, Psychiatry 109:294-9, 1963.

16] Pfeiffer, Carl C, <u>Mental and Elemental Nutrients</u>. Keats, New Canaan, CN, 1975

17] Quillin, Patrick PhD, RD, <u>Healing Nutrients</u>. Contemporary Books, Chicago, 1987.

18] Rebec, GE,, et al. <u>Ascorbic acid and the behavioural response to haloperidol: Implications for the action of antipsychotic drugs</u>. Science, 227:438-40: 1985

19] Suboticanec, K <u>Vitamin C status in schizophrenia</u>. Bibl. Nutr. Dieta 38: 173-81, 1986.

20] Suboticanec K et al. <u>Vitamin C and schizophrenia</u>. Acta Med Iugosl, 38(5):299-308,1984.

21] Suboticanec K, et al., <u>Plasma levels and urinary C excretion in schizophrenic patients</u>. Hum. Nutr. Clin. 40C;421-28, 1986

22] Tolbert, L.C., et al., <u>Effect of ascorbic acid on neurochemical, behavioural, and physiological symptoms mediated by catecholamines</u>. Life Sci., 25:2189- 95; 1979.

23] Tolbert, L.C., et al., <u>Ascorbate affects conversion of tyrosine to dopamine in mouse brain</u>. Abst., Trans. Am. Sot. Neurochem. 1979.

24] VanderKamp H., <u>A biochemical abnormality in schizophrenics involving ascorbic acid</u>. Intl. J of Neuropsychiatry. , 2(3):204-6, 1966


**Vitamin C and Antioxidant Effects**

25] Rose, R. C. <u>Ascorbic acid protection against free radicals</u>. In: Third Conference on Vitamin C. 1987. Annals of the New York Academy of Sciences. Volume 498, 1987.

26] Vayda, W. <u>Prevention of aging: How to keep your cells younger, longer</u>. Australian Wellbeing. 9:33-42, 1985.

## Vitamin C and Immunity

27] Anderson, R., Oosthuizen, R., Theron, A. & Van Rensburg. <u>The effects of increasing weekly doses of ascorbate on certain cellular and humoral immune functions in normal volunteers</u>. American Journal of Clinical Nutrition. 33:71, 1980.

28] Anderson, R. <u>Assessment of oral ascorbate in three children with chronic granulomatous disease and defective neutrophil motility over a two-year period</u>. Clinical and Experimental Immunology. 43:180-188, 1981.

29] Bates, C. J. <u>Vitamin C intake and susceptibility to the common cold - invited commentaries</u>. British Journal of Nutrition. 78(5):857-859, 1997.

30] Boxer, L. A., et al. <u>Correction of leukocyte function in Chediak-Higashi syndrome by ascorbate</u>. New England Journal of Medicine 295:1041-1045, 1976.

31] Boxer, L. A., et al. <u>Enhancement of chemotactic response and microtubule assembly in human leukocytes by ascorbic acid</u>. Journal of Cellular Physiology. 100:119-126, 1979.

32] Carr, A. B., et al. <u>Vitamin C and the common cold: Using identical twins as controls</u>. Medical Journal of Australia. 2:411-412, 1981.

33] Carr, A. B., et al. <u>Vitamin C and the common cold: A second MZ cotwin control study</u>. Acta Geneticae

34] Dalton, W. L. <u>Massive doses of vitamin C in the treatment of viral disease</u>. J Indiana State Med Assoc. 55:1151-1154, 1962.

35] Dahl, H., et al. <u>The effect of ascorbic acid on production of human interferon and the antiviral activity in vitro</u>. Acta Pathologica et Microbiologica Scandinavia. 84(5):280-284, 1976

36] Destro, R. L., et al. <u>An appraisal of vitamin C in adjunct therapy of bacterial and viral meningitis</u>. Clin Ped. 16:936, 1977.

37] Frei, B., et al. <u>Ascorbate is an outstanding antioxidant in human blood plasma</u>. Proceedings of the National Academy of Sciences USA. 86:6377-6381, 1989.

38] Gerber, W. F., et al. <u>Effect of ascorbic acid, sodium salicylate, and caffeine on the serum interferon level in response to viral infection</u>. Pharmacology. 13:228, 1975.

39] Goodman, K. J., et al. <u>Nutritional factors and Helicobacter pylori infection in Colombian children</u>. J Pediatr Gastroenterol Nutr. 25(5):507-515, 1997

40] Haas, Elson M. <u>Staying Healthy with Nutrition</u>. Celestial Arts, Berkeley, California, USA. 1992:144.

41] Hemila, H. <u>Does vitamin C alleviate the symptoms of the common cold? - A review of current evidence</u>. Scand J Infect Dis. 26(1):1-6, 1994.

42] Hemila, H. <u>Vitamin C and the common cold: A retrospective analysis of Chalmer's review</u>. J Am Coll Nutr. 14(2):116-123, 1995.

43] Hemila, H. <u>Vitamin C and the common cold</u>. Br J Nutr. 67:3-16, 1992.

44] Hemila, H. <u>Vitamin C and common cold incidence: A review of studies with subjects under heavy physical stress</u>. International Journal of Sports Medicine. 17(5):379-383, 1996.

45] Holden, M., et al. <u>In vitro action of synthetic crystalline vitamin C (ascorbic acid) on herpes virus</u>. Journal of Immunology. 31:455-462, 1936.

46] Holden, M., et al. <u>Further experiments on inactivation of herpes by vitamin C (l-ascorbic acid)</u>. Journal of Immunology. 33:251-257, 1936.

47] Horrobin, D. F., et al. <u>The nutritional regulation of T lymphocyte function</u>. Medical Hypotheses. 5:969-985, 1979.

48] Hovi, T., et al. <u>Topical treatment of recurrent mucocutaneous herpes with ascorbic acid-containing solution</u>. Antiviral Research. 27:263-270, 1995.

49] Jungeblut, C. W. <u>Inactivation of poliomyelitis virus by crystalline vitamin C</u>. Journal of Experimental Medicine. 62:517-521, 1935.

50] Jungeblut, C. W. <u>Further observations on vitamin C therapy in experimental poliomyelitis</u>. Journal of Experimental Medicine. 65:127-146, 1937.

51] Jungeblut, C. W. <u>A further contribution to the vitamin C therapy in experimental poliomyelitis</u>. Journal of Experimental Medicine. 70:327, 1939.

52] Klenner, F. R. The treatment of poliomyelitis and other virus diseases with vitamin C. J Southern Med Surg. 111:210-214, 1949.

53] Levy, R., et al. Vitamin C for the treatment of recurrent furunculosis in patients with impaired neutrophil functions. J Infect Dis. 173(6):1502-1505, 1996.

54] Linder, M. C. Nutrition and metabolism of vitamins. In: Nutritional Biochemistry and Metabolism, 2nd Edition. Maria C. Linder (editor). Simon & Schuster, Connecticut, USA, 1991:146.

55] Pauling, L. Ascorbic acid and the common cold. Medical Tribune. 24:1, 1976.

56] Pauling, L. Vitamin C, the Common Cold and the Flu. W. H. Freeman & Company, San Francisco, USA. 1976.

57] Prinz, W. The effect of ascorbic acid supplementation on some parameters of human immunological defence system. International Journal of Vitamin and Nutritional Research. 47:248-256, 1977.

58] Renker, K., et al. Vitamin C-Prophylaxe in der Volkswertf Stralsund. Deutsche Gesundheitswesen. 9:702-706, 1954.

59] Rudolph, M. The immunity factor. The Energy Times. 5(6):20-25, 1995.

60] Schorah, C. J. Vitamin C intake and susceptibility to the common cold - invited commentaries. British Journal of Nutrition. 78(5):859-861, 1997.

61] Schwerdt, P. R., et al. Effect of ascorbic acid on rhinovirus in WI-38 cells. Proc Soc Biol Med. 148:1237, 1975.

62] Sirsi, M. Antimicrobial action of vitamin C on M. tuberculosis and some other pathogenic organisms. Indian J Med Sci. 6:252-255, 1952.

63] Thomas, W. R., et al. Vitamin C and immunity: an assessment of the evidence. Clinical Experimental Immunology. 32:370-379, 1978.

64] Vallance, S. Relationships between ascorbic acid and serum proteins of the immune system. British Medical Journal. 2:437-438, 1977.

65] Washko, P., et al. Ascorbic acid and human neutrophils. American Journal of Clinical Nutrition. 54:1221S-7S, 1991

66] White, L. Cold sores be gone. Nutrition Science News. March 1999.

67] Yonemoto, R. H., et al. Enhanced lymphocyte blastogenesis by oral ascorbic acid. Proceedings of the American Association for Cancer Research. 17:288, 1976.

## Vitamin C and Cancer

68] Anderson, R. Effects of ascorbate on normal and abnormal leukocyte functions. Vitamin C: New Clinical Applications in Immunology. Lipid Metabolism and Cancer. 1-178, 1982.

69] Bandera E. V., et al. Diet and alcohol consumption and lung cancer risk in the New York State Cohort. Cancer Causes Control. 8(6):828-840, 1997.

70] Bram, S., et al. Vitamin C preferential toxicity for malignant melanoma cells. Nature. 284:629-631, 1980.

71] Bruemmer, B., et al. Nutrient intake in relation to bladder cancer among middle-aged men and women. American Journal of Epidemiology. 144(5):485-495, 1996.

72] Burke, E. R. Vitamins C & E cut risk of prostate cancer cell growth. Muscular Development. 36(11):54, 1999.

73] Byers, R., et al. Epidemiologic evidence for vitamin C and vitamin E in cancer prevention. Am J Clin Nutr. 62(Supplement):1385S-1392S, 1995.

74] Graham, S., et al. Dietary factors in the epidemiology of cancer of the larynx. American Journal of Epidemiology. 113(6):675-680, 1981.

75] Greenblatt, M. Brief communication: Ascorbic acid blocking of aminopyrine nitrosation in NZO-B1 mice. Journal of the National Cancer Institute. 50(4):1055-1056, 1973.

76] Howe, G. R., et al. Dietary factors and risk of breast cancer: Combined analysis of 12-case control studies. Journal of the National Cancer Institute. 82:561-569, 1990.

77] Kurbacher, C. M., et al. Ascorbic acid (vitamin C) improves the antineoplastic activity of doxorubicin, cisplatin, and paclitaxel in human breast carcinoma cells in vitro. Cancer Letters. 103-119, 1996.

78] Maurer, K. <u>Vitamins may prevent bladder cancer recurrence</u>. Family Practice News. 15 December 1995:12.

79] O'Connor, H. J., et al. <u>Effect of increased intake of vitamin C on the mutagenic activity of gastric juice and intragastric concentrations of ascorbic acid</u>. Carcinogenesis. 6(11):1675-1676, 1985.

80] Pierson, H. F., et al. <u>Sodium ascorbate enhancement of carbidopa-levodopa methyl ester anti-tumor activity against pigmented B16 melanoma</u>. Cancer Research. 43:2047-2051, 1983.

81] Reed, P. I. <u>Vitamin C, Helicobacter pylori infection and gastric carcinogenesis</u>. Int J Vitamin Nutr Res. 69(3):220-227, 1999.

82] Shamaan, N. A., et al. <u>Vitamin C and Aloe Vera supplementation protects from chemical hepatocarcinogenesis in the rat</u>. Nutrition 14 (11-12):846-852, 1998

83] Schiffman, M. H. <u>Diet and faecal genotoxicity</u>. Cancer Surv. 6:653-672, 1987.

84] Taper, H. S., et al. <u>Non-toxic potentiation of cancer chemotherapy by combined C and K3 vitamin pre-treatment</u>. Int J Cancer. 40:575-579, 1987.

85] Vermeer, I. T., et al. <u>Effect of ascorbic acid and green tea on endogenous formation of N-nitrosodimethylamine and N-nitrosopiperidine in humans</u>. Mutation Research. 16;428(1-2):353-361, 1999.

86] Zhang, H. M., et al. <u>Vitamin C inhibits the growth of a bacterial risk factor for gastric carcinoma: Helicobacter pylori</u>. Cancer. 80(10):1897-1903, 1997.

87] Zheng, W., et al. <u>Retinol, antioxidant vitamins, and cancers of the upper digestive tract in a prospective cohort study of postmenopausal women</u>. American Journal of Epidemiology. 142(9):955-960, 1995.

In all the time I was in medical school, no one ever mentioned magnesium. All we heard about was sodium, potassium, calcium and a bit about iron. After researching the mineral's role in human biochemistry, it turns out that it is probably the most important ion in the body. So I make no apologies for taking extreme detail in discussing its role.

## Summary of the functions of Magnesium

**Magnesium deficiency/blockade causes fatigue.** The details of why will become apparent by the time you have finished this chapter.

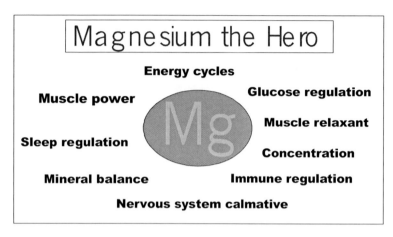

Let's look at the contributors to the symptoms.

Magnesium's ionic role and modulating Calcium
Antioxidant and sleep enhancer.
Magnesium and energy cycles.
Magnesium and Muscles
Magnesium and tubes.
Magnesium and depression.
Magnesium and Neuromuscular excitability
Cardiac effects of low magnesium
Magnesium, digestion and blood sugar
Sources of Magnesium
Absorption of Magnesium
Antagonism of Magnesium
Loss of Magnesium
Magnesium and bone density
Magnesium and calcium deposition
Magnesium and immunity

> Low brain magnesium gives unrefreshed sleep easy fatigue poor concentration daytime sleepiness

**Figure 1**

| 11 | 12 |
|---|---|
| Sodium | Magnesium |
| 19 | 20 |
| Potassium | Calcium |

**Figure 2**

## Ionic role of Magnesium

The periodic table of elements is immensely helpful in understanding the role of elements and anti-nutrients in Nutritional Medicine. At the top left lie four important minerals (atomic numbers shown)

An important feature is apparent regarding the balance of Cations. Sodium and potassium determine membrane charge and are in the same column. Calcium and magnesium determine release of neurotransmitter and muscle contraction status and are also in the same column.

Magnesium is mostly intracellular. We store about 25,000mg of magnesium in our body and only 1% of it is in the blood. So most of it is in the **tissues**. It demonstrates the features of most intracellular ions, in that you can become depleted *without it showing up in a blood test*. Intracellular levels are upwards of 25 Meq/L depending on the tissues. Fig 3 shows the scale of tissue magnesium levels. Astute readers will make the connection the cancer rates seem to be much higher in tissues that ordinarily have lower magnesium concentrations. The connection may be related to the efficiency of energy cycles within the cells. Energy cycles help to ensure Apoptosis occurs when it should. That is, when all the functions of the cell are working properly, abnormalities in DNA should be detected by the internal cell "auditors", the Apoptosis "button" is pressed and the cell stops dividing. This concept of energy normalisation has lead to some exciting new work in cancer.

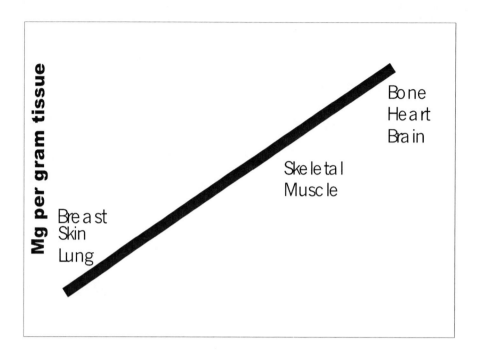

Figure 3

## As a modulator of Calcium.

The best example of this is muscle contraction. Fig 4 shows the relationship of Calcium:Magnesium ratio in determining muscle contraction. Excess calcium, low magnesium or blockade of magnesium (by copper or cadmium) will make it difficult to complete the relaxation phase of the muscle cycle.

**Figure 4**

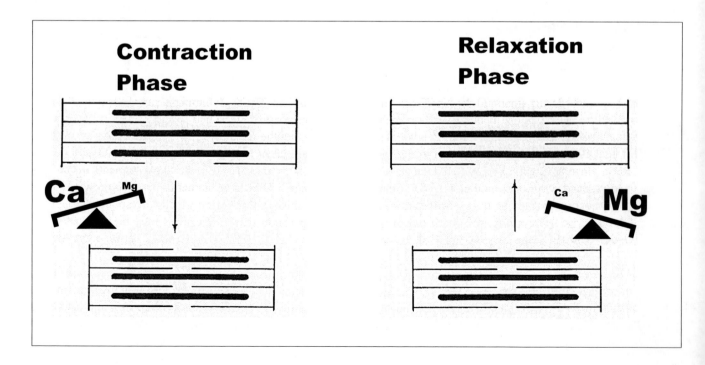

This has several clinical effects.

In terms of cardiac muscle this will reduce time for diastole and will reduce stroke volume. The effect is dyspnoea especially on exertion.

In terms of skeletal muscle, this will give the feeling of muscle weakness and foster a tendency to muscle cramp and spasm. In Fig 5, limb movement relies upon synchronisation of flexor and extensor. The flexor must be in a high Calcium:Magnesium state, and the extensor in a high Magnesium:Calcium state. In magnesium deficiency, the extensor cannot relax, rather like a tug of war, and this makes movement seem difficult and uses much more energy (which the TCA cycle may not cope with due to the low Magnesium).

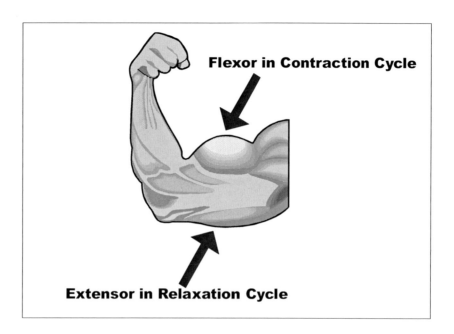

**Figure 5**

In the case of circular smooth muscle, the effects are quite variable, but may be summarised in the graphic on the following pages. This is why magnesium has been used in hypertension. When confronted about the intracellular effects of Calcium channel blockers, most doctors will eventually concede that these drugs could lead to an increase in the effect of magnesium (as a muscle relaxant) and hence lower the blood pressure. When I ask them if they had considered *just giving magnesium*, they would often reply, "Can you do that?". Check the references to see just how many people actually *have* done that.

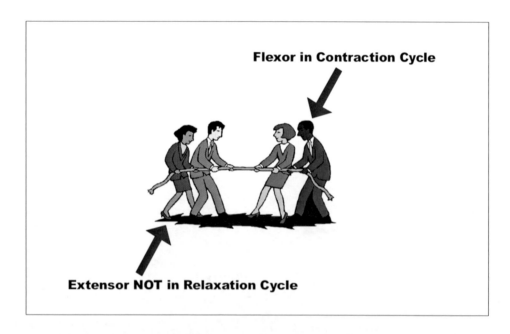

## Magnesium and tubes.

A circular muscle, is a muscle which is attached to itself, creating a tube. Therefore contraction causes a reduction in the diameter of the tube, reducing flow.

One very practical application is in asthma. Magnesium has been given by nebuliser and intravenously for status asthmaticus, but it could be useful in the prevention of symptoms, not just at the last minute.

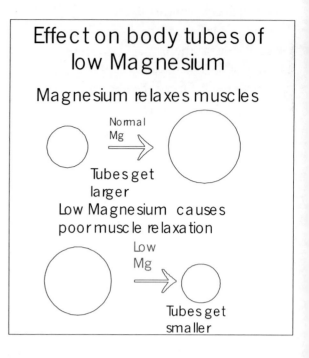

Figure 6

The effect of magnesium deficiency or blockade on smooth muscle is shown in figure 7 below. Magnesium is required for the full dilatation of smooth muscle and hence affects diameter of tubes formed from such muscles.

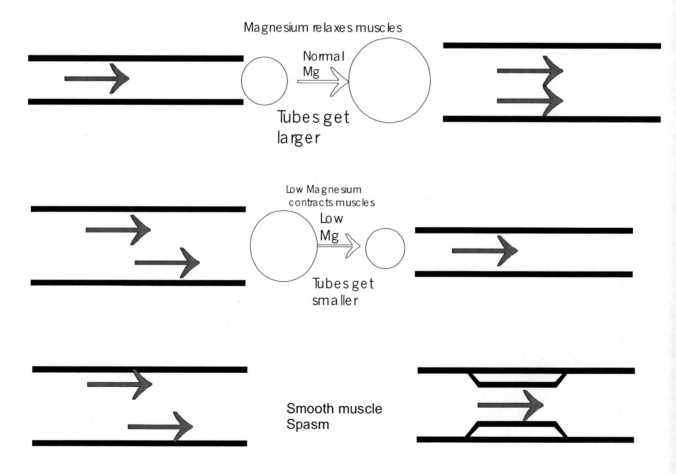

**Figure 7**

Imagine a smorgasbord of various organs that have smooth or cardiac muscle.

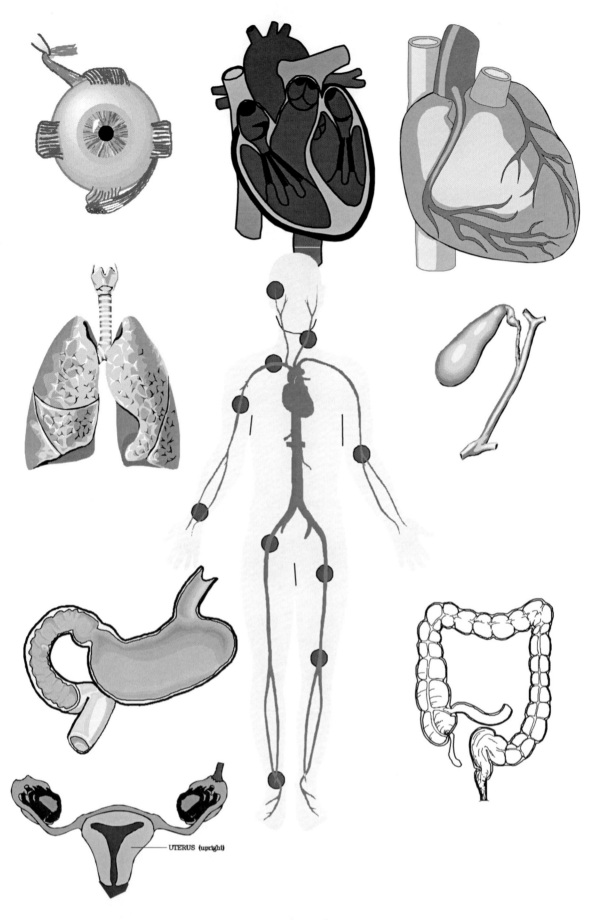

**Figure 8**

Now envisage the diversity of symptoms that result from magnesium deficiency or blockade in the tissues.

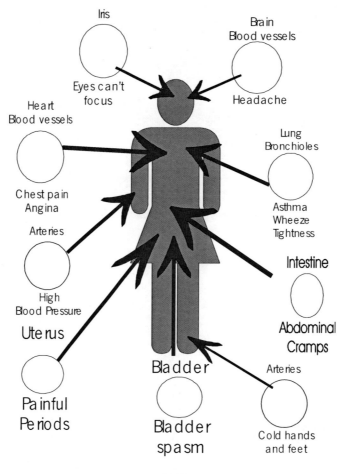

**Figure 9**

## Antioxidant and sleep enhancer.

Generally, one does not consider Magnesium as an antioxidant, but there is one important example. That example is melatonin. Fig 10 shows the pathway of melatonin synthesis from proteins to melatonin. To synthesis the co-factor S-adenosylmethionine (SAMe), magnesium is required also.

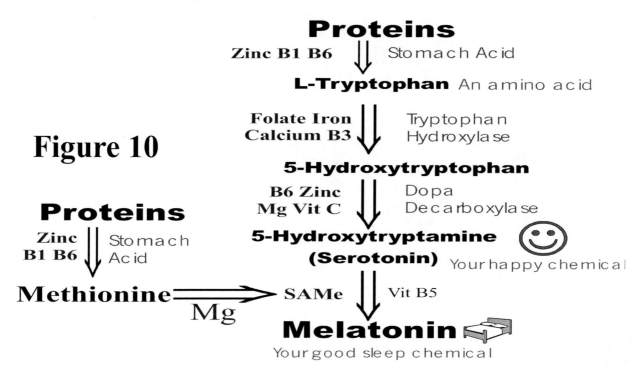

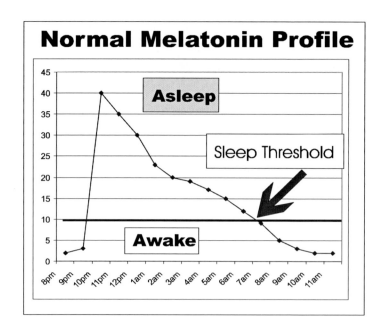

**Figure 11**

Humans have an innate clock cycle of 24 hours and 40 minutes. So, if we don't "reset" every night, we get out of synchronisation with the rest of the world. The perfect analogy is the ATM's. Every day, at 4 pm (annoying as this is), all the ATM's synchronise and confirm that it is now the next working day. No arguments. Our reset chemical is melatonin. Fig 11 shows the melatonin profile at night.

A pulse of this is made an hour before we go to sleep, like an intravenous bolus of anaesthetic. Magnesium is involved in two ways. Firstly, we need it to manufacture melatonin. Secondly, magnesium is melatonin's private chaperone. The higher the magnesium level, the longer melatonin lasts in the body. The higher the magnesium, the better the recharge we get during our sleep. There's only one problem: magnesium falls at night. It hits rock bottom at 5 am (this is why the blood pressure is highest at this time). Add the problem of low magnesium levels create the recipe for insomnia (pattern 1 &2) poor sleep quality, unrefreshed sleep, poor concentration, daytime sleepiness and easy fatigue.

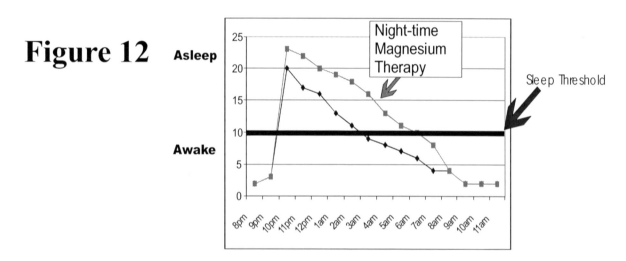

**Figure 12**

Fig 12 shows the profile for magnesium deficiency. Note the lower peak melatonin level. Magnesium if given at night in appropriate dose (say 300mg) will improve sleep by buoying the melatonin level longer into the sleep cycle.

## Magnesium and energy cycles.

Magnesium is involved in energy cycles. To convert glucose to ATP (the energy currency), we have three main steps: Glycolysis, the Krebs cycle and oxidative phosphorylation. Magnesium is needed in 12 of the 22 steps. Hence the tendency for lactic acid to build up in muscles and cause pain. Figs 13 &14 show the importance of Magnesium in glycolysis, the Krebs cycle. You cannot create ATP without these pathways. Magnesium also helps the "tail" of ATP to curl around a bit like a scorpion so that it packs into a smaller space.

With regards to oxidative phosphorylation, Fig 15 depicts the importance in the final step. In general Magnesium is needed in all ATPase reactions.

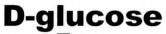
# D-glucose

Mg ⬇ Hexokinase/glucokinase

**Glucose-6-phosphate**

⬇ Phosphoglucose isomerase

**Fructose-6-phosphate**

Mg K ⬇ Phosphofructokinase-1

**Fructose-1,6-biphosphate**

⬇ Aldolase

**Glyceraldehyde-3-phosphate**

B3 ⬇ Gylceraldehyde-3-phosphate dehydrogenase

**1,3 biphosphoglycerate**

Mg ⬇ Phosphoglycerate kinase

**3- phosphoglycerate**

Mg ⬇ Phosphoglycero mutase

**2- phosphoglycerate**

Mg or Mn ⬇ Enolase

**Phosphoenolpyruvate**

Mg ⬇ Pyruvate kinase

# Pyruvate

## Figure 13

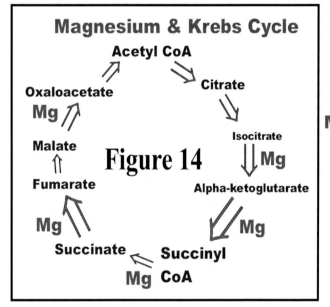

**Magnesium & Krebs Cycle**

Figure 14

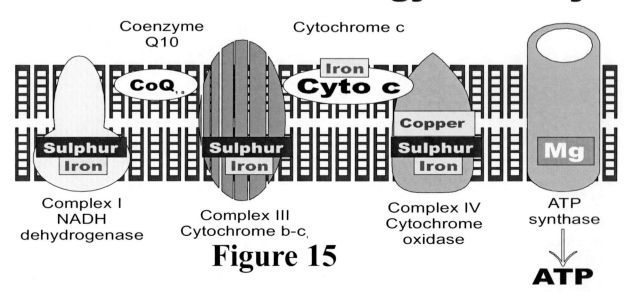

# Mitochondrial Energy Pathway

Coenzyme Q10

Cytochrome c

CoQ₁₀

Iron
Cyto c

Copper

Sulphur Iron — Sulphur Iron — Sulphur Iron — Mg

Complex I
NADH
dehydrogenase

Complex III
Cytochrome b-c₁

Complex IV
Cytochrome
oxidase

ATP
synthase
⬇
**ATP**

## Figure 15

## Magnesium and depression.

Fig 16 shows the pathway of Serotonin synthesis and the need for magnesium by Dopa Decarboxylase.

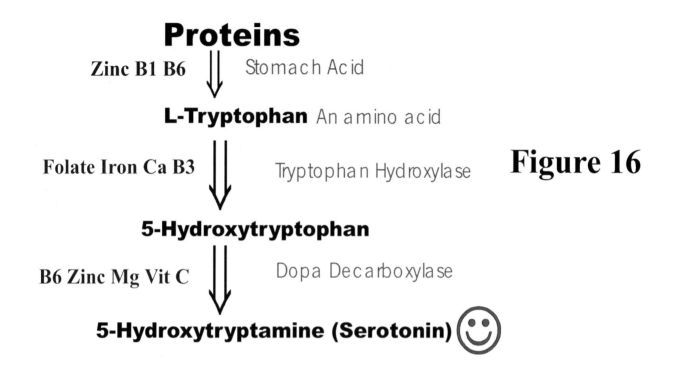

Figure 16

## Magnesium and Neuromuscular excitability.

Fig 23 shows the spectrum of excitability states that may be caused by magnesium deficiency or blockade. The reason for this is that the Calcium: Magnesium ratio strongly affects the threshold behaviour of excitable membranes (see figures 17, 18, 19 and 20)

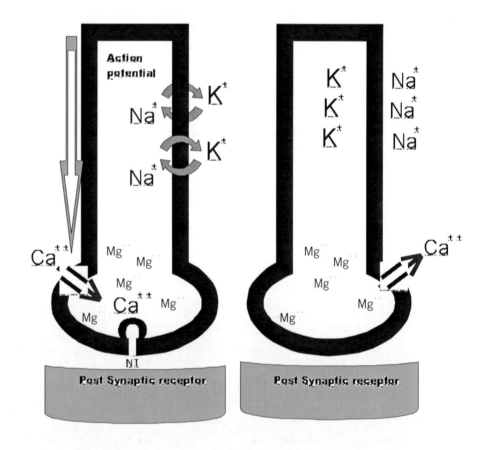

Figure 17

In the simple process of one nerve releasing a neurotransmitter, the course of the action potential is propagated by the influx of sodium into the axon and the efflux of potassium out of the axon. This action potential reaches a point near the end of the nerve, which allows calcium to flow into the terminal neuron. This influx of calcium stimulates the massive release of neurotransmitter in to the synaptic cleft. The major ion in this area is magnesium. Most of the mitochondria are in this area and wherever you find mitochondria you find lots of magnesium. The reason should be very obvious from the above description of magnesium and energy cycles. Therefore when calcium flows into the cell it disturbs the equilibrium. In the resting state, magnesium is in abundance. In the NT release state, calcium is in abundance. Therefore NT release depends upon Calcium: Magnesium ratio.

In resting muscle, small fluctuations in membrane potential occur at the end-plate region. These are called miniature end-plate potentials (MEPP's). They are produced by spontaneous releases of Acetylcholine from the motor nerve ending. Magnesium reduces the number of packets released by affecting MEPP's and during depolarisation. Lack of it causes twitching of muscles and nerve irritability.

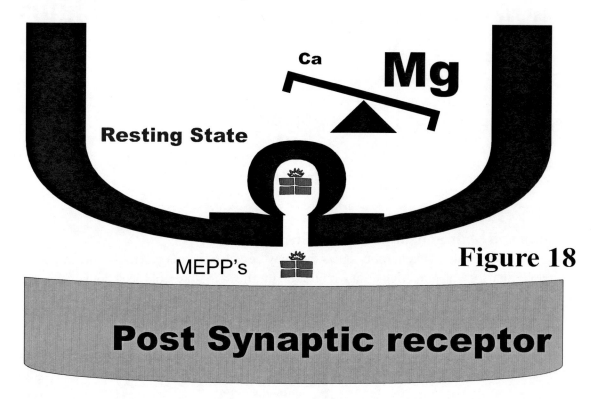

Figure 18

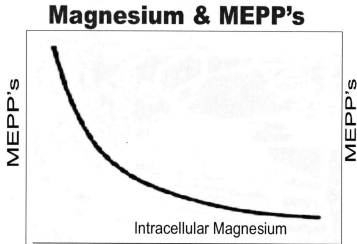

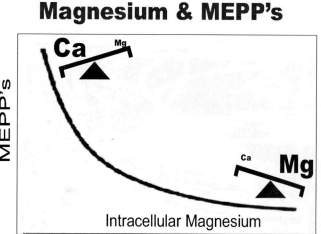

Figures 19 & 20

The mechanism of tinnitus is related to nerve cell damage in the organ of hearing. The layout of the cochlea is that each nerve responds to a set frequency. When one of the nerves is damaged, it fires spontaneously at its frequency causing the pure tone tinnitus. The propensity of this discharge is dependent upon the MEPP rate. The MEPP rate is dependent upon Calcium: Magnesium ratio. Hence the use of magnesium in tinnitus.

**Mineral balance and Tinnitus**

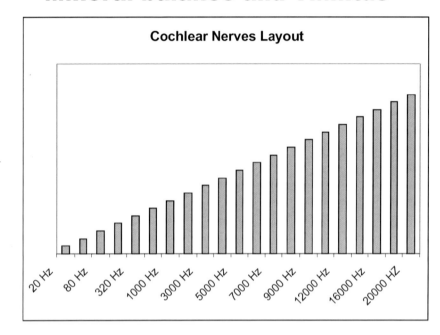

**Figure 21**

The mechanism of vertigo is similar to tinnitus in those hair cells that are damaged or excessively calcified, fire position sense information incorrectly. The propensity to send this inappropriate information is dependent upon calcium: magnesium ratio.

In summarising the CNS hyperexcitability symptoms, little imagination is required to explain the set of symptoms that I call "Nerves behaving badly".

**Mineral balance and Vertigo**

**Figure 22**

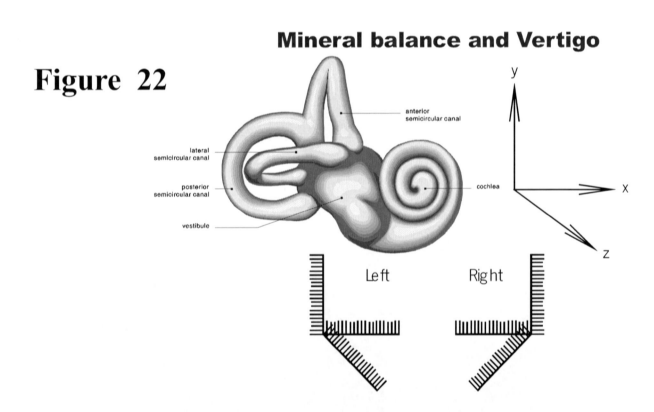

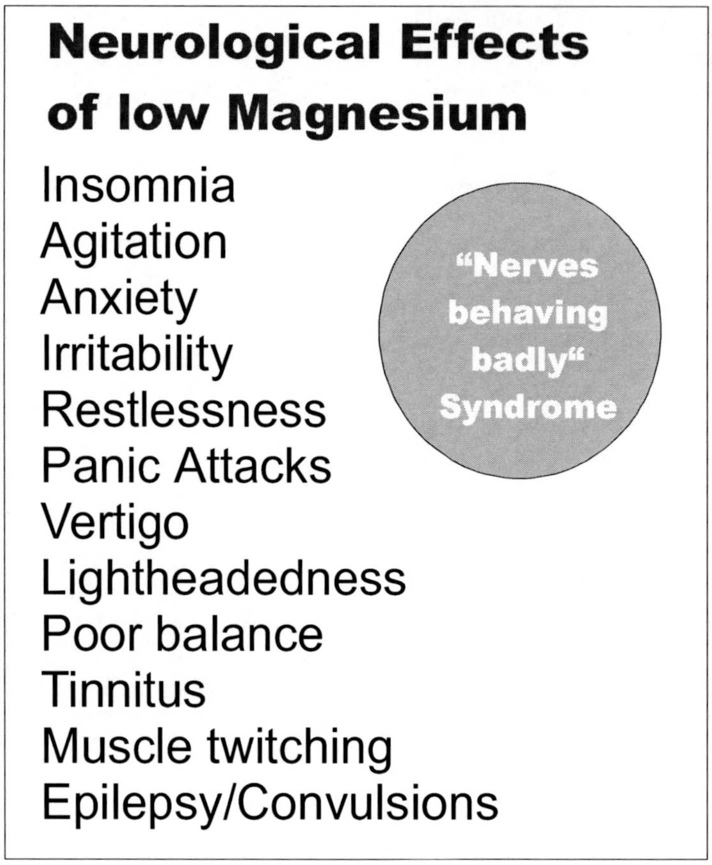

**Neurological Effects of low Magnesium**

Insomnia
Agitation
Anxiety
Irritability
Restlessness
Panic Attacks
Vertigo
Lightheadedness
Poor balance
Tinnitus
Muscle twitching
Epilepsy/Convulsions

"Nerves behaving badly" Syndrome

**Figure 23**

**Cardiac effects of Magnesium deficiency or Blockade**

Fig 24 shows the spectrum of problems caused by magnesium deficiency or blockade. These may be paroxysmal and the first symptoms often start at night. It is a good example of when muscle meets nerve in one tissue. The Gut is another one.

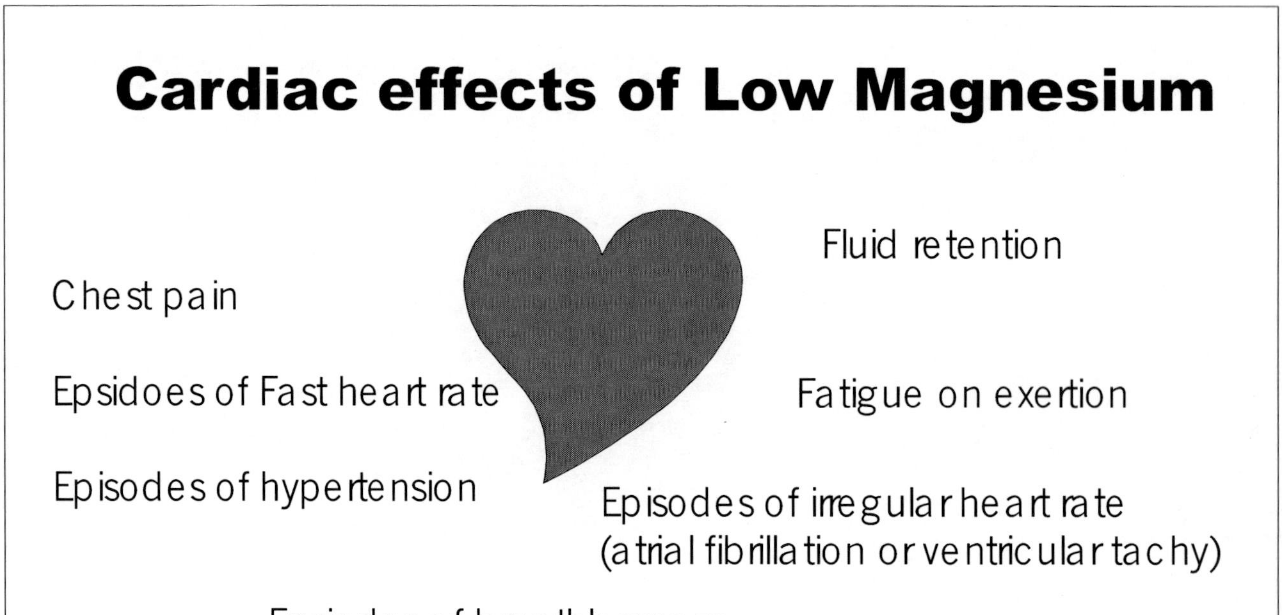

**Cardiac effects of Low Magnesium**

Chest pain

Epsidoes of Fast heart rate

Episodes of hypertension

Epsiodes of breathlessness

Fluid retention

Fatigue on exertion

Episodes of irregular heart rate
(atrial fibrillation or ventricular tachy)

**Figure 24**

## Foods that contain magnesium.

The table below of magnesium foods has the highest to lowest sources ranked in columns from left to right. Broad acre farming has seen a drop in magnesium intake. Fig 26 depicts the apparent fall in dietary magnesium plotted against the use of fertilisers. Comparisons of Organic and supermarket fruit and vegetables show that organic produce has about 4 times the amount of magnesium for (say) green beans.

### Sources of Magnesium

| Excellent | Good | Fair |
| --- | --- | --- |
| kelp, soya bean lima bean, rice bran, white bean, wheat bran, mung bean, cowpea peas, pinto beans red beans, pidgeon peas, pistachios, chestnuts, wheat germ chick peas, NZ spinach lentils, almonds, raisins parsley, sesame seeds brazil nuts, hazel nuts peanuts, dates, figs watercress, avocado pecans parsnip, garlic | Rye, cashews, walnuts millett, mushroom potato, collard, fennel broccoli, kale, banana brussel sprouts, leek blackcurrants, wheat sorghum, carrot, celery pumpkin, beetroot, peas radish, barley, endive cauliflower, nectarines guava, apricot, turnip sweet corn, asparagus macadamias | lettuce, coconut, melon rock melon, rhubarb chives, okra, tomato sweet potato, green beans kumquat, papaya, cabbage onions, wild rice, eggplant mung bean sprouts rice, capsicum, grapes peaches, oranges, figs black raspberry, cherry blackberry, loganberry cucumber, gooseberry pineapple, lemons, pear lychees, strawberry |

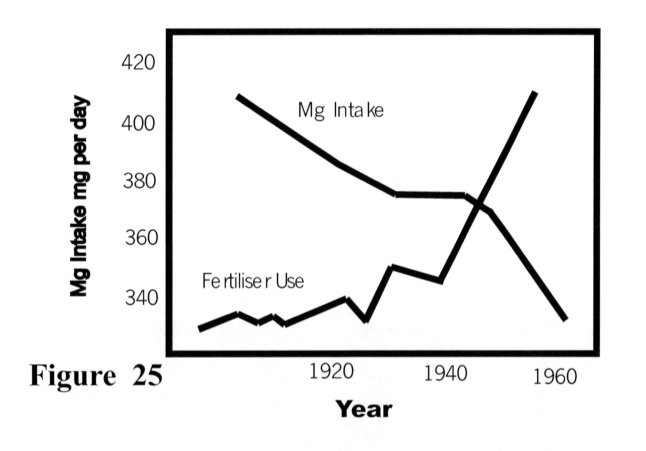

**Figure 25**

## Absorption of magnesium.

Magnesium needs to be in the charged divalent form to be absorbed easily. This requires hydrochloric acid (stomach acid). The production of stomach acid needs Zinc, Vitamin B1 and Vitamin B6. Fig 27 depicts the connection.

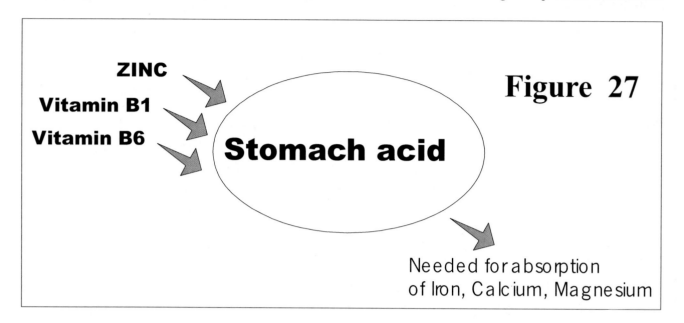

## Magnesium and Glucose Control.

Fig 28 depicts the contributors in the correct management of dietary and liver made glucose. There are several important points to make. The synchrony between intestinal absorption and appropriate insulin release. The appropriate production of glucose (gluconeogenesis) by the liver during fasting. The role of Glucose tolerance factor in aiding the effect of insulin (Chromium, Vanadium and Vitamin B3). The importance of Zinc, Sulphur and Manganese in the production of insulin. Contrary to the popular dichotomous classification of either IDDM or NIDDM, one can plainly see that deficiency (or blockade) of Zinc, Selenium, Manganese, Chromium, or Vanadium will also cause hyperglycaemia. Magnesium acts like the tap that releases insulin into the blood. It is also important for gluconeogenesis. Hence magnesium deficiency (or blockade) will cause unstable blood sugars, which result in periodic fatigue.

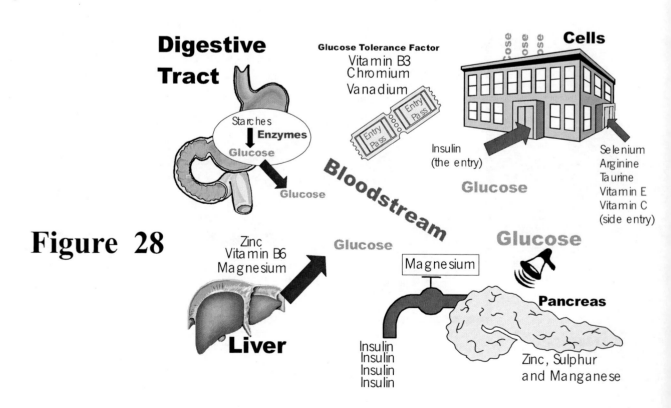

## Antagonism of Magnesium

Magnesium can be severely blocked in cells by copper and cadmium. This explains why blood tests may not fully reveal the extent of magnesium symptoms. Take the example of RBC Magnesium. Clearly, some patients have magnesium deficiency symptoms, but may be within the normal range. Fig 30 shows the probability of symptoms versus the RBC Mg level. This can be determined by a questionnaire. The more symptoms reported of magnesium deficiency the higher the probability of a deficiency. The problem comes when explaining why symptoms occur while still in the reference range (figure 31). The explanation is that there are unseen antagonists of magnesium which must also be measured.

## Spectrum of intracellular magnesium deficiency

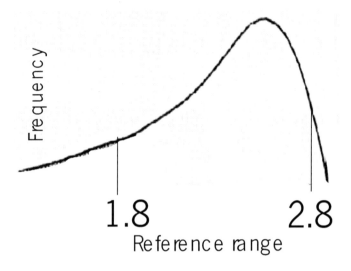

### Red Blood Cell Magnesium level

Frequency

1.8          2.8

Reference range

## Figure 29

## Figures 30 & 31

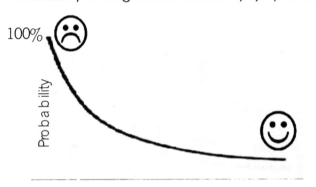

Probability of Magnesium deficiency symptoms

100%

Probability

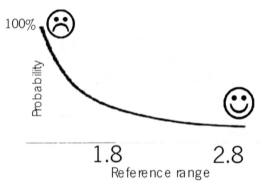

Probability of Magnesium deficiency symptoms

100%

Probability

1.8          2.8

Reference range

The most reliable form of testing is by tissue mineral analysis. Two examples are shown below. **Both** have magnesium deficiency symptoms. The low level is easy to imagine. The second example will give magnesium deficiency symptoms even though it is "high" because this level of magnesium will be totally blocked by the high level of tissue copper.

**NUTRITIONAL ELEMENTS**

| Ca | Mg | Na | K | Cu | Zn | P | Fe | Mn | Cr | Se | B | Co | Mo | S |
|----|----|----|----|----|----|----|----|----|----|----|----|----|----|----|
| 28 | 1.0 | 29 | 20 | 3.2 | 15 | 12 | 0.5 | .005 | 0.05 | 0.04 | 0.30 | .001 | .003 | 3904 |

**TOXIC ELEMENTS**

| Sb | U | As | Be | Hg | Cd | Pb | Al |
|----|----|----|----|----|----|----|----|
| .001 | .0016 | .005 | .0010 | 0.04 | .003 | 0.20 | 1.6 |

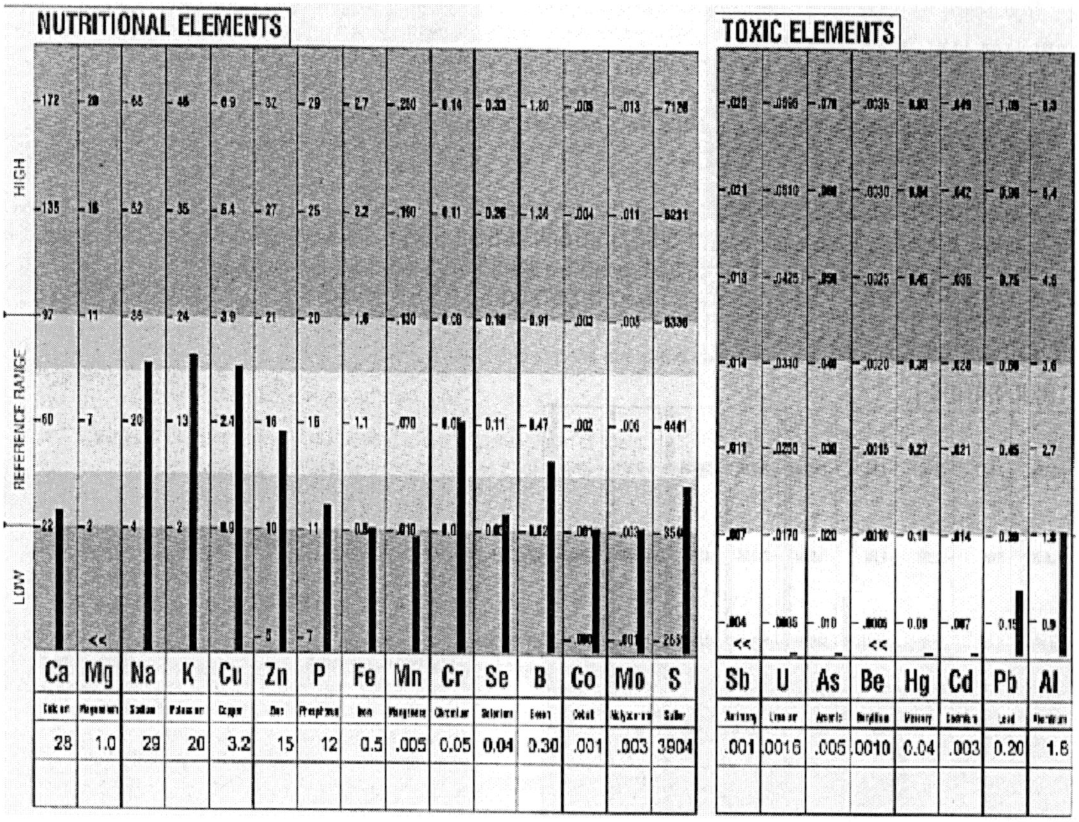

**Figure 33**

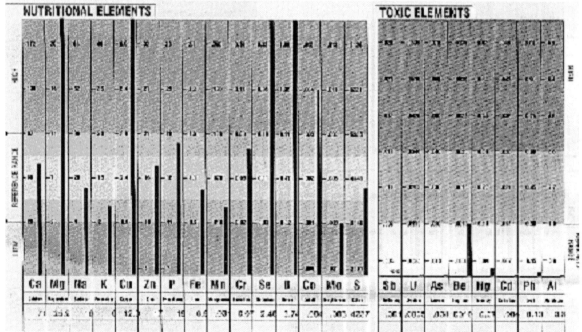

**Figure 34**

### Loss of Magnesium.

Magnesium is lost through the sweat and urine (increased by Alcohol and coffee). Stress hormones like cortisol and adrenalin deplete magnesium. The oral contraceptive pill, HRT and Pregnancy are associated with magnesium deficiency. Diuretics, ACE inhibitors and Beta blockers deplete magnesium.

### Magnesium and bone density

Fig 35 shows the team effort required to make bone. You can see that calcium is *not the most important* factor involved. Magnesium's role is probably stronger, but generally not acknowledged by the Medical profession.

## Nutrients needed for Bone Production

Magnesium
Calcium
Phosphorus
Manganese
Zinc
Molybdenum
Boron
Potassium

Vitamin D
Vitamin C
Parathyroid Hormone
Progesterone
Calcitonin

**Figure 35**

### Magnesium and calcium deposition.

An underrated role of magnesium is to prevent inappropriate deposition of calcium in tissues. The following experiment illustrates magnesium's role. With the progressive addition of calcium salts to row of beakers, eventually calcium will spontaneously precipitate. The addition of magnesium to the solution delays the point of precipitation.

## Calcium salt precipitation point

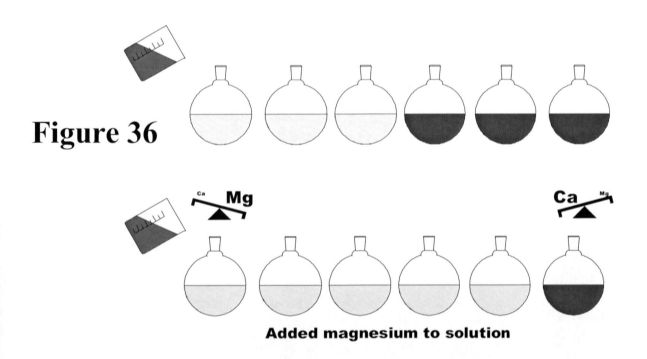

**Figure 36**

**Added magnesium to solution**

98

Figure 37 below is a list of calcium deposition sites seen in clinical practice and on X-rays. The importance of magnesium in the prevention of stone formation has been well documented, but the information is rarely used in practice.

## Calcium deposition sites

**Figure 37**

1] Kidneys

2] Bile

3] Tendon insertions and ligaments

4] Blood vessels (eg coronary arteries)

5] Pineal gland

6] Salivary glands

7] Pancreas

8] Cochlea Semicircular canals

## Magnesium and immunity.

A very little known feature of magnesium is its role in the regulation of the immune system. It plays "DNA replication auditor" by binding to phosphate groups. This enhances genomic stability.

**Figure 38**

## Magnesium and Immunity
DHEA production
Melatonin production
Antibody synthesis
DNA auditor

**References:**

1] Abbott L. et al. Magnesium deficiency in alcoholism: possible contribution to osteoporosis and cardiovascular disease in alcoholics. Alcoholism: Clinical and Experimental Research. 18(5):1076-1082, 1994

2] Abraham G.E., et al. Effect of vitamin B6 on plasma red blood cell magnesium levels in premenopausal women. Ann Clin Lab Sci. 11(4):333-336, 1981

3] Abraham G.E., Lubran MM. Serum and red cell magnesium levels in-patients with premenstrual tension. Am J Clin. Nutrition; 34(11)2364-66, 1981

4] Abraham GE et al. A total dietary program emphasising magnesium instead of calcium. Effect on the mineral density of calcaneous bone in postmenopausal women on hormonal therapy. J Reprod Med. 35:5 503-7, 1990

5] Abraham et al. Hypothesis: Management of fibromyalgia: rationale for the use of magnesium and malic acid. J Nutr Med. 3:49-59, 1992

6] Adaniya H., et al. Effects of magnesium on polymorphic ventricular tachycardia induced by aconite. Journal of Cardiovascular Pharmacology. 24:721-729, 1994

7] Agarwal O.P. Role of magnesium in development of spontenous atherosclerosis in pigs. Indian J Exp Biol. 20(3):262-263, 1982

8] Ahlborg H., et al. Effect of potassium-magnesium aspartate on the capacity for prolonged exercise in man. Acta Physiologica Scandinavia. 74:238-245, 1968

9] Alamoudi O.S. Hypomagnesesmia in chronic stable asthmatics: prevalence, correlation with severity and hospitalisation. Eur Resp. J 16:427-431, 2000

10] Al-Ghamdi, Saeed M.G., et al. Magnesium Deficiency: Pathophysiologic and Clinical Overview. American Journal of Kidney Diseases, November; 24(5): 737-752, 1994

11] Altura B.M., et al. Role of magnesium in the pathogenesis of hypertension updated: relationship to its action on cardiac, vascular smooth muscle, and endothelial cells. In: Laragh, J., Brenner, B. M. (editors). Hypertension: Pathophysiology, Diagnosis, and Management, 2nd Edition. Raven Press, New York, USA. :1213-1242, 1995

12] Altura B.M., et al. Mg, Na, and K interactions and coronary heart disease. Magnesium; 1:241-265, 1982

13] Altura B.M., et al. The role of magnesium in Etiology of strokes and cerebrovasospasm. Magnesium; 1:277-291, 1982

14] Altura B.M; Altura B.T. Magnesium ions and contraction of vascular smooth muscles: Relationship to some vascular diseases. Fed Proc; 40(12):2672-9, 1981

15] Altura B.M; Altura B.T. Interactions of Mg and K on blood vessels: Aspects in view of hypertension. Magnesium; 3(4-5) :175-94, 1984

16] Altura B. M., et al. Magnesium deficiency and hypertension: correlation between magnesium- deficient diets and microcirculatory changes in situ. Science. 223(4642):1315-1317, 1984

17] Altura B. M., et al. New perspectives on the role of magnesium in the pathophysiology of the cardiovascular system. Magnesium. 4:226-244, 1985

18] Altura B.T., et al. Biochemistry and pathophysiology of congestive heart failure: Is there a role for magnesium? Magnesium. 5(3-4):134-143, 1986

19] Altura B.M. Ischemic heart disease and magnesium. Magnesium. 7:57-67, 1988

20] Altura B.M., et al. Cardiovascular risk factors and magnesium: relationships to atherosclerosis, ischemic heart disease and hypertension. Magnes Trace Elem. 10(2-4):182-192, 1991-92

21] Altura B.M., et al. Magnesium: Growing in Clinical Importance. Patient Care, January 15; 130-136, 1994

22] Altura B.M., et al. Role of magnesium and calcium in alcohol-induced hypertension and strokes as probed by in vivo television microscopy, digital image microscopy, optical spectroscopy, 31P-NMR, spectroscopy and a unique magnesium ion-selective electrode. Alcohol Clin Exp Res. 18(5):1057-1068, 1994

23] Anast C.S. Impaired release of parathyroid hormone in magnesium deficiency. J Clin Endocrin Metab. 42: 707, 1976

24] Anderson T.W., et al. Ischemic heart disease, water hardness and myocardial magnesium. Canadian Medical Association Journal. 113:199, 1975

25] Ascherio A., et al. Intake of potassium, magnesium, calcium, and fiber and risk of stroke among US men. Circulation. 98:1198-204, 1998

26] Ascherio A. et al. A prospective study of nutritional factors and hypertension among US men. Circ. 86:5. 1475-84, 1992

27] Atar D., et al. Effects of magnesium supplementation in a porcine model of myocardial ischemia and reperfusion. J Cardiovasc Pharmacol. 24(4):603-611, 1994

28] Attias J., et al. Oral magnesium intake reduces permanent hearing loss induced by noise exposure. Am J Otolaryngol. 15:26-32, 1994

29] Baker S. Magnesium in primary care. Magnesium and Trace Elements. 10:251-5, 1994

30] Baker J.C., et al. Dietary antioxidants and magnesium in type I asthma Case control study. Thorax. 54(2) 115-8, 1999

31] Banki C. M., et al. Cerebrospinal fluid magnesium and calcium related to amine metabolites, diagnosis, and suicide attempts. Biol Psychiatry. 20(2):163-71, 1985

32] Barbagallo M., et al. Effects of vitamin E and glutathione on glucose metabolism: role of magnesium. Hypertension. 34(4 Part 2):1002-1006, 1999

33] Bashir Y., et al. Effects of long-term oral magnesium chloride replacement in congestive heart failure secondary to coronary artery disease. Am J Cardiol. 72:1156-1162, 1993

34] Benga I., et al. Plasma and cerebrospinal fluid concentrations of magnesium in epileptic children. J Neurol Sci. 67(1):29-34, 1985

35] Beyers E. Occurrence and Correction of Micro-element and Magnesium Deficiencies in the Deciduous Orchards and Vineyards in the Union of South Africa. Plant Analysis & Fertilizer Problems (I.R.H.O., Paris). 1956

36] Bhargava B., et al. Adjunctive magnesium infusion therapy in acute myocardial infarction. Int J Cardiol. 52(2):95-99, 1995

37] Bjorum N. Electrolytes in blood in endogenous depression. Acta Scand Psych. 48:59-68, 1972

38] Bloch H., et al. Intravenous magnesium sulfate as an adjunct in the treatment of acute asthma. Chest. 107(6):1576-1581, 1995

39] Blondell J.M. The anticarcinogenic effect of magnesium. Med Hypotheses. 6: 863-871, 1980

40] Blum M., et al. Oral contraceptive lowers serum magnesium. Harefuah. 121(10):363-364, 1991

41] Bohmer T., et al. Magnesium deficiency in chronic alcoholic patients uncovered by an intravenous loading test. Scand J Clin Lab Invest. 42:633, 1982

42] Briggs S. Magnesium - a forgotten mineral. Health & Nutrition Breakthroughs. November 1997

43] Brilla L. R., et al. Effect of magnesium supplementation on strength training in humans. J Am Coll Nutr. 11:326-329, 1992

44] Brisco A.M. & Regan, C. Effects of Magnesium on Calcium Metabolism in Man. Am J Clin Nutr. 19, 1966

45] Britton et al. Dietary magnesium, lung function, wheezing and airway hyperreactivity in a random adult population sample. Lancet. 344:357-362, 1994

46] Brodsky M.A. Magnesium, Myocardial Infarction and Arrhythmias. Journal Am Coll of Nutr, 11(5): 607/Abstract 36, 1992

47] Brodsky M.A., et al. Magnesium Therapy in New-Onset Atrial Fibrillation. The Am J of Cardiol. 15; 73:1227-1229, 1994

48] Cairns C.B., et al. Magnesium attenuates the neutrophil respiratory burst in adult asthmatic patients. Acad Emerg Med. 3(12):1093-1097, 1996

49] Cappuccio F, Markandu N, Beynon G., et al. Lack of effect of oral magnesium on high blood pressure. BMJ 1985; 291:235-238

50] Casscells W. Magnesium and Myocardial Infarction. Lancet, April 2; 343:808-809, 1994

51] Cernak I., et al. Alterations in magnesium and oxidative status during chronic emotional stress. Magnesium Research. 13(1):29-36, 2000

52] Chipperfield B., et al. Magnesium and the heart. American Heart Journal. 93:679, 1977

53] Ciarallo L et al. Intravenous magnesium therapy for moderate to severe pediatric asthma: results of a randomized, placebo-controlled trial. J Pediatr. 129(6):809-814, 1996

54] Ciarallo L et al. Higher dose intravenous magnesium therapy for children with moderate to severe acute asthma. Arch Pediatr Adolesc medicine. 154 979-983, 2000

55] Clague et al. Intravenous magnesium loading in chronic fatigue syndrome. Letter Lancet. 340:124-125, 1992

56] Classen HG et al. The clinical importance of magnesium The indications for supplementation and therapy. Fortschr Med. 108 (10): 198-200 1990

57] Clauw D. J., et al. Magnesium deficiency in the eosinophilia-myalgia syndrome. Arth Rheum. 9:1331-1334, 1994

58] Corica F, Allegra A, Di Benedetto A, et al. Effects of oral magnesium supplementation on plasma lipid concentrations of patients with non-insulin-dependent diabetes mellitus. Magnes Res. 7:43-47, 1994

59] Corica F., et al. Changes in plasma, erythrocyte, and platelet magnesium levels in normotensive and hypertensive obese subjects during oral glucose tolerance test. American Journal of Hypertension. 12(2 Part 1):128-136, 1999

60] Cohen L Infrared spectroscopy and magnesium content in bone mineral in osteoporotic women. J Med Sci. 17: 1123-5, 1981

61] Cohen L., et al. Magnesium sulphate and digitalis-toxic arrhythmias. JAMA. 249:2808-2810, 1983.

62] Cohen L, et al. Magnesium sulfate in the treatment of variant angina. Magnesium. 3:46-49, 1984

63] Cohen L., et al. Prompt termination and/or prevention of cold-pressor-stimulus-induced vasoconstriction of different vascular beds by magnesium sulfate in patients with Prinzmetal's angina. Magnesium. 5:144-149, 1986

64] Cohen N., et al. Metabolic and clinical effects of oral magnesium supplementation in furosemide-treated patients with severe congestive heart failure. Clin Cardiol. 23(6):433-436, 2000

65] Cox et al. Red Blood cell magnesium and chronic fatigue syndrome. Lancet 337:757-760, 1991

66] Curry D.L., et al. Magnesium modulation of glucose-induced insulin secretion by the perfused mouse pancreas. Endocrinology. 101:203, 1977

67] Dahle et al. The effect of oral magnesium substitution on pregnancy induced leg cramps. AM J Obstet Gynecol. 173:1 175-80, 1995

68] Davis W. H., et al. Monotherapy with magnesium increases abnormally low high density lipoprotein cholesterol: A clinical essay. Clin Ther Res. 36:341-346, 1984

69] Demirkaya et al. Efficacy of intravenous magnesium sulfate in the treatment of acute migraine attacks. Headache. 41 171-177, 2001

70] De Swart P.M., et al. The interrelationship of calcium and magnesium absorption in idiopathic hypercalciuria and renal calcium stone disease. Journal of Urology. 159(3):669-772, 1998

71] Deulofeu et al. Magnesium and chronic fatigue syndrome. Letter Lancet 338: 66, 1991

72] Deuster P.A., et al. Responses of plasma magnesium and other cations to fluid replacement during exercise. J Am Col Nutr. 12(3):286-293, 1993

73] Dipalma J.R. Magnesium replacement therapy. Am Fam Physician. 42 (1): 173-6, 1990

74] Ditmar R.,et al. The significane of magnesium in orthopaedics Magnesium in osteoporosis. Acta Chir Orthoop Traumatol Cech. 56(2): 143-59, 1989

75] Dominguez L. J., et al. Magnesium responsiveness to insulin and insulin-like growth factor I in erythrocytes from normotensive and hypertensive subjects. J Clin Endocrinol Metab. 83:4402-4407, 1998

76] Domingez et al. Bronchial reactivity and intracellular magnesium: a possible mechanism for the brochodilating effect of magnesium in asthma. Clin Sci. 95:137-142, 1998

77] Dorup I. Magnesium and potassium deficiency. Its diagnosis, occurrence and treatment in diuretic therapy and its consequences for growth, protein synthesis and growth factors. Acta Physiol Scand. 618(Supplement):1-55, 1994

78] Drach G.W. Contribution to therapeutic decisions of ratios, absolute values and other measures of calcium, magnesium, urate or oxalate balance in stone formers. Journal of Urology. 116(3):338-340, 1976

79] Dubey A., et al. Magnesium, myocardial ischaemia and arrhythmias: The role of magnesium in myocardial infarction. Drugs. 37:1-7, 1989

80] Durlach J., et al. The Control of Central Neural Hyperexicability in Magnesium Deficiency. Nutrients and Brain Function Karger Publishers. 48-71, 1987

81] Durlach J. Magnesium depletion and pathogenesis of Alzheimer's disease. Magnesium Research . 3(3):217-218, 1990

82] Durlatch J. New trends in international magnesium research. Magnesium Research. 5: 23-27, 1992

83] Dyckner T., et al.  Intracellular potassium after magnesium infusion.  British Medical Journal.  1:882, 1978

84] Dyckner T., et al.  Aggravation of thiamine deficiency by magnesium depletion.  Acta Med Scand.  218:129-131, 1985

85] Dyckner T., et al.  Effect of magnesium on blood pressure.  British Medical Journal.  286(6381):1847-1849, 1983

86] Eisinger J., et al.  Selenium and magnesium status in fibromyalgia.  Magnesium Research.  7(3-4):285-288, 1994

87] Emelianova et al.  Magnesium sulfate in management of bronchial asthma.  Klin Med.  47:8 55-8, 1996

88] Facchinetti F., et al.  Magnesium prophylaxis of menstrual migraine: effects on intracellular magnesium.  Headache, 31:5, 298-301, 1991

89] Facchinetti F., et al.  Oral magnesium successfully relieves premenstrual mood changes.  Obstet Gynecol.78:2,177-81, 1991

90] Feillet-Coudray et al.  Exchangeable magnesium pool masses in healthy women: effects of magnesium supplementation.–American Journal of Clinical Nutrition, Vol. 75, No. 1, 72-78, January 2002

91] Fernandes J. S., et al.  Therapeutic effect of a magnesium salt in patients suffering from mitral valve prolapse and latent tetany.  Magnesium.  4:283-289, 1985

92] Ferrara L, Iannuzzi R, Castaldo A, et al.  Long-term magnesium supplementation in essential hypertension.  Cardiology.  81:25-3, 1992

93] Fiaccadori E., et al.  Muscle and serum magnesium in pulmonary intensive care unit patients.  Crit Care Med.  16(8):751-760, 1988

94] Flink E.B.  Magnesium deficiency in alcoholism.  Alcoholism.  10(6):590-594, 1986

95] Fontana-Klaiber H., et al.  Therapeutic effects of magnesium in dysmenorrhea.  Schweiz Rundsc Med Prax 79(16): 491-4, 1990

96] Fourman P. & Morgan D.B.  Chronic Magnesium Deficiency in Man.  Clin Sci Nutr 26, 1973

97] Frizel D., et al.  Plasma calcium and magnesium in depression.  British Journal of Psychiatry.  115:1375-1377, 1969.

98] Fugii S, Takemura T, Wada M., et al.  Magnesium levels in plasma, erythrocyte, and urine in patients with diabetes mellitus.  Horm Metab Res.  14:161-162, 1982

99] Gallai V., et al.  Red blood cell magnesium levels in migraine patients.  Cephalalgia.  13:2, 94-81, 1993

100] Galland L. D., et al.  Magnesium deficiency in the pathogenesis of mitral valve prolapse.  Magnesium.  5:165-174, 1986

101] Gantz N.M.  Magnesium and chronic fatigue.  Letter Lancet.  338 66, 1991

102] Gaspar A.Z., et al.  The influence of magnesium on visual field and peripheral vasospasm in glaucoma.  Ophthalmologica.  209(1):11-13, 1995

103] Gatewood J. W., et al.  Mental changes associated with hyperparathyroidism.  Am J Psychiat.  132(2):129-132, 1975

104] Gawaz M.  Antithrombotic effectiveness of magnesium.  Fortschr Med.  114: 329-332, 1996

105] Glick L.J.  The role of magnesium deficiency and an hypothesis concerning the pathogenesis of Alzheimer's disease.  Medical Hypotheses.  31(3):211-225, 1990

106] Gorges L.F., et al.  Effect of magnesium on epileptic foci.  Epilepsia.  19(1):81-91, 1978

107] Goto et al.  Magnesium deficiency detected by intravenous loading dose test in variant angina pectoris.  Am J Cardiol. 15 65: 709-12, 1990

108] Gottlieb S. S.  Importance of magnesium in congestive heart failure.  Am J Cardiol.  63:39G-42G, 1989

109] Gottlieb S. S., et al.  Prognostic importance of serum magnesium concentration in patients with congestive heart failure.  J Am Coll Cardiol.  16:827-831, 1990

110] Gottlieb S., et al.  Effects of Intravenous Magnesium Sulfate on Arrhythmias in Patients With Congestive Heart Failure.  American Heart Journal, June; 125:1645-1649, 1993

111] Gueux E., et al.  The effect of magnesium deficiency on glucose stimulated insulin secretion in rats.  Horm Metab Res.  15:594-597, 1983

112] Gullestad L., et al.  Oral magnesium supplementation improves metabolic variables and muscle strength in alcoholics.  Alcohol Clin Exp Res.  16(5):986-990, 1992

113] Gums I.J.  Clinical Significance of Magnesium.  Intell Clin Pharm.  21:240-46, 1987

114] Haga H.  Effects of dietary magnesium supplementation on diurnal variations of blood pressure and plasma sodium, potassium-ATPase activity in essential hypertension.  Jpn Heart J.  33:785-800, 1992

115] Hall R. C. W., et al.  Hypomagnesemia:  physical and psychiatric symptoms.  Journal of the American Medical Association.  224:1749-1751, 1973

116] Hallson P., et al.  Magnesium reduces calcium oxalate crystal formation in human whole urine.  Clin Sci.  62:17-19, 1982

117] Hampton E. M., et al.  Intravenous magnesium therapy in acute myocardial infarction.  Ann Pharmacother.  28:212-219, 1994

118] Hanna S & MacIntyre, I.  Influence of Aldosterone on Magnesium Metabolism.  Lancet. 2, 1960

119] Harari et al.  Magnesium in the management of acute and chronic treatments and Deutsches Medizinisches Zentrum's (DMZ's) clinical experience at the dead sea.  J Asthma. 35:525-536, 1998

120] Hartwig  A Role for Magnesium in genomic stability.  Mutat Res. 475 (1-2) 113-21 2001-11-21

121] Hashimoto et al.  Assessment of magnesium status in patients with bronchial asthma.  J Asthma. 37:489-496, 2000

122] Hattori K., et al.  Intracellular magnesium deficiency and effect of oral magnesium on blood pressure and red cell sodium transport in diuretic-treated hypertensive patients.  Jpn Circ J.  52(11):1249-1256, 1988

123] Haury V.G.  Blood serum magnesium in bronchial asthma and its treatment by the administration of magnesium sulfate.  The Journal of Laboratory and Clinical Medicine.  26:340-344, 1940

124] Hauser S.P., et al.  Intravenous magnesium administration in bronchial asthma.  Scweiz Med Wochenschr. 199(46) 1633-1635, 1989

125] Henderson D.G., et al.  Effect of magnesium supplementation on blood pressure and electrolyte concentrations in hypertensive patients receiving long term diuretic treatment.  British Medical Journal.  293(6548):664-665, 1986

126] Henrotte J.G.  Type A behavior and magnesium metabolism.  Magnesium.  5:201-210, 1986

127] Herzog W.R., et al. How magnesium therapy may influence clinical outcome in acute myocardial infarction: review of potential mechanisms. Coron Artery Dis. 7(5):364-370, 1996

128] Hinds et al. Normal red cell magnesium concentrations and magnesium loading tests in patients with chronic fatigue syndrome. Ann Clin Biochem. 31:459-461, 1994

129] Hill et al. Investigation of the effect of short-term change in dietary magnesium intake in asthma. Eur Respir J. 10:2225-2229, 1997

130] Howard J. M. H. Magnesium deficiency in peripheral vascular disease. Journal of Nutrition and Medicine. 1:39-49, 1990

131] Humphries S., et al. Low dietary magnesium is associated with insulin resistance in a sample of young, nondiabetic Black Americans. Am J Hypertens. 12:747-756, 1999

132] Hwang D.L., et al. Insulin increases intracellular magnesium transport in human platelets. J Endocrinol Metab. 76:549-553, 1993

133] Ichihara A. Effects of magnesium on the renin-angiotensin-aldosterone system in human subjects. J Lab Clin Med. 112(4):432-440, 1993

134] Iseri L.T. Magnesium and cardiac arrhythmias. Magnesium. 5:111-126, 1986

135] Iseri L.T., et al. Magnesium for intractable ventricular tachyarrhythmias in normomagnesemic patients. Western Journal of Medicine. 138(6):823-828, 1983

136] ISIS-4 Collaborative Group. Fourth international study of infarct survival: protocol for a large simple study of the effects of oral mononitrate, oral captopril, and of intravenous magnesium. Am J Cardiol. 68:87-100, 1991

137] Itoh K., et al. The effects of high oral magnesium supplementation on blood pressure, serum lipids and related variables in apparently healthy Japanese subjects. Br J Nutr. November; 78:5, 737-50, 1997

138] Izenwasser S.E., et al. Stimulant-like effects of magnesium on aggression in mice. Pharmacol Biochem Behav. 25(6):1195-9, 1986

139] Jing M.A., Folsom A.R., Melnick S.L., et al. Associations of serum and dietary magnesium with cardiovascular disease, hypertension, diabetes, insulin, and carotid arterial wall thickness: the ARIC study. J Clin Epidemiol. 48:927-940, 1995

140] Joffres M.R., et al. Relationship of magnesium intake and other dietary factors to blood pressure: the Honolulu heart study. Am J Clin Nutr 45:2,469-75, 1987

141] Johansson G., et al. Biochemical and clinical effects of the prophylactic treatment of renal calcium stones with magnesium hydroxide. Journal of Urology. 124(6):770-774, 1980

142] Johansson G., et al. Magnesium metabolism in renal stone disease. Invest Urol. 18(2):93-96, 1980

143] Johansson G., et al. Effects of magnesium hydroxide in renal stone disease. Journal of the American College of Nutrition. 1(2):179-185, 1982

144] Johansson G. Magnesium and renal stone disease. Acta Med. Scand. (supplement). 661:13-18, 1982

145] Johnson C. J., et al. Myocardial tissue concentrations of magnesium and potassium in men dying suddenly from ischemic heart disease. American Journal of Clinical Nutrition. 32:967, 1979

146] Johnson S., et al. The multifaceted and widespread pathology of magnesium deficiency. Medical Hypotheses. 56(2):163-170, 2001

Jooste, P. L., et al. Epileptic-type convulsions and magnesium deficiency. Aviat. Space Environ. Med. 50(7):734-735, 1979

147] Jorgensen F. S. The urinary excretion and serum concentration of calcium, magnesium, sodium and phosphate in male patients with recurring renal stone formation. Scand J Urol Nephrol. 9(3):243-248, 1975

148] Kantak K. M. Magnesium deficiency alters aggressive behavior and catecholamine function. Behav Neurosci. 102(2):304- 11, 1988.

149] Karkkainen P., et al. Alcohol intake correlated with serum trace elements. Alcohol. 23:279-282, 1988

150] Kawano Y., Matsuoka H., Takashita S., et al. Effects of magnesium supplementation in hypertensive patients: assessment by home, office, and ambulatory blood pressures. Hypertension ;32:260-265, 1998

151] Keynes et al. Nerve & Muscle. Cambridge Uni Press. 1991

152] Kh R., et al. Effect of oral magnesium supplementation on blood pressure, platelet aggregation and calcium handling in deoxycorticosterone acetate induced hypertension in rats. Journal of Hypertension. 18(7):919-926, 2000

153] Kirov G.K., et al. Magnesium, schizophrenia and manic-depressive disease. Neuropsychobiology. 23(2):79-81, 1990

154] Klevay et al. Low dietary magnesium increases supraventricular ectopy. American Journal of Clinical Nutrition. Vol. 75, No. 3, 550-554, March 2002

155] Kozielec T., et al. Assessment of magnesium levels in children with attention deficit hyperactivity disorder (ADHD). Magnesium Research. 10(2):143-148, 1997

156] Kysters K., Spieker C., Tepel M., et al. New data about the effects of oral physiological magnesium supplementation on several cardiovascular risk factors. Magnes Res. 6:355-360, 1993

157] Labeeuw M., et al. [Role of magnesium in the physiopathology and treatment of calcium renal lithiasis.] La Presse Medicale. 16(1):25-27, 1987

158] Landon et al. Role of magnesium in regulation of lung function. J Am Diet Assoc. 93:674-677, 1993

159] Leary W.P., et al. Magnesium and deaths ascribed to ischaemic heart disease in South Africa. A preliminary report. S Afr Med J. 64(20):775-776, 1983

160] Leclercqu-Meyer et al. Effect of Calicium and Magnesium on Glucagon Secretion. Endocrinol. 93, 1973

161] Lefebvre P.J., et al. Magnesium and glucose metabolism. Therapie. 49:1-7, 1994

162] Lelord G., et al. Effects of pyridoxine and magnesium on autistic symptoms - Initial observations. J Autism Dev Disorders. 11:219-230, 1981

163] Lemke M.R. Plasma magnesium decrease and altered calcium/magnesium ratio in severe dementia of the Alzheimer type. Biol Psychiatry. 37(5):341-343, 1995

164] Lichodziejewska B., et al. Clinical symptoms of mitral valve prolapse are related to hypomagnesemia and attenuated by magnesium supplementation. American Journal of Cardiology. 79(6):768-772, 1997

165] Lind L., Lithell H., Landsberg L Blood pressure response during long-term treatment with magnesium is dependent on magnesium status. Am J Hypertens. 4:674-679, 1991

166] Lindeman R. D., et al. Magnesium in Health and Disease. SP Medical and Scientific Books, Jamaica, NY. 1980:236-245

167] Linder J., et al. Calcium and Magnesium concentrations in affective disorder: Difference between plasma and serum in relation to symptoms. Acta. Psych Scand 80:527-37, 1989

168] Ma J. Associations of serum and dietary magnesium with cardiovascular disease, hypertension, diabetes ,insulin and carotid arterial wall thickness: the ARIC study Atherosclerosis Risk in Communities. J Clin Epidem 48:7 927-40, 1995

169] MacIntyre I., et al. Intracellular Magnesium Deficiency in Man. Clin Sci 20, 1961

170] Malpuech-Brugere C., et al. Early morphological and immunological alterations in the spleen during magnesium deficiency in the rat. Magnesium Research. 11(3):161-169, 1998

171] Marlow M., et al. Decreased magnesium in the hair of autistic children. J Orthomol Psychiat. 13(2):117-122, 1984

172] Martineau J., et al. Vitamin B6, magnesium, and combined vitamin B6-Mg: Therapeutic effects in childhood autism. Biol Psychiat. 20:467-478, 1978

173] Martineau J., et al. The effects of combined pyridoxine plus magnesium administration on the conditioned evoked potentials in children with autistic behavior. Curr Top Nutr Dis. 19:357-362, 1988

174] Maruer J.R. Role of environmental magnesium in cardiovascular disease. Magnesium. 1:266-276 1982 and 2:57-61, 1983

175] Marx A & Neutra R. Magnesium in drinking water and ischemic heart disease. Epidemiol Rev.19:258-272, 1997

176] Mather H. M., et al. Hypomagnesemia in diabetes. Clin Chem Acta. 95:235-242, 1979

177] Matz R. Magnesium: Deficiencies and Therapeutic Uses. Hospital Practice. April 30, 79-72, 1993

178] Mauskop A., et al. Intravenous magnesium sulfate rapidly alleviates headaches of various types. Headache. 36:154-160, 1996

179] Mauskop A. & Altura B.M. Role of magnesium in the pathogenesis and treatment of migraines. Clin Science 89(6):633-636, 1995

180] Mauskop A., et al. Role of magnesium in the pathogenesis and Treatment of migraine. Clin Neurosciences. 5:24-27, 1998

181] McCarty M.F. Magnesium taurate and fish oil for prevention of migraine. Med Hypotheses. 47: 461-466, 1996

182] McLean R.M. Magnesium and its therapeutic uses: a review. American Journal of Medicine. 96(1):63-76, 1994

183] McNair P., et al. Hypomagnesemia, a risk factor in diabetic neuropathy. Diabetes. 27:1075-1077, 1978

184] McNair P., Christensen M.S., Christiansen C., et al. Renal hypomagnesemia in human diabetes mellitus: its relation to glucose homeostasis. Eur J Clin Invest ; 12:81-85, 1982

185] Melnick I., et al. Magnesium therapy of recurrent calcium oxalate urinary calculi. I Urol. 105:119, 1978

186] Mishima et al. Platelet ionised magnesium, cyclic AMP and cyclic GMP levels in migraine and tension type headache. Headache. 37:561-564, 1997

187] Moore M.P., Redman C.W. Case-control study of severe pre-eclampsia of early onset. Br Med J. 287:580-83, 1983

188] Moore T.J. The role of dietary electrolytes in hypertension. J Am Coll Nutr, 8 Suppl S. 68S-80S, 1989

189] Moorkens et al. Magnesium deficit in a sample of the Belgian population presenting with chronic fatigue. Magnes Res. 10:329-337, 1997

191] Motoyama T., et al. Oral magnesium supplementation in patients with essential hypertension. Hypertension. 13(3):227-232, 1989

192] Muenzenberg et al. Mineralogic apects in the treatment of osteoporosis with magnesium. J Am Coll Nutr. 8(5): 461, 1989

193] Muir K.W., et al. Dose optimization of intravenous magnesium sulfate after acute stroke. Stroke. 29:918-923, 1998

194] Muneyvirci-Delale O., et al. Sex steroid hormones modulate serum ionized magnesium and calcium levels throughout the menstrual cycle in women. Fertil Steril. 69(5): 958-62, 1998

195] Nadler J.L., et al. Magnesium deficiency produces insulin resistance and increased thromboxane synthesis. Hypertension. 21:1024-1029, 1993

196] Nowson C & Morgan T. Magnesium supplementation in mild hypertensive patients on a moderately low sodium diet. Clin Exp Pharmacol Physiol. 16:299-302, 1989

197] O'Brien P., et al. Progesterone, Fluid and Electrolytes in Premenstrual Syndrome. Brit Med Journal. (1) 1161-1163, 1980

198] Okayama H., et al. Bronchodilating effect of intravenous magnesium sulfate in bronchial asthma. JAMA. 257(8):1076-1078, 1987

199] Olhaberry J., Reyes A., Acousta-Barrios T., et al. Pilot evaluation of the putative antihypertensive effect of magnesium. Magnes Bull. 9:181-184, 1987

200] Omu A. E., et al. Magnesium in human semen: possible role in premature ejaculation. Arch Androl. 46(1):59-66, 2001

201] Paolisso G., et al. Daily magnesium supplements improve glucose handling in elderly subjects. American Journal of Clinical Nutrition. 55:1161-1167, 1992

202] Paolisso G., et al. Improved insulin response and action by chronic magnesium administration in aged NIDDM subjects. Diabetes Care. 12(4):265-269, 1989

203] Paolisso G., et al. Magnesium and glucose homeostasis. Diabetologia. 33(9):511-514, 1990

204] Paolisso et al. Changes in glucose turnover parameters and improvement of glucose oxiation after 4-week magnesium administrataion in elderly non-insulin dependent diabetic patients. J Clin Endocrin Metab. 78:6 1510-4, 1994

205] Paolisso et al. Hypertension, diabetes and insulin resistance: the role of intracellular magnesium. Am J Hypertens. 10:3 346-55, 1997

206] Peikert A., et al. Prophylaxis of migraine with oral magnesium: results from a prospective, multi- centre, placebo-controlled and double-blind randomized study. Cephalalgia. June, 16:4, 257-63, 1996

207] Perticone F., et al. Antiarrhythmic short-term protective magnesium treatment in ischemic dilated cardiomyopathy. J Am Coll Nutr. 9:492-499, 1990

208] Picado M., de la Sierra A., Aguilera M., et al. Increased activity of the magnesium-sodium exchanger in red blood cells for essential hypertensive patients. Hypertension; 23(part 2):987-991, 1993

209] Poenaru S., et al. Magnesium and monoaminergic neurotransmitters: Elements of human and experimental pathaphysiology. In: Magnesium in Health and Disease. Itakawa Y., and Durlach, J. London. :291-297, 1989

210] Popoviciu L., et al. Parasomnias (non-epileptic nocturnal episodic manifestations) in patients with magnesium deficiency. Romanian Journal of Neurology and Psychiatry. 28(1):19-24, 1990

211] Porta S., et al. Significant inhibition of the stress response with magnesium supplementation in fighter pilots. Magnesium-Bulletin. 16,2:54-58, 1994

212] Purvis J. R., et al. Magnesium disorders and cardiovascular disease. Clin Cardiol. 15:556-568, 1992

213] Purvis J.R., Cummings D.M., Landsman P., et al. Effect of oral magnesium supplementation on selected cardiovascular risk factors in non-insulin-dependent diabetics. Arch Fam Med. 3:503-508, 1994

214] Ralo J. Magnesium: Another metal to bone up on. Science News. 154:134, 1998

215] Ramadan et al. Low brain magnesium in migraine. Headache. 29:590-593, 1989

216] Rasmussen H. S., et al. Intravenous magnesium in acute myocardium infarction. The Lancet. 1:234-235, 1986

217] Rasmussen H. S., et al. Influence of magnesium substitution therapy on blood lipid composition in patients with ischemic heart disease. Archives of Internal Medicine. 149:1050-1053, 1989

218] Regan R. R., et al. Magnesium deprivation decreases cellular reduced glutathione and causes oxidative neuronal death in murine cortical cultures. Brain Res. 890(1):177-183, 2001

219] Resnick L. M., et al. Intracellular free magnesium in erythrocytes of esential hypertension: Relation to blood pressure and serum divalent cations. Proceedings of the National Academy of Sciences. 81:6511, 1984

220] Resnick L. Magnesium in the pathophysiology and treatment of hypertension and diabetes mellitus: where are we in 1997? Am J Hypertension. 10:368-370, 1997

221] Reynolds I. J. Intracellular calcium and magnesium, critical determinants of excitotoxicity. Prog Brain Res. 116:225-243, 1998

222] Rheinhart R.A. Clinical correlates of the molecular and cellular actions of magnesium on the cardiovascular system. Am Heart J. 121 (5): 1513-21, 1991

223] Robinson J.B.D. & Chenery E.M. Magnesium Deficiency in Coffee with Special Reference to Mulching. Emp. J. exp. Agric. 26:259-73, 1958

224] Rolla G., et al. Acute effect of intravenous magnesium sulfate on airway obstruction of asthmatic patients. Annals of Allergy. 61:388-391, 1988

225] Romano T.J. Magnesium deficiency in systemic lupus erythematosis. Journal of Nutritional & Environmental Medicine. 107-111, 1997

226] Ruddell H., et al. Effect of magnesium supplementation in patients with labile hypertension. Journal of the American College of Nutrition. 6:445, 1987

227] Rude R. K., et al. Magnesium deficiency: possible role in osteoporosis associated with gluten-sensitive enteropathy. Osteoporos Int. 6(6):453-461, 1996

228] Rude R. Low serum concentrations of 1,25-dihyroxyvitamin D in human magnesium deficiency. J Clin Endocirn Metab. 61: 933-40, 1985

229] Rude R. Magnesium Metabolism and Deficiency. Endocrin & MetabClin N America, June. 22(2): 377-395, 1993

230] Rude R. K., et al. Magnesium deficiency induced osteoporosis in the rat: uncoupling of bone formation and bone resorption. Magnesium Research. 12:257-267, 1999

231] Rudnicki M., et al. Comparison of magnesium and methyldopa for the control of blood pressure in pregnancies complicated with hypertension. Gynecol Obstet Invest. 49(4):231-235, 2000

232] Russell R. I. Magnesium requirements in patients with chronic inflammatory disease receiving intravenous nutrition. J Am Coll Nutr. 4(5):553-558, 1985

233] Ryan M. P., et al. The role of magnesium in the prevention and control of hypertension. Ann Clin Res. 16(Supplement 43):81-88, 1984

234] Saito K., Hattori K., Omatsu T., et al. Effects of oral magnesium on blood pressure and red cell sodium transport in patients receiving long-term thiazide diuretics for hypertension. Am J Hypertens. 1:71S-74S, 1988

235] Sanjuliani A. F., et al. Effects of magnesium on blood pressure and intracellular ion levels of Brazilian hypertensive patients. Int J Cardiol. 56(2):177-183, 1996

236] Saris N.E.L., et al. Magnesium: an update on physiological, clinical and analytical aspects. Clinica Chimica Acta. 294:1-26, 2000

237] Satake et al. Relation between severity of magesuim deficiency and frequency of anginal attacks in men with variant angina. J Am Coll Cardiol. 28:4 897-902, 1996

238] Schecter M., Hod H., Marks N., et al. Beneficial effect of magnesium sulfate in acute myocardial infarction. Am J Cardiol. 66:271-274, 1990

239] Schecter M., et al. The rationale of magnesium supplementation in acute myocardial infarction. A review of the literature. Arch Intern Med. 152:2189-2196, 1992

240] Schoenen, J., et al. Blood Magnesium levels in Migraine. Cephalalgia. 11(2) 97-99, 1991

241] Seelig M.S. Interrelationship of magnesium and estrogen in cardiovascular and bone disorders, eclampsia, migraine and premenstrual syndrome. J Am Coll Nutr Aug. 12(4): 442-58, 1933

242] Seelig M. Human requirements of magnesium: factors that increase needs. In: First International Symposium on Magnesium Deficiency in Human Pathology. Springer Verlag, Paris. 1971:11

243] Seelig M., et al. Magnesium interrelationships with ischemic heart disease: A review. American Journal of Clinical Nutrition. 27:59-79, 1974

244] Seelig M.S. Magnesium Deficiency in the pathogenesis of Disease. Plenum Pub N.Y. 1980

245] Seelig M.S.,et al. Low Magnesium: A Common Denominator in Pathologic Process in Diabetes Mellitus, Cardiovascular Disease and Eclampsia. Journal of the American College of Nutrition, October; 11(5): 608/Abstr 39, 1992

246] Seifert B., et al. Magnesium a new therapeutic alternative in primary dysmenorrhoea. Zentrabl Gynakol. 111 (11): 755-60, 1989

247] Shechter M. Magnesium For Acute MI: Although the Mechanisms of its Therapeutic Effects Are Still Being Debated, The Element Seems Likely to Secure a Place in The Armamentarium Against Myocardial Infarction. Em Med, May. 135-139, 1993

248] Sherwood R.A., Rocks B.F., et al. Magnesium and the premenstrual syndrome. Ann Clin Biochem. 23:667-70, 1986

249] Singh et al. Is Verapamil a better Magnesium agonist rather than a calcium antagonist? A Hypothesis? Med Hypotheses. 24:1 1-9, 1987

250] Singh R.B. Effect of dietary magnesium supplementation in the prevention of coronary heart disease and sudden cardiac death. Magnes Trace Elements; 9:141-151, 1990

251] Singh A., et al. Biochemical indices of selected trace minerals in men: effect of stress. Am J Clin Nut. 53(1):126-131, 1991

252] Sjogren A., et al. Oral administration of magnesium hydroxide to subjects with insulin dependent diabetes mellitus. Magnesium. 121:16-20, 1988

253] Sjogren A., et al. Oral administration of magnesium hydroxide to subjects with insulin-dependent diabetes mellitus: effects on magnesium and potassium levels and on insulin requirements. Magnesium. 7(3):117-122, 1988

254] Sjogren A., et al. Magnesium deficiency in coronary artery disease and cardiac arrhythmias. Journal of Internal Medicine. 226:213-222, 1989

255] Skobeloff E.M., et al. Intravenous magnesium sulfate for the treatment of acute asthma in the emergency department. Journal of the American Medical Association. 262(9):1210-1213, 1989

256] Smetana R., et al. Stress and magnesium metabolism in coronary artery disease. Mag Bulletin. 13(4):125-127, 1991

257] Soldatovic D., et al. Compared effects of high oral Mg supplements and of EDTA chelating agent on chronic lead intoxication in rabbits. Magnesium Research. 10:127-133, 1997

258] South J. Magnesium - the underappreciated mineral of life. Part 1. Vitamin Research News. September 1997

259] Sparkman D. Magnesium helps prevent bone loss: equal to calcium in fighting osteoporosis. All Natural Muscular Development. 36(2):34, 1999

260] Specter M.J., et al. Studies on magnesium's mechanism of action in digitalis-induced arrhythmias. Circulation. 52:1001, 1975

261] Starobrat-Hermelin B., et al. The effects of magnesium physiological supplementation on hyperactivity in children with attention deficit hyperactivity disorder (ADHD). Positive response to magnesium oral loading test. Magnes Res. 10:149-156, 1997

262] Stebbing J.B., et al. Reactive hypoglycemia and magnesium. Mag Bull. 2:131-134, 1982

263] Stendig-Lindberg G., et al. Changes in serum magnesium concentration after strenuous exercise. Journal of the American College of Nutrition. 6(1):35-40, 1987

264] Stendig-Lindberg et al. Trabecular bone density in a two year controlled trial of peroral magnesium in osteoporosis. Mag Res. 6;2 155-63, 1993

265] Sueta C.A., et al. Effect of actur magnesium administration on the frequency of ventricular arrhythmia in patients with heart failure. Circulation. 89(2):660-666, 1994

266] Swain R., Kaplan-Machlis B. Magnesium for the next millennium. South Med J Nov; 92(11): 1040-7, 1999

267] Swanson D.R. Migraine and Magnesium: Eleven neglected connections. Pespect Biol Med. 31:526-557, 1988

268] Szelenyi I., et al. Effect of magnesium orotate and orotic acid on induced blood pressure elevation and cardiopathogenic changes of the myocardium in animal experiments. Dtsch Med J.; 21(22):1405-1412, 1970

269] Taubert K. Magnesium in Migraine. Results from a multicenter pilot study. Fortschr Med. 112 (24) 328-330, 1994

270] Teo K.K., et al. Effects of intravenous magnesium in suspected acute myocardial infarction: overview of randomized trials. British Medical Journal. 303:1499-1503, 1991

271] Teo K.K., et al. Role of magnesium in reducing mortality in acute myocardial infarction. A review of the evidence. Drugs. 46:347-359, 1993

272] Teragawa H. et al. The preventive effect of magnesium on coronary spasm in patients with vasospastic angina. Chest. 118(6) 1690-95 2000

273] Theodore H. et al. Magnesium and the pancreas. Am J Clin Nutr. 26, 1973

274] Tinker P.B.H. & Bull R.A. Some Effects of Variations in Soil Potassium and Magnesium on Yield Responses and Deficiency Symptoms in Oil Palms. Proc. W. African Soils and Plant Nutrition Conference. 72-90, 1957

275] Touyz R M. Magnesium supplementation as an adjuvant to synthetic calcium channel antagonists in the treatment of hypertension. Medical Hypotheses. 36:140-141, 1991

276] Touyz R., Schiffrin E. The effect of angiotensin II on platelet intracellular free magnesium and calcium ionic concentrations in essential hypertension. J Hyperten. 11:551-558, 1993

277] Turlapaty P., et al. Magnesium deficiency produces spasms of coronary arteries: Relationship to etiology of sudden death ischemic heart disease. Science. 208:199-200, 1980

278] Turnlaud J.R., et al. Vitamin B6 depletion followed by repletion with animal- or plant-source diets in calcium and magnesium metabolism in young women. The American Journal of Clinical Nutrition 56:905-10, 1992

279] Wacker W.E. & Vallee B.L. Magnesium Metabolism. NEJM 254, 1958

280] Wallach S. Effects of magnesium on skeletal metabolism. Magnes Trace Elem. 9(1): 1-14,1990

281] Watts D.L. The Assessment of Hypertensive Tendencies from Trace Element Analysis. Chiro Econ March. 1986

282] Watts D.L. Trace Elements and Neuropsychological problems as reflected in tissue mineral analysis (TMA) patterns. J Ortho Med. 5(3) 159-166, 1990

283] Weaver K. Magnesium and its role in vascular reactivity and coagulation. Contemp Nutr. 12(3), 1987

284] Weaver K. Magnesium in Health and Disease. Spectrum Pubs. p. 833, 1980

285] Welshman S.G., et al. The relationship of the urinary cations, calcium, magnesium, sodium and potassium, in patients with renal calculi. British Journal of Urology. 47(3):237-242, 1975

286] Wester P.O., Dyckner T. Magnesium and hypertension. J Am Coll Nutr; 6(4):321-28, 1987

287] Weston P.G., et al. Magnesium sulfate as a sedative. Am J Med Sci. 165:431–33, 1923

288] Whang R., et al. Hypomagnesemia and hypokalemia in 1,000 treated ambulatory hypertensive patients. J Am Coll Nutr. 1:317-322,1982

289] Whang R., et al. Magnesium homeostasis and clinical disorders of magnesium deficiency. Ann Pharmacother. 28:220-225, 1994

290] Whelton P., Klag M.J. Magnesium and blood pressure: Review of the epidemiologic and clinical trial experience. Am J Cardiol. 63(14):26G-30G,1989

291] Widman L., Webster P., Stegmayr B., et al. The dose-dependent reduction in blood pressure through administration of magnesium. Am J Hypertens. 6:41-45, 1993

292] Winterkorn J.M. The influence of magnesium on visual field and peripheral vasospasm in glaucoma. Surv Ophthalmol. 40(1):83-84,1995

293] Wirell M., Webster P., Stegmayr B. Nutritional dose of magnesium in hypertensive patients on beta blockers lowers systolic blood pressure: a double-blind cross-over study. J Intern Med . 236:189-195, 1994

294] Wittman J., et al. Reduction of blood pressure with oral magnesium supplementation in women with mild to moderate hypertension. Am J Clin Nutr. 60:129-135, 1994

295] Wittman J.C., et al. A prospective study of nutritional factors and hypertension among US women. Circulation, November. 80:5, 1320-7, 1989

296] Wong E.T., Rude R.K., Singer F.R., et al. A high prevalence of hypomagnesemia in hospitalized patients. Am J Clin Pathol. 79:348-352,1983

297] Woods K.L., et al. Intravenous magnesium sulphate in suspected acute myocardial infarction: results of the second Leicester Intravenous Magnesium Intervention Trial (LIMIT-2). The Lancet. 339:1553-1558, 1992

298] Wright J.V. Magnesium can relieve migraine (and other magnesium-related matters). AAEM Nwsletter, Winter, p.14, 1989

299] Wunderlich W. Aspects of the influence of magnesium ions on the formation of calcium oxalate. Urol Res. 9:157-160, 1981

300] Yasui M., et al. Magnesium concentration in brains from multiple sclerosis patients. Acta Neurology Scandinavia. 81(3):197-200,1990

301] Yeh J.K., et al. Effect of physical activity on the metabolism of magnesium in the rat. Journal of the American College of Nutrition. 10(5):487-493,1991

302] Yu-Yahiro J.A. Electrolytes and their relationship to normal and abnormal muscle function. Orthop Nurs. 13(5):38-40, 1994

303] Zehender M., et al. Antiarrhythmic effects of increasing the daily intake of magnesium and potassium in patients with frequent ventricular arrhythmias. J Am Coll Cardiol. 29:1028-1034, 1997

304] Zorbas Y.G., et al. Magnesium loading effect on magnesium deficiency in endurance-trained subjects during prolonged restriction of muscular activity. Biol Trace Elem Res. 63(2):149-166, 1998

The effects of zinc deficiency on the immune system have been recognised for over 100 years, but the other functions of zinc are relatively recent discoveries.

The human body is topologically like a torus. To protect us from the outside world, we have zinc. It protects us from stress, infections and toxins.

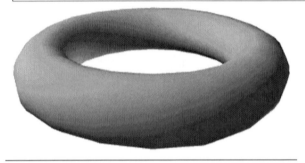

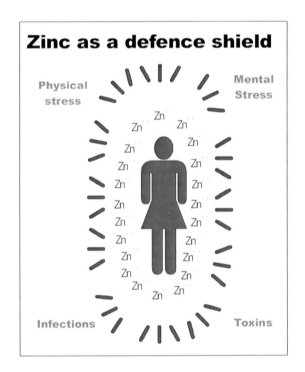

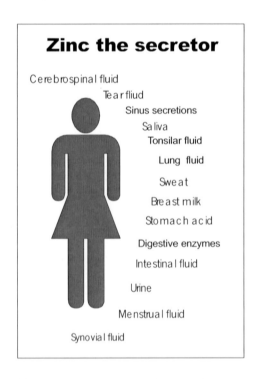

Part of the defence against excessive metal absorption (esp copper, mercury and cadmium) is related to a protein called Metallothionine. This protein is made up mostly of the amino acid cysteine and contains seven zinc atoms. The sites of this metalloprotein suggest its important as a filter for toxins, but also it plays a part in learning and socialisation. Defects of this protein cause Autism, copper overload, dysbiosis, skin problems and gastritis with wheat and dairy intolerance.

# Metallothionine Structure

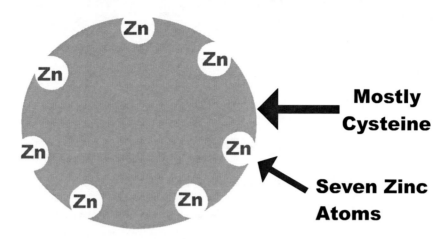

Mostly Cysteine

Seven Zinc Atoms

## Sites of Metallothionine

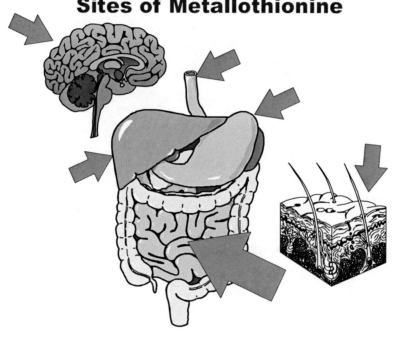

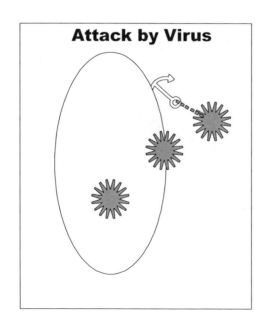

**Attack by Virus**

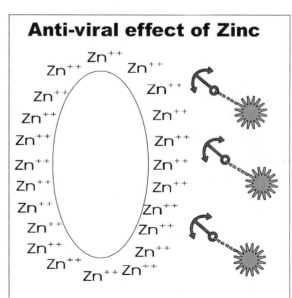

**Anti-viral effect of Zinc**

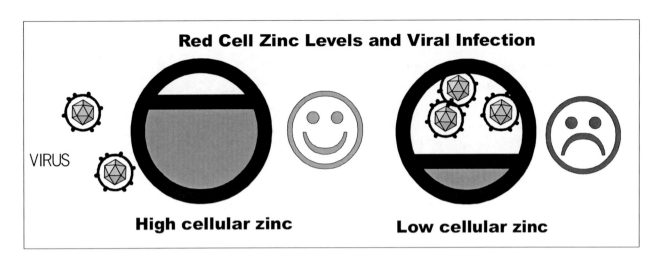

**Red Cell Zinc Levels and Viral Infection**

VIRUS

**High cellular zinc**

**Low cellular zinc**

## Zinc and secretions.

Zinc is secreted by every cavity and orifice, because it is a lubricant and an antiseptic. Impressive studies have shown that zinc blocks cytadherance by viruses that would like to invade us.

This explains several interesting phenomenon. Low zinc levels are associated with vaginal thrush after menstruation. Zinc is supposed to be secreted in vaginal fluid to "disinfect" the vagina while the cervix is open. Candida likes blood and will flourish if there is no zinc to kill it off.

## Zinc and immunity.

Zinc is required for white cell production. Low zinc levels will allow viruses to penetrate and infect cells. Very low zinc's will allow chronic infection by intracellular organisms like Mycoplasma, Rickettsia's and Chlamydia.

## Zinc and DNA synthesis.

Zinc is required for correct DNA transcription. The Mechanism appears to be related to zinc's ability to bind two amino acids. This binding causes a finger-like structure to be formed, hence the term "zinc finger".

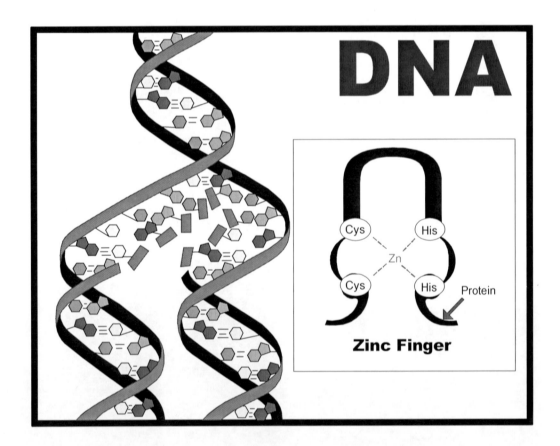

**DNA**

Cys His

Zn

Cys His

Protein

**Zinc Finger**

## Zinc and digestion

Zinc, Vitamin B1 and Vitamin B6 are needed for production of stomach acid. Stomach acid levels stimulate pancreatic secretion of picolinic acid. This is the prime binder for trace elements like zinc, selenium, chromium, manganese, boron, molybdenum and vanadium. If you don't make stomach acid, you don't absorb zinc. And if you don't absorb zinc, you don't make stomach acid! Zinc has been used in the treatment of Helicobacter.

Zinc is required for the secretion of stomach acid and the protective layer that coats the acid exposed areas. Lack of zinc will cause atrophy and hypochlorhydria. Proton pump inhibitors may reduce pain but they do not correct digestion. Zinc is required for the digestive enzymes Carboxypeptidase and Aminopeptidase.

Zinc is secreted into the intestinal fluid to help control intestinal flora populations. High dose zinc can correct many cases of wind, bloating and intestinal hurry.

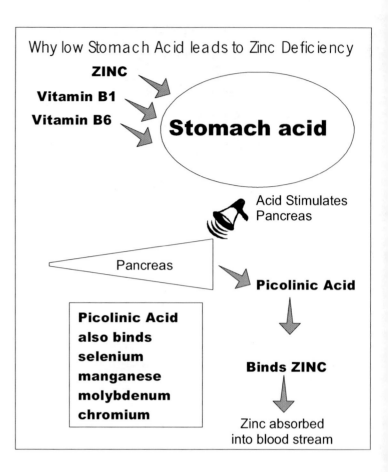

Normal Gastric lining

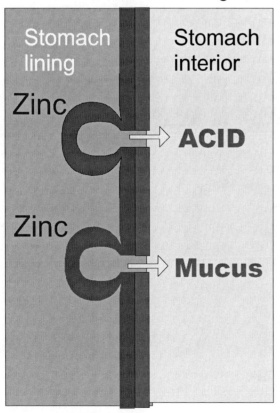

Atrophic lining in Zinc deficiency

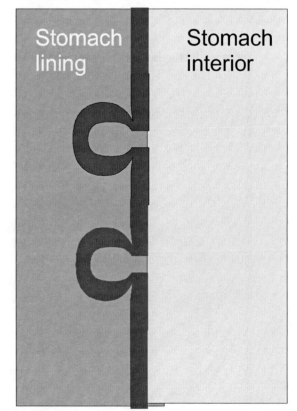

# Zinc secretion

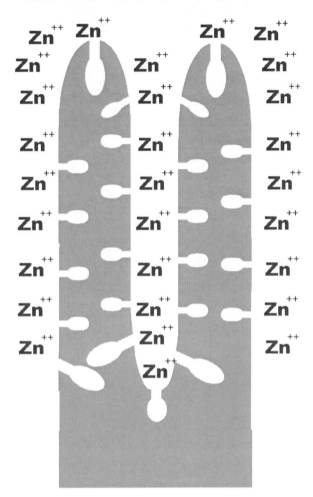

$Zn^{++}$  $Zn^{++}$  $Zn^{++}$  $Zn^{++}$
$Zn^{++}$  $Zn^{++}$  $Zn^{++}$
$Zn^{++}$  $Zn^{++}$  $Zn^{++}$
$Zn^{++}$  $Zn^{++}$  $Zn^{++}$
$Zn^{++}$  $Zn^{++}$  $Zn^{++}$
$Zn^{++}$  $Zn^{++}$  $Zn^{++}$
$Zn^{++}$  $Zn^{++}$  $Zn^{++}$
$Zn^{++}$  $Zn^{++}$  $Zn^{++}$
$Zn^{++}$  $Zn^{++}$

## Zinc and pH regulation.

Zinc is required for the enzyme carbonic anhydrase. This enzyme allows the correct excretion of water and carbon dioxide from the body through the lung and kidneys.

# Carbonic Anhydrase

**Glucose or Lactate**

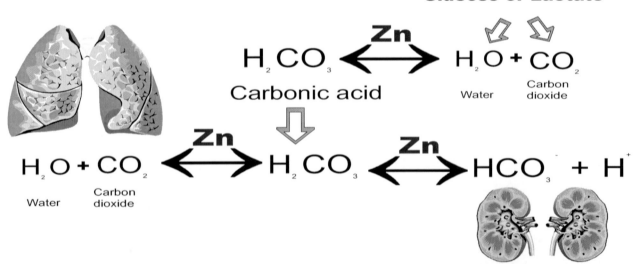

$$H_2CO_3 \xleftrightarrow{\ Zn\ } H_2O + CO_2$$

Carbonic acid          Water    Carbon dioxide

$$H_2O + CO_2 \xleftrightarrow{\ Zn\ } H_2CO_3 \xleftrightarrow{\ Zn\ } HCO_3^- + H^+$$

Water  Carbon dioxide

## Zinc and liver function.

Liver function. Zinc is required for enzymes such as alcohol dehydrogenase, lactate dehydrogenase, and alkaline phosphatase. Pyruvate is converted to lactate and zinc is required within lactate dehydrogenase, the short term gain of 2 ATP must be repaid with interest by the liver. The cost is 6 ATP. The lactate returns to the liver where it can be converted to pyruvate.

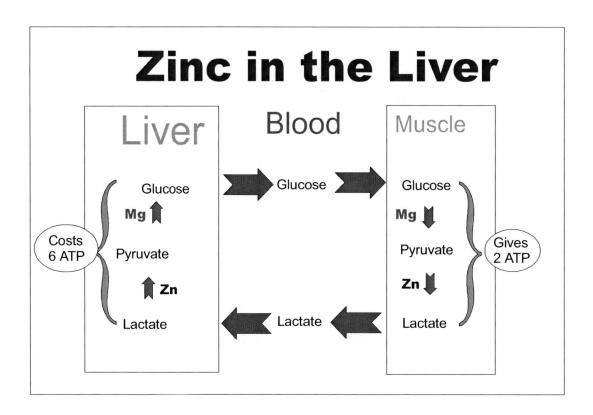

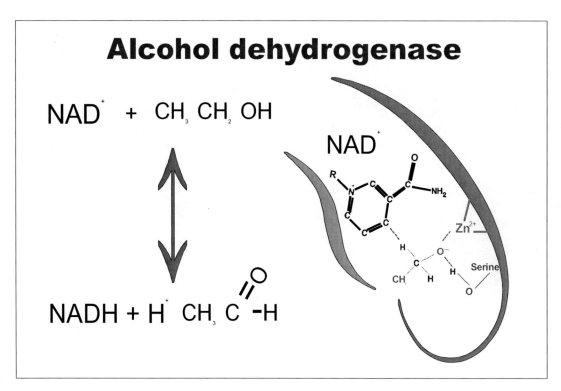

## Zinc and the brain.

Zinc is important for several aspects of brain function. Alertness can be affected in two ways. Hypoglycaemia is common with zinc deficiency and zinc blockade. The problem arises every 2-3 hours. This is called postprandial hypoglycaemia and will never be picked up on fasting BSL.

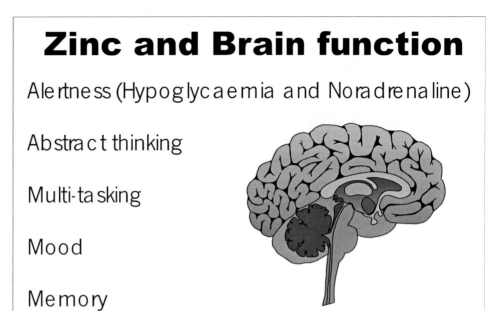

# Zinc and Brain function

Alertness (Hypoglycaemia and Noradrenaline)

Abstract thinking

Multi-tasking

Mood

Memory

## Zinc Levels and Glucose control

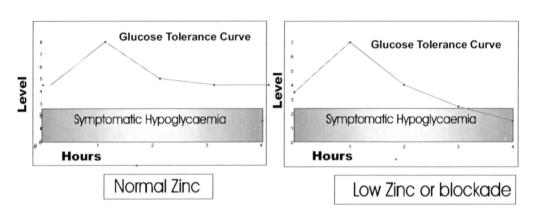

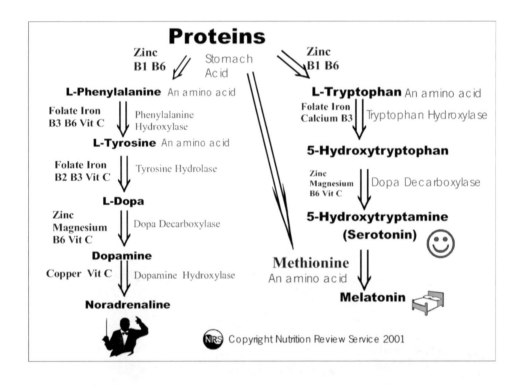

114

Zinc and Neurotransmitters.
Zinc is required for serotonin and melatonin, dopamine and noradrenaline synthesis. Hence sleep disturbance and depression with low zincs. The requirement for zinc begins with stomach acid to digest proteins. Then zinc is needed for Dopa Decarboxylase. Reduction of noradrenaline reduces alertness and signal processing by the brain. Lack of noradrenaline is the lesion in ADD.

The best analogy for noradrenaline would be as a conductor of an orchestra. If he waves softly, not much noise comes out of the orchestra pit and the audience falls asleep. If he waves wildly, the orchestra blares and wake up the all of those in the auditorium. The neurotransmitter responsible for this is noradrenaline.

**Zinc and language**
In order to learn language, one must be able to abstract concepts. This is required in order to learn nouns. Nouns are the basis of all human language. Take the example of a glass. The model must cater for full, partially full or empty glasses of all shapes. This is a zinc function.

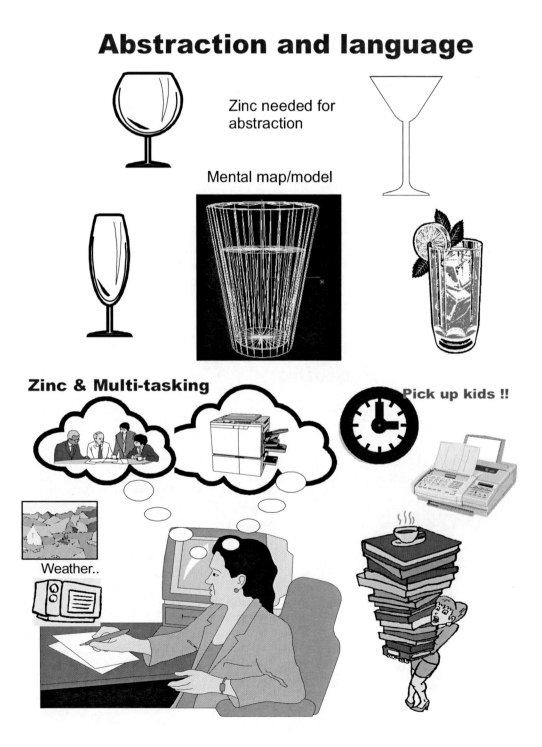

# Abstraction and language

Zinc needed for abstraction

Mental map/model

**Zinc & Multi-tasking**

Pick up kids !!

Weather..

In order to multitask, each task must be abstracted. The current task is dealt with and then put on hold while another is dealt with. Then this task is put on hold. This mental juggling is a zinc effect. Those with low zincs or with zinc blockade cannot handle multiple tasks. They can do one at a time and do not take interruptions well.

## Zinc and hormones.

Zinc turns up several times in steroidal hormone pathways. You can see why zinc deficiency is associated with infertility. Zinc is also important for preventing unnecessary conversion of Androgens to Estrogens; Zinc has a negative feedback on the enzyme aromatase and is much cheaper than the drugs sanctified by the PBS.

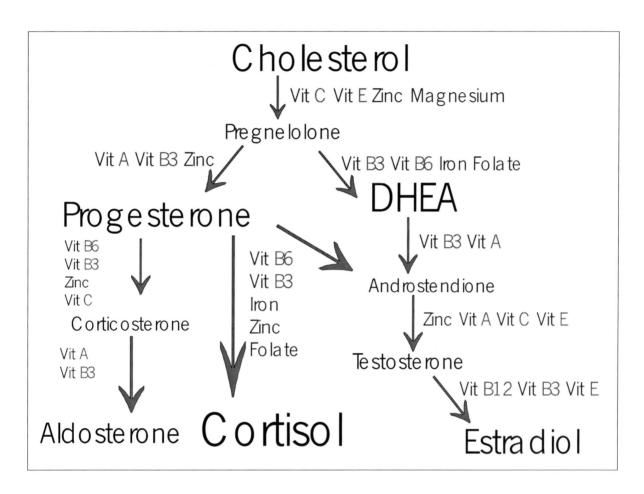

## Non-adrenal Aromatase activity

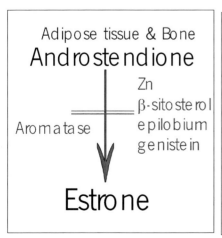 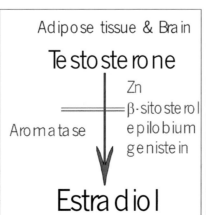 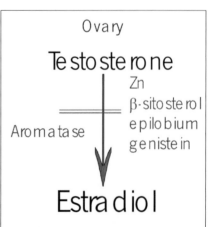

**Zinc and Cholesterol Metabolism**
Many Nutrients are required for the correct metabolism of cholesterol. Low zinc or zinc: copper imbalance will cause the cholesterol to rise.

## Nutrients needed for correct Cholesterol control

Manganese    Vitamin B3

Chromium    Vitamin B5

Zinc    Vitamin C

Selenium    Vitamin E

Molybdenum

Those affected by Zinc:Copper imbalance

## Zinc and allergies.

Many allergic phenomena (especially those causing histamine release) are associated with abnormalities with zinc. This makes the patient "allergic", but not necessarily to anything in particular. They just seem to release histamine with little provocation.

## Factors involved with Allergies

1. Low Zinc
2. High Copper
3. Low Zinc:Copper ratio
4. Low Molybdenum
5. Low Vitamin C
6. Digestive problems
7. Helicobacter stomach infection
8. Candida overgrowth
9. Hormone imbalance

Those affected by Zinc:Copper imbalance

## Zinc and joints.
Zinc is required to make synovial fluid of correct viscosity. Zinc is needed for repair of tissues including daily wear and tear. Low zinc would allow chronic infections of synovia and cartilage.

## Zinc and arthritis.
Zinc is important in the prevention and repair of joint damage. It keeps the synovial fliud viscous so that it cushions impact better.

### Nutrients important in Osteoarthritis

Zinc *Cu⚖Zn*
Boron
Molybdenum
Selenium
Folic acid *Cu⚖Zn*

Niacinamide [B3] *Cu⚖Zn*
B5 B6 B12 *Cu⚖Zn*
Vitamin C *Cu⚖Zn*
Vitamin D
Vitamin E *Cu⚖Zn*
MSM

Those affected by Zinc:Copper imbalance *Cu⚖Zn*

Osteoarthritis

### Nutrients important in Rheumatoid Arthritis

Boron
Copper *Cu⚖Zn*
Germanium
Manganese
Molybdenum
Selenium
Zinc *Cu⚖Zn*
Sulphur

Niacinamide [B3] *Cu⚖Zn*
B5 B6 *Cu⚖Zn*
Vitamin C *Cu⚖Zn*
Vitamin K
Vitamin E *Cu⚖Zn*
Vitamin A

Those affected by Zinc:Copper imbalance *Cu⚖Zn*

**Rheumatoid Arthritis**
A Zinc: Copper imbalance features highly in the genesis of rheumatoid arthritis. It turns out that Zinc copper balance determines Th1:Th2 balance of helper lymphocyte subsets.

---

# Skin Conditions associated with Zinc/Copper imbalance

| Dermatitis | Psoriasis | Tinea |
| Dry Skin | Pimples | Thrush |
| Eczema | Hair loss | Warts |

---

Zinc and the skin.

| Excellent | Good | Fair |
|---|---|---|
| oysters, beef, veal brazil nuts, almonds cashews, hazel nuts walnuts, rice, barley sunflower seeds, rye wheat, olives herring, liver | pumpkin seeds, oats wheat bran, garlic wheat germ, lettuce millet, soya beans brewer's yeast asparagus | brussel sprouts, peas blackberries banana, oranges peaches, tomato cucumber, spinach avocado, artichoke |

Zinc is important for activating Vitamin A. Many skin conditions respond to zinc.

**Foods that contain zinc**

Zinc Blockade.
High copper, and the presence of mercury, cadmium, aluminium, and antimony will block the function of zinc within tissues. This effect does not show up on blood testing. Only tissue mineral analysis will pick this up. Many practitioners are unaware that 1 mercury molecule will block 1000 zinc ions. One cadmium molecule will block 100 zinc ions. The patient does not need to be toxic for these effects to occur. As a passing point toxicity is defined by industry, not medicine. Industry will pick the least sensitive method of defining toxicity, hence the use of blood and urine for this purpose.

**Zinc References**

1] Abbassi A.A., et al. Experimental zinc deficiency in man. Effect on testicular function. J Lab Clin Med. 96(3):544, 1980
**2] Aliaga A. Psoriasis: clinical trial of an aerosol for topical use formulated with zinc pyrithione at 0.2% and sodium methyl ethyl sulfate at 0.1%. Hospital General, Valencia.1982**
3] Al-Nakib W., et al. Prophylaxis and treatment of rhinovirus colds with zinc gluconate lozenges. J Antimicrob Chemother.

20(6):893-901, 1987

4] Amer M., et al. <u>Serum zinc in acne vulgaris.</u> Int J Dermatol. 21(8):481-482, 1982

5] Ananda S., et al. <u>Duration of symptoms and plasma cytokine levels in patients with the common cold treated with zinc acetate.</u> Annals of Internal Medicine. 133(4):245-252, 2000

6] Anderson R.A., Roussel A-M, Zouari N. et al. <u>Potential antioxidant effects of zinc and chromium supplement in people with type II diabetes mellitus.</u> J Am Coll Nutr. 20(3):212-218, 2001

7] Apisariyakulm A., et al. <u>Zinc monoglycerolate is effective against oral herpetic sores.</u> Med J Aust. 152(1):54, 1990

8] Arnold et al. <u>Does hair zinc predict amphetamine improvement of ADD/hyperactivity?</u> Int J Neuroscience. 50:103-107, 1990

9] Bakan R. <u>The role of zinc in anorexia nervosa: Etiology and treatment.</u> Medical Hypotheses. 5:731-736, 1979

10] Bakan R., et al. <u>Dietary Zinc Intake of Vegetarian and Nonvegetarian Patients with Anorexia Nervosa.</u> Int. J. Eat. Disord. 13:229-233, 1993

11] Balogh Z., et al. <u>Plasma zinc and its relationship to clinical symptoms and drug treatment in rheumatoid arthritis.</u> Ann Rheum Dis. 39(4):329032, 1980

12] Barbarino F., et al. <u>Effects of zinc-aspartate and zinc-glycinate in healthy rats and on reserpine-induced gastric lesions.</u> Biol Trace Elem Res. 16(3):253-267, 1988

13] Barrie S.A., et al. <u>Comparative absorption of zinc picolinate, zinc citrate and zinc gluconate in humans.</u> Agents and Actions. 5:1-6, 1986

14] Baum M.K., et al. <u>Zinc status in human immunodeficiency virus infection.</u> Journal of Nutrition. 130(5):1421S-1423S, 2000

15] Beach, R.S., et al. <u>Altered thymic structure and mitogen responsiveness in postnatally zinc-deprived mice.</u> Dev Comp Immunol. 3:725-738, 1979

16] Bekaroglu M., et al. <u>Relationships between serum free fatty acids and zinc, and attention deficit hyperactivity disorder: a research note.</u> J Child Psychol Psychiatry. 37(2):225-227, 1996

17] Bellanti J. A., et al. <u>ADHD: Causes and Possible Solutions Conference.</u> Arlington, VA, USA. Nov 4-7, 1999

18] Bhutta A., et al. <u>Prevention of diarrhea and pneumonia by zinc supplementation in children in developing countries: pooled analysis of randomized controlled trials.</u> Zinc Investigators' Collaborative Group. J Pediatr. 135(6):689-697, 1999

19] Blechman S., et al. <u>Zinc: low levels restrict aerobic capacity.</u> Muscular Development. 36(12):53, 1999

20] Birmingham C.L., et al. <u>Controlled trial of Zinc Supplementation in Anorexia Nervosa.</u> Int. J. Eat. Disord. 15:251-255, 1994

21] Birdsall T. C. <u>Zinc picolinate: Absorption and supplementation.</u> Alt Med Rev. 1:26-30, 1996

22] Bradshaw A.D. <u>Populations of Agrostis tenuis Resistant to Lead and Zinc Poisoning.</u> Phytopath. Z. 12:, HF. 1:1-112, 1939

23] Brandao-Neto J., et al. <u>Zinc acutely and temporarily inhibits adrenal cortisol secretion in humans.</u> A preliminary report. Biol. Trace Elem. Res. 24:83-89, 1990

24] Bresink I., et al. <u>Zinc changes AMPA receptor properties: results of binding studies and patch clamp recordings.</u> Neuropharmacology. 35(4):503-509, 1996

25] Brewer G.J., Johnson V.D., Dick R.D. et al. <u>Treatment of Wilson's disease with zinc.</u> XVII: Treatment during pregnancy. Hepatology 31, 364-370, 2000

26] Brody I. <u>Topical treatment of recurrent herpes simplex and post-herpetic erythema multiforme with low concentrations of zinc sulphate solution.</u> British Journal of Dermatology. 104:191, 1981

27] Browning J.D., et al. <u>Reduces Food Intake in Zinc Deficient Rats is normalized by Megestrol Acetate but not by Insulin-like growth factor-1.</u> J. Nutr. 128:136-142, 1998

28] Bryce-Smith D. & Simpson R.I. <u>Case of Anorexia Nervosa responding to Zinc Sulphate.</u> Lancet. 2:350, 1984

29] Bryce-Smith D. <u>Prenatal zinc deficiency.</u> Nursing Times. 1985

30] Buamah P.K., et al. <u>Maternal zinc status: a determination of central nervous system malformation.</u> Br J Obstet Gynaecol. 91(8):788-790, 1984

31] Bulbena EG. <u>Zinc compounds, a new treatment in peptic ulcer.</u> Drugs under Experimental and Clinical Research.15(2):83-89 1989

32] Bush I.M., et al. <u>Zinc and the prostate.</u> Presented at the annual meeting of the American Medical Association. Chicago, 1974

33] Calhoun N.R., et al. <u>The effects of zinc on ectopic bone formation.</u> Oral Surg. 39(5):698-706, 1975

34] Caruthers R. <u>Oral zinc in cutaneous healing.</u> Drugs. 6:164. 1973

35] Cass Smith W.P. & Harvey H.L. <u>Zinc Deficiency of Flax.</u> J. Dep. Agric. W. Aust. 25:136-42, 1948

36] Castillo-Duran C., et al. <u>Controlled trial of Zinc Supplementation during recovery from Malnutrition: Effects on Growth and immune Function.</u> Am. J. Clin. Nutr. 45:602-608, 1987

37] Chan S., et al. <u>The role of copper, molybdenum, selenium, and zinc in nutrition and health.</u> Clin Lab Med. 18(4):673-685, 1998

38] Chauser A. <u>Zinc, Insulin and Diabetes.</u> J of American College of Nutrition. 17(2):109-115, 1998

39] Chen M-D, Lin P-Y. <u>Zinc-induced hyperleptinaemia relates to the amelioration of sucrose-induced obesity with zinc repletion.</u> Obesity Res. 8(7), 525-529, 2000

40] Chester C.G.C. & Robinson G.N. <u>The Role of Zinc in Plant Metabolism.</u> Biol. Rev. 26:239-52, 1951

41] Chiricolo M., et al. <u>Enhanced DNA repair in lymphocytes of Down syndrome patients: The influence of zinc nutritional supplementation.</u> Mutat Res Dnaging Genet Instab Aging (Netherlands). 295(3):105-111, 1993

42] Christian P., et al. <u>Zinc supplementation might potentiate the effect of vitamin A in restoring night vision in pregnant</u>

Nepalese women. American Journal of Clinical Nutrition. 73(6):1045-1051, 2001

43] Chuong C.J. & Dawson E.B. Zinc and copper levels in premenstrual syndrome. Fert. Steril. Aug 62:2, 313-20 1994

44] Cohen C. Zinc sulphate and bed sores. Br Med J. 2:561,1968

45] Collip P.J., et al. Zinc deficiency: improvement in growth and growth hormone levels with oral zinc therapy. Ann Nutr Metab. 26(5):287-290, 1992

46] Cordova A., et al. Behavior of zinc and physical exercise: A special reference to immunity and fatigue. Neuroscience and Behavioral Reviews. 19(3):439-444, 1995

47] Cordova A, et al. Effect of training on zinc metabolism: changes in serum and sweat zinc concentrations in sportsmen. Ann Nutr Metab. 42(5):274-282, 1998

48] Costello L.C., et al. Novel role of zinc in the regulation of prostate citrate metabolism and its implications in prostate cancer. Prostate. 35(4):285-296, 1998

49] Cunliff W.J., et al. A double-blind trial of a zinc sulphate/zinc citrate complex and tetracycline in the treatment of acne. British Journal of Derm. 101:321-325, 1979

50] Demetree J.W., et al. The effect of zinc on sebum secretion rate. Acta Dermatovenerol. 60(2):166-169, 1980

51] Dinsmore W.W., et al. Zinc Absorption in Anorexia Nervosa. Lancet 1:1041-1042, 1985

52] Donadini A., et al. Plasma levels of Zn, Cu and Ni in healthy controls and in psoriatic patients. Acta Vitamin Enzymol. 1:9-16, 1980

53] Dreno B., et al. Low doses of zinc gluconate for inflammatory acne. Acta Derm Venereol. 69:541-543, 1989

54] Duchateeau J., et al. Influence of oral zinc supplementation on the lymphocyte response to mitogens of normal subjects. Am J Clin Nutr. 34:88-93, 1981

55] Duchateau J., et al. Beneficial effects of oral zinc supplementation on the immune response of old people. Am J Med. 70:1001-1004, 1981

56] Duncan J., et al. Thymidine kinase and DNA polymerase activity in normal and zinc deficient developing rat embryos. Proc Soc Exp Biol Med. 159:39-43, 1978

57] Eby G.A., et al. Reduction in duration of common colds by zinc gluconate lozenges in a double-blind study. Antimicrobial Agents and Chemotherapy. 25:20, 1984

58] Eby G. Use of topical zinc to prevent recurrences of orolabial and genital herpetic infections: Review of literature and suggested protocols. Medical Hypotheses. 17(2):157-165, 1985

59] Editor Another look at Zinc. Br Medical Journal. 282:1098-99, 1981

60] Eggleton W.G. The Zinc Content of Epidermal Structures in Beri-beri. Biochem. J. 33(i): 403-6, 1939

61] Elcoate P.V., et al. The Effect of Zinc Deficiency on the Male Genital System. J. Physiol. 129:53, 1955

62] Esca S.A., et al. Kwashiorkor-like zinc deficiency syndrome in anorexia nervosa. Acta Derm Venereol. Stockholm. 59:361-364, 1979

63] Evans G.W., et al. Effect of iron, vitamin B-6 and picolinic acid on zinc absorption in the rat. Journal of Nutrition. 111(1):68-75, 1981

64] Fabris N., et al. AIDS, zinc deficiency and thymic hormone failure. Journal of the American Medical Association (Letter). 259:839-840, 1988

65] Fabris N., Mocchegiani E., Muzzoli M., and Provinciali M. Role of zinc in neuroendocrine-immune reactions during aging. In: Physiological Senescence and its Postponement. Annals of the New York Academy of Sciences, Volume 621, by Walter Pierpaoli and Nicola Fabris (editors). 314-326, 1991

66] Fahim M., et al. Zinc treatment for the reduction of hyperplasia of the prostate. Federation Proceedings. 35(3):361, 1976

67] Federico A., Lodice P., Federico P. et al. Effects of selenium and zinc supplementation on nutritional status in patients with cancer of digestive tract. Eur J Clin Nutr. 55 (4):293-7, 2001

68] Fernandes G., et al. Impairment of cell-mediated immune function by dietary Zn deficiency in mice. Proceedings of the National Academy of Sciences, USA. 76:457-461, 1979

69] Ferrigno D., et al. Serum copper and zinc content in non-small cell lung cancer: abnormalities and clinical correlates. Monaldi Arch Chest Dis (Italy), Jun. 54(3):204-8, 1999

70] Finnerty E. F. Topical zinc in the treatment of herpes simplex. Cutis. 37(2):130-131, 1986

71] Fischer P.W.F., et al. The effect of dietary zinc on intestinal copper absorption. American Journal of Clinical Nutrition. 34(9):1670-1675, 1981

72] Fong L.Y.Y., et al. Zinc deficiency and the development of oesophageal and forestomach tumours in Sprague-Dawley rats fed precursors of N-nitroso-N-benzylmethylamine. Journal of the National Cancer Institute. 72:419-425, 1984

73] Frank J. Zinc and your skin. Australian Wellbeing. 10:69-71, 1985

74] Fraker P.J., et al. Interrelationships between zinc and immune function. Fed Proc. 45:1474-1479, 1986

75] Fraker P.J. The dynamic link between the integrity of the immune system and zinc status. Journal of Nutrition. 130 (5S Supplement). 1399S-1406S, 2000

76] Freeland-Graves J.H., et al. Effect of zinc supplementation on plasma high-density lipoprotein cholesterol and zinc. American Journal of Clinical Nutrition. 35(5):988-992, 1982

77] Frithiof L., et al. The relationship between marginal bone loss and serum zinc levels. Acta Med Scand. 207(1):67-70, 1980

78] Frommer D.J. The healing of gastric ulcers by zinc sulphate. Medical Journal of Australia. 2:793, 1975

79] Gao Y., et al. Zinc enhancement of genistein's anabolic effect on bone components in elderly female rats. Gen Pharmac. 31(2):199-202, 1998

80] Garfinkel D. Is aging inevitable? The intracellular zinc deficiency hypothesis of aging. Med Hypotheses. 19(2):117-137, 1986

81] Gersdorff M., et al. [The zinc sulfate overload test in patients suffering from tinnitus associated with low serum zinc. Preliminary report]. Acta Otorhinolaryngol Belg. 41(3):498-505, 1987

82] Godfrey J.C., et al. Zinc for treating the common cold: review of all clinical trials since 1984. Alternative Therapies in Health & Medicine. 2(6):63-72, 1996

83] Golik A., et al. Effects of captopril and enalapril on zinc metabolism in Hypertension Subjects. J. of Am College of Nutrition. 17(1): 75-78, 1998

84] Gong H., et al. Optic nerve changes in zinc-deficient rats. Exp Eye Res. 72(4):363-369, 2001

85] Goransson K., et al. Oral zinc in acne vulgaris: a clinical and methodological study. Acta Derm Venereol. 58(5):443-8, 1978

86] Goto T., et al. Long-term zinc deficiency decreases taste sensitivity in rats. Journal of Nutritiion. 131(2):305-310, 2001

87] Greaves M.W., et al. Double-blind trial of zinc sulphate in the treatment of chronic venous leg ulceration. Brit Jour of Derm. 87:63251,1972

88] Hadden J.W. The treatment of zinc deficiency is an immunotherapy. International Journal of Immunopharmacology. 17(9):697-701, 1995

89] Hagino N. & Kobayashi J. Strange Osteomalacia "Itaiitai" Disease in the Jintsu River Basin, Polluted with Zinc, Lead and Cadmium I. Private Communication, 1960

90] Haglund et al. Evidence of a relationship between childhood onset type 1 diabetes and low groundwater concentration of zinc. Diabetes Care Aug. 19:8 873-5, 1996

91] Hambridge K.M., et al. Zinc nutritional status during pregnancy: a longitudinal study. Am J Clin Nutr. 37:429-42, 1983

92] Hartoma T.R., et al. Zinc, plasma androgens and male sterility. Letter to the Editor. The Lancet. 3:1125-1126, 1977

93] Hasegawa H., et al. Effects of zinc on the reactive oxygen species-generating capacity of human neutrophils and on the serum opsonic activity in vitro. Luminescence. 15(5):321-327, 2000

94] Hess F.M., et al. Zinc excretion in young women on low zinc intakes and oral contraceptive agents. J Nutr. 107, 1977

95] Heyneman C.A. Zinc deficiency and taste disorders. Ann Pharmacotherapy Feb. 30:2 186-7, 1996

96] Higashi A., et al. A prospective survey of serial zinc levels and pregnancy outcome. J Ped Gastro. 7:430-33, 1988

97] Hillstrom L., et al. Comparison of oral treatment with zinc sulfate and placebo in acne vulgaris. British Journal of Dermatology. 97:679-684, 1977

98] Hirt M., et al. Zinc nasal gel for the treatment of common cold symptoms: a double-blind, placebo-controlled trial. Ear, Nose, & Throat Journal. 79(10):778-782, 2000

**99] Horning M. S., et al. Endogenous mechanisms of neuroprotection: role of zinc, copper, and carnosine. Brain Res. 852(1):56-61, 2000**

100] Huang X., Cuajungco M.P.,.Atwood C.S., et al. Alzheimer's disease, beta-amyloid protein and zinc. J Nutr. 130, 1488S-1492S, 2000

101] Humphries L., et al. Zinc deficiency and eating disorders. Journal of Clinical Psychiatry. 50(12):456-459, 1989

102] Humphries L.L., et al. Anorexia Nervosa, Zinc Supplementation and weight gain. In: Anderson H, ed. Biology of Feast and Famine: Relevance to Eating Disorders, Symposium on Nutrition Research. Toronto: University of Toronto. 124-136, 1990

103] Hunt C.D., et al. Effects of dietary zinc depletion on seminal volume and zinc loss, serum testosterone concentrations, and sperm morphology in young men. Am J Clin Nutr. 56(1):148-157, 1992

104] Iitaka M. et al. Induction of apoptosis and necrosis by zinc in human thyroid cancer cell lines. J Endocrinol. 169(2):417-24, 2001

105] Jackson E.A. Are zinc acetate lozenges effective in decreasing the duration of symptoms of the common cold? J Fam Pract. 49(12):1153, 2000

106] Joseph C.E., et al. Zinc deficiency changes in the permeability of rabbit periodontium to 14 C-phenytoin and 14 C-albumin. J Periodontol. 53:251-256, 1982

107] Karayalcin S., et al. Zinc plasma levels after oral zinc tolerance test in nonalcoholic cirrhosis. Dig Dis Sci. 33:1096-1102, 1988

108] Katz R.L., et al. Zinc deficiency in anorexia nervosa. J Adolesc Health Care. 8(5):400-406, 1987

109] Kneist W., et al. Clinical double-blind trial of topical zinc sulfate for herpes labialis recidivans. Arzneimittelforschung. 45:524-526, 1995

110] Kobayashi J. & Hagino N. Strange Osteomalacia "Itaiitai" Disease in the Jinsu River Basin Polluted with Zinc, Lead and Cadmium II. Private Communication, 1960

111] Koo S.I. & Turk D.E. Effect of Zinc Deficiency on the Ultrastructure of the Pancreatic Acinar Cell and Intestinal Epithelium in the Rat. J. Nutr. 107:896-908, 1977

112] Korant B.D., et al. Zinc ions inhibit replication of rhinoviruses. Nature. 248:588-590, 1974

113] Korant B.D., et al. Inhibition by zinc of rhinovirus protein cleavage: Interaction of zinc with capsid polypeptides. J Virol. 18:298-306, 1976

114] Krieger I., et al. Tryptophan deficiency and picolinic acid: effect on zinc metabolism and clinical manifestations of pellagra.

American Journal of Clinical Nutrition. 46:511-517, 1987

115] Krotkiewski M., et al. Zinc and muscle strength and endurance. Acta Physiol Scandinavia. 116(3):309-311, 1982

116] Kruis W. et al. Zinc deficiency as a problem in patients with Crohn's disease and fistula formation. Hepatogastroenterol. 32(3):133-134, 1985

117] Kugelmas M. Preliminary observation: oral zinc sulfate replacement is effective in treating muscle cramps in cirrhotic patients. J Am Coll Nutr. 19(1):13-15, 2000

118] Lally E.V., et al. An element of uncertainty: The clinical significance of zinc deficiency in rheumatoid arthritis. Int Medicine. 8(1):98-107, 1987

119] Larue J.P., et al. [Zinc in the human prostate]. Journal of Urology (Paris). 91(7):463-468, 1985

120] Lask B., et al. Zinc Deficiency and childhood-onset Anorexia Nervosa. J. Clin. Psychiatry. 54:63-66, 1993

121] Leake A., et al. Subcellular distribution of zinc in the benign and malignant human prostate: evidence for a direct zinc androgen interaction. Acta Endocrinol (Copenhagen). 105:281-288, 1984

122] Leissner K.H., et al. Concentration and content of zinc in the human prostate. Investigative Urology. 18:32-35, 1980

123] Liang J.Y., et al. Inhibitory effect of zinc on human prostatic carcinoma cell growth. Prostate. 40(3):200-207, 1999

124] Lin D.D., et al. Zinc-induced augmentation of excitatory synaptic currents and glutamate receptor responses in hippocampal CA3 neurons. J Neurophysiol. 85(3):1185-1196, 2001

125] Loneragen J.F. The Effect of Applied Phosphate on the Uptake of Zinc by Flax. Aust. J. Sci. Res. Ser. B,4:108-14, 1951

126] Macknin M.L. Zinc lozenges for the common cold. Cleveland Clin J Med. 66:27-32, 1999

127] Mantzoros C.S., et al. Zinc may regulate serum leptin concentrations in humans. J. Am. Coll. Nutr. 17:270-275, 1998

128] Marchesini G., et al. Zinc supplementation improves glucose disposal in patients with cirrhosis. Metabolism. 47:792-798, 1998

129] Marone G. et al. Physiological concentrations of zinc inhibit the release of histamine from human basophils and lung mast cells. Agents Actions. 18:103-106, 1986

130] Marshall S. Zinc gluconate and the common cold. Review of randomized controlled trials. Canadian Family Physician. 44:1037-1042, 1998

131] Mattingley P.C., et al. Zinc sulphate in rheumatoid arthritis. Annals of the Rheumatic Diseases. 41:456-457, 1982

132] Mawson C.A. & Fischer M.I. The Occurrence of Zinc in the Human Prostate Gland. Canad. J. Med. Sci. 30:336-9, 1952

133] Mawson C.A. & Fischer M.I. Zinc and Carbonic Anhydrase in Human Semen. Biochem. J. 55:696, 1953

134] McCarthy M. Zinc Lozenges shorten duration of common cold. Lancet. 348:184, 1996

135] McClain C.J., et al. Zinc-deficiency-induced retinal dysfunction in Crohn's disease. Dig Dis Sci. 28:85, 1983

136] McClain C.J., et al. Zinc deficiency in the alcoholic: A review. Alcoholism: Clin Exp. 7:5, 1983

137] McClain C.J., et al. Zinc status before and after zinc supplementation of eating disorder patients. Journal of the American College of Nutrition. 11(6):694-700, 1992

138] McLoughlin I.J., et al. Zinc in depressive disorder. Acta Psychiatrica Scandinavica. 82(6):451-453, 1990

139] Mechegiani E., et al. Zinc-dependent low thymic hormone level in type I diabetes. Diabetes. 12:932-937, 1989

140] Merialdi M., et al. Adding zinc to prenatal iron and folate tablets improves fetal neurobehavioral development. Am J Obstet Gynecol. 180(2 Partt 1):483-490, 1999

141] Merluzzi V.J., et al. Evaluation of zinc complexes on the replication of rhinovirus 2 in vitro. Res Commun Chem Pathol Pharmacol. 66(3):425-440, 1989

142] Michaelsson G., et al. Effects of oral zinc and vitamin A in acne. Archives of Dermatology. 113:31-36, 1977

143] Michaelsson G., et al. Serum zinc and retinol-binding protein in acne. British Journal of Dermatology. 96:283-286, 1977

144] Michaelsson G., et al. A double blind study of the effect of zinc and oxytetracycline in acne vulgaris. British Journal of Dermatology. 97:561-565, 1977

145] Miller M.J., et al. The Effect of Dietary Zinc Deficiency on the Reproductive System of Male Rats. Rev. Canad. de Biol. 13 No.5, 1954

146] Millikan C.R. Effect of Phosphates on the Development of Zinc Deficiency Symptoms in Flax. J. Dept. Agric. Victoria. 45: 273-8, 1947

147] Mocchegiani E., et al. The zinc-melatonin interrelationship: A working hypothesis. Ann NY Acad Sci. 719:298-307, 1994

148] Mocchegiani E., et al. Therapeutic application of zinc in human immunodeficiency virus against opportunistic infections. Journal of Nutrition. 130(5S Supplement):1424S-1431S, 2000

149] Mocchegiani E., at al. The immuno-reconstituting effect of melatonin or pineal grafting and its relation to zinc pool in aging mice. J Neuroimmunol. 53:189-201, 1994.

150] Moran J., et al. A study to assess the plaque inhibitory action of a new zinc citrate toothpaste formulation. J Clin Periodontol. 28(2):157-161, 2001

151] Mossad S.B., et al. Zinc gluconate lozenges for treating the common cold. A randomized, double-blind, placebo-controlled study. Ann Int Med. 125(2):81-88, 1996

152] Munoz N., et al. Effect of riboflavin, retinol, and zinc on the micronuclei of buccal mucosa and of esophagus: A randomized double-blind intervention study in China. J Nat Cancer Inst. 79:687-691, 1987

153] Nakamura T., et al. Kinetics of zinc status in children with IDDM. Diabetes Care. 14:553-557, 1991

154] Nason A., et al. Changes in Enzymatic Constitution in Zinc Deficient Neurospora. J. Biol. Chem. 188:397-406, 1951

155] Neil F., et al. Neurobiology of zinc-influenced eating behavior. Journal of Nutrition. 130(5 Supplement):1493S-1499S, 2000

156] Netter A., et al. Effect of zinc adminisration on plasma testosterone, dehydrotestosterone and sperm count. Archives of Andrology. 7(1):69-73, 1981

157] Newsome D.A., et al. Oral zinc in macular degeneration. Arch Ophthalmol. 106(2):192-198, 1988

158] Newsome D.A., et al. Zinc uptake by primate retinal pigment epithelium and choroid. Current Eye Research. 11(3):213-217, 1992

159] Niewoener C.B., et al. Role of zinc supplementation in type II diabetes mellitus. Am J Med. 63-68, 1988

160] Nishi Y. Zinc Status in various diseases. Hiroshima J. Med. Sci. 29:69-74, 1980

161] Nishida K., et al. [A study on a low serum zinc level in Crohn's disease]. Nippon Shok Gakkai Zasshi. 82(3):424-433, 1985

162] Nishiyama S., et al. Zinc supplementation alters thyroid hormone metabolism in disabled patients with Zinc deficiency. J Am Col Nut 13(1):62-67, 1994

163] Novick S.G., et al. How does zinc modify the common cold? Clinical observations and implications regarding mechanisms of action. Medical Hypotheses. 46(3):295-302, 1996

164] Novick S.G., et al. Zinc-induced suppression of inflammation in the respiratory tract, caused by infection with human rhinovirus and other irritants. Medical Hypotheses. 49(4):347-357, 1997

165] Ochi K., et al. [The serum zinc level in patients with tinnitus and the effect of zinc treatment]. Nippon Jibiinkoka Gakkai Kaiho. 100(9):915-919, 1997

166] Om A.S. & Chung K.W. Dietary Zinc Deficiency alters 5 alpha-reduction and Aromatization of Testosterone and Androgen and Estrogen receptors in Rat Liver. J. Nutr. 126:842-848, 1996

167] Osendarp S.J., et al. Zinc supplementation during pregnancy and effects on growth and morbidity in low birthweight infants: a randomised placebo controlled trial. Lancet. 357(9262):1080-1085, 2001

168] Pandley S.P., et al. Zinc in rheumatoid arthritis. Indian Journal of Medical Research. 81:618-620, 1985

169] Park J.S., et al. Zinc finger of replication protein A, a non-DNA binding element, regulates its DNA binding activity through redox. J Biol Chem. 274(41):29075-29080, 1999

170] Petrus E.J., et al. Randomized, double-masked, placebo-controlled clinical study of the effectiveness of zinc acetate lozenges on common cold symptoms in allergy-tested subjects. Curr Ther Res. 59:595–607, 1998

171] Pfeiffer C. Zinc and other micronutrients New canan CT Keats. 1978

172] Pidduck H.G., et al. Hyperzincuria of diabetes mellitus and possible genetic implications of this observation. Diabetes. 19:240-247, 1970

173] Pilerard-Franchimont C., et al. A double-blind controlled evaluation of the sebosuppressive activity of topical erythromycin-zinc complex. European Journal of Clinical Pharmacology. 1-2(49):57-60, 1995

174] Pohit J., et al. Zinc status of acne vulgaris patients. Journal of Applied Nutrition. 37(1):18-25, 1985

175] Pories W.J.et al. Acceleration of wound healing in man with zinc sulphate given by mouth. The Lancet. 1:1069, 1969

**176] Powell S.R. The antioxidant properties of zinc. Journal of Nutrition. 130(5):1447S-1454S, 2000**

177] Prasad A Trace elements in human health and disease. Vol 1 Zinc and Copper. New York Academic press.1976

178] Prasad A.S., et al. Experimental zinc deficiency in humans. Ann Intern Med. 89:483, 1978

179] Prasad A.S. Clinical, Endocrinological and Biochemical Effects of Zinc Deficiency. Clin. Endocrinol Metab. 14:567-589, 1985

**180] Prasad et al. Biochemistry of Zinc. New York Plenum press. 1993**

181] Prasad A.S., et al. Trace elements in head and neck cancer patients: zinc status and immunologic functions. Otolaryngol Head Neck Surg Jun. 116(6 Pt 1):624-9, 1997

182] Prasad A.S., et al. Duration of symptoms and plasma cytokine levels in patients with the common cold treated with zinc acetate: a randomized, double-blind, placebo-controlled trial. Ann Intern Med. 133(4):245-252, 2000

183] Prout T.E., et al. Zinc Metabolism in Patients with Diabetes Mellitus. Metabolism. 9:109-17. 1960

184] Rao K.V.R., et al. Effect of zinc sulfate therapy on control and lipids in type I diabetes. JAPI. 35:52, 1987

185] Rapisarda E., et al. [Effects of zinc and vitamin B 6 in experimental caries in rats.] Minerva Stomatol. 30(4):317-320, 1981

186] Record I. R., et al. Protection by zinc against UVA- and UVB-induced cellular and genomic damage in vivo and in vitro. Biol Trace Elem Res. 53:15-19, 1996

187] Reed H.S. The Relation of Zinc to Seed Production. J. Agric. Res. 64:635-44, 1942

188] Ripa S., et al. Zinc and the elderly. Minerva Med. (6):275-278, 1995

189] Rogers L.H. & Wu C.H. Zinc Uptake by Oats as Influenced by Applications of Lime and Phosphate. J. Amer. Soc. Agron. 40:563-6, 1948

190] Rogers S.A. Zinc deficiency as a model for developing chemical sensitivity. Int Clin Nutr Rev. 10(1):253-59, 1990

191] Romics I., et al. Spectrographic determination of zinc in the tissues of adenoma and carcinoma of the prostate. Int Urol Nerphol. 15(2):171-176, 1983

192] Russell R.M., et al. Zinc and the special senses. Ann Int Med. 99:227-229, 1983

193] Safai-Kutti S., et al. Zinc and anorexia nervosa. Annals of Internal Medicine. 100(2):317-318, 1984

194] Safai-Kutti S. Oral Zinc Supplementation in Anorexia Nervosa. Acta. Psychiatr. Scand. Suppl. 361:14-17, 1990

195] Saha K.C. Therapeutic value of zinc in acne. Indian J Dermatol. 23(2):25-31, 1978

196] Sakai F., et al. [Therapeutic efficacy of zinc picolinate in patients with taste disorders]. Nippon Jibiinkoka Gakkai Kaiho. 98:(7)1135-1139, 1985

197] Salvin S.B., et al. The effect of dietary zinc and prothymosin a on cellular immune responses of RF/J mice. Clin Immunol Immunopathol. 43:281-288, 1987

198] Salvin S.B., et al. Resistance and susceptibility to infection in inbred murine strains. IV. Effects of dietary zinc. Cellular Immunol. 87(2):546-552, 1984

199] Sandstrom B. et al. Absorption of zinc from soy protein meals in humans. J Nutr. 117 321-327, 1987

200] Sanstead H.H. W.O. Atwater memorial lecture. Zinc: Essentiality for Brain Development and Function. Nutr. Rev. 43:129-137, 1985

201] Sanstead H.H. Zinc in Human Nutrition: Disorders of mineral metabolism. Vol 1. Academic press N.Y. 1981

202] Saxton C.A., et al. The effect of dentifrices containing zinc citrate on plaque growth and oral zinc levels. J Clin Periodontol. 13(4):301-306, 1986

203] Sayeg Porto M.A., et al. Linear growth and zinc supplementation in children with short stature. J Pediatr Endocrinol Metab. 13(8):1121-1128, 2000

204] Sazawal S., et al. Zinc supplementation reduces the incidence of acute lower respiratory tract infections in infants and preschool children: a double-blind controlled trial. Pediatrics. 102:1-5, 1998

205] Schauss A.G., et al. Evidence of zinc deficiency in anorexia nervosa and bulimia nervosa. In: Nutrients and brain function. Essman, W. B. (editor). Basel:Karger, 151-162, 1987

206] Schauss A. & Costin C. Zinc as a Nutrient in the Treatment of Eating Disorders. Am. J. Nat. Med. 4:8-13, 1997

207] Scholmerich J., et al. Zinc and vitamin A deficiency in liver cirrhosis. Hepatogastroenterol. 30:119-125, 1983

208] Schoelmerich J., et al. Zinc and vitamin A deficiency in patients with Crohn's disease is correlated with activity but not with localization or extent of the disease. Hepatogastroenterology. 32(1):34-38, 1985

209] SchÜtte K.H. The Influence of Zinc upon the Stomata of Citrus Leaves. Unpublished. 1962

210] Scott D.A. & Fisher A.M. Insulin and Zinc Content of Bovine Pancreas. J. Clin. Invest. 17:725, 1938

211] Scott M.E., et al. Zinc deficiency impairs immune responses against parasitic nematode infections at intestinal and systemic sites. Journal of Nutrition. 130(5 Supplement): 1412S-1420S, 2000

212] Sempertegui F., et al. Effects of short-term zinc supplementation on cellular immunity, respiratory symptoms, and growth of malnourished Equadorian children. Eur J Clin Nutr. 50(1): 42-46, 1996

213] Seri S., et al. Effects of dietary tryptophan bioavailability on zinc absorption in rats. IRCS Medical Science. 12:452-453, 1984

214] Shambaugh G.E. Zinc: the neglected nutrient. Am J Otol. 10(2):156-160, 1989

215] Shankar A.H., et al. Zinc and immune function: the biological basis of altered resistance to infection. American Journal of Clinical Nutrition. 68(Supplement):447S-463S, 1998

216] Shay N.F., Mangian H.F. Neurobiology of zinc-influenced eating behaviour. J Nutr 130, 1493S1499S, 2000

217] Simkin P.A. Treatment of rheumatoid arthritis with oral zinc sulfate. Agents and Actions. (Suppl.) 8:587-595, 1981

218] Simkin P.A. Oral zinc sulphate in rheumatoid arthritis. The Lancet. 2:539, 1976

219] Singh R.B., et al. Current zinc intake and risk of diabetes and coronary artery disease and factors associated with insulin resistance in rural and urban populations of North India. J Am Coll Nutr. 17:564-570, 1998

220] Singh K.P., et al. Effect of zinc on immune functions and host resistance against infection and tumor challenge. Immunopharmacol Immunotoxicol. 14:813-840, 1992

221] Singh R.B., et al. Current zinc intake and risk of diabetes and coronary artery disease and factors associated with insulin resistance in rural and urban populations of North India. J Am Coll Nutr. 17:564-570, 1998

222] Sjogren A., et al. Magnesium, potassium and zinc deficiency in subjects with type II diabetes mellitus. Acta Med Scand. 224(5):461-466, 1988

223] Solomons N.W., et al. Zinc deficiency in Crohn's disease. Digestion. 16:87, 1977

224] Song M.K., et al. Effects of Bovine Prostate Powder on Zinc, Glucose and Insulin Metabolism in Old Patients with Non-insulin-dependent Diabetes Mellitus. Metabolism. 47:39-43, 1998

225] Sparkman D. Zinc: lower risk of heart disease, diabetes. Muscular Development. 36(6):44, 1999

226] Staker E.V. Progress Report on the Control of Zinc Toxicity in Peat Soils. Soil Sci. Amer. Proc. 7:387-92, 1943

227] Sterling M. New zinc resarch reveals more applications. Nutrition Science News. July 2001

228] Svenson K.L., et al. Reduced zinc in peripheral blood cells from patients with inflammatory connective tissue diseases. Inflammation. 9(2):189-199, 1985

229] Swanson C.A. & King J.C. Zinc and pregnancy outcome. AM J Clin Nutr. 46(5): 763-71, 1987

230] Takeda A., et al. Zinc homeostasis in the brain of adult rats fed zinc-deficient diet. J Neurosci Res. 63(5):447-452, 2001

231] Takihara H., et al. Zinc sulfate therapy for infertile males with or without variococelectomy. Urology. 29(6):638-641, 1987

232] Tang, X-h., et al. Zinc has an insulin-like effect on glucose transport mediated by phosphoinositol-3-kinase and akt in 3t3-l1 fibroblasts and adipocytes. Journal of Nutrition. 131(5):1414-1420, 2001

233] Terhune M.W., et al. Decreased RNA polymerase activity in mammalian zinc deficiency. Science. 177:68-69, 1972

234] Terwolbeck K., et al. Zinc in lymphocytes-the assessment of zinc status in patients with crohn's disease. Journal of Trace Element, Electrolytes, Health and Disease. 6(2):117-121, 1992

235] Tikkiwal M., et al. Effect of zinc administration on seminal zinc and fertility of oligospermic males. Indian J Physiol Pharmacol. 31(1):30-34, 1987

236] Toke G.B.& Dhamne B.K. A study of serum copper, serum zinc and Cu/Zn ratio as diagnostic and prognostic index in cases of head, neck and face tumors. Indian J Pathol Microbiol Apr. 33(2):171-4, 1990

237] Tuormaa T.E. Adverse effect of zinc deficiency: A review from the literature. J Orthomol Med. 10(3):149-162, 1995

238] Tvedt K.E., et al, Intracellular distribution of calcium and zinc in normal, hyperplastic, and neoplastic human prostate: x-ray microanalysis of freeze-dried cryosections. Prostate. 15:41-51, 1989

239] Van Binsbergen C.J., et al. Nutritional Status in Anorexia Nervosa: Clinical Chemistry, vitamins, iron and zinc. Eur. J. Clin. Nutr. 42:929-937, 1988

240] Van Campen D.R. Zinc interference with copper absorption in rats. Journal of Nutrition. 91:473, 1967

241] Vasquez A. Zinc treatment for reduction of hyperplasia of prostate. Townsend Letter for Doctors & Patients. 100,1996

242] Vega Robledo G.B., et al. Effect of zinc on Entamoeba histolytica pathogenicity. Parasitol Res. 85:487-492, 1999

243] Verm K.C., et al. Oral zinc sulphate therapy in acne vulgaris: A double-blind trial. Acta Dermatovener. 60:337-340, 1980

244] Voelker R. Zinc reduces pneumonia. Journal of the American Medical Association. 283(2), 2000

245] Wallace E.C. Diabetic epidemic. Energy Times. 9(4):24-28, 1999

246] Walsh C.T., et al. Zinc health effects and research priorities for the 1990's. Environ Health Perspect. 102:5-46, 1994

247] Wapnir R.A. Zinc Deficiency, Malnutrition and the Gastrointestinal Tract. J. Nutr. 130:1388S-1392S, 2000

248] Ward N., et al. The influence of the chemical additive tartrazine on the zinc status of hyperactive children, a double blind placebo controlled study. J Nut Med. 1: 51-57, 1990

249] Watts D. The Nutritional relationships of Zinc. J Ortho Med. 2: 99-108, 1989

250] Wear J.I. Effect of Soil pH and Calcium on the Uptake of Zinc by Plants. Soil Sci. 81:311-15, 1956

251] Weimar V., et al. Zinc sulphate in acne vulgaris. Arch Dermatol. 114(12):1776-1778, 1978

252] Wilkinson E.A.J., et al. Does oral zinc aid the healing of chronic leg ulcers? A systematic literature review. Arch Dermatology. 134(12):1556-1560, 1998

253] Wood J.G. & Silby P.M. Carbonic Anhydrase Activity in Plants in Relation to Zinc Content. Aust. J. Sci. Res. B, 5:244-55, 1952

254] Wood R.J. Assessment of Marginal Zinc Status in Humans. J. Nutr. 130:1350S-1354S, 2000

255] Wray D.W. A double blind trial of systemic zinc sulfate in recurrent aphthous stomatitis. Oral Surg. 53(5):469, 1982

256] Wright J.V. Treatment of benign prostate hypertrophy with zinc. Townsend Letter for Doctors & Patients. 82, April 1996

257] Yamaguchi H., et al. Anorexia Nervosa responding to Zinc Supplementation: a case report. Gastroenterol Jpn. 27:554-558, 1992

**Molybdenum: The unpronounceable, yet precious metal.**

"What on earth is molybdenum?" Molybdenum is a secret metal only known to farmers, vets, metallurgists and bicycle salespersons. Ironically it turns out to be a pivotal mineral in the copper-zinc balance. Even more unbelievable is that the Western Australian copper-zinc-molybdenum problem has been known about for 75 years. I guess it takes time for this sort of thing to filter down to the medical profession.

The average human body contains about 9,000 mg of Molybdenum. Molybdenum is an antioxidant and is important in the defence against cancer and carcinogens. Part of this defence is to keep pH at optimum levels.

It has a defence role within the gastrointestinal tract by detoxifying compounds that cause cancer. It forms a balance with zinc and copper to control the release and breakdown of histamine. Molybdenum is important for kidney function and helps excrete heavy metals like mercury.

## Molybdenum helps detox the following

### 1] Aldehydes

### 2] Nitrates & Nitrosamines

### 3] Petrochemicals

### 4] Sulphites & sulphurs

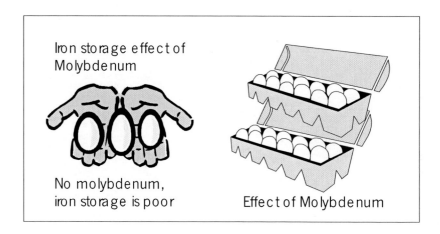

Iron storage effect of Molybdenum

No molybdenum, iron storage is poor

Effect of Molybdenum

Molybdenum is often found with iron in relation to energy cycles. The brain and nervous system rely on molybdenum to keep the peace. This is why molybdenum deficiency causes anxiety and irritability. Molybdenum is necessary for the metabolism of dietary fats.

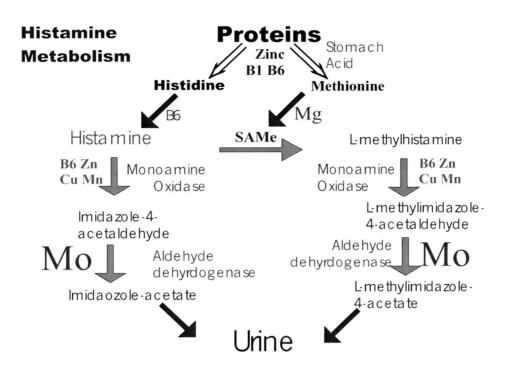

## Histamine Release affected by Zn:Cu:Mo balance

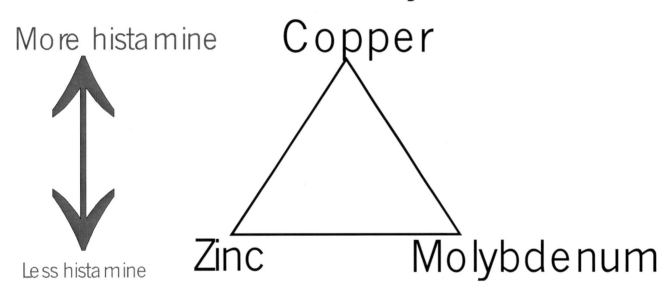

It has been used in many forms of arthritis with success. It is necessary for the formation of tooth enamel and hence helps prevent tooth decay. It is needed for the following enzymes Xanthine Oxidase, Aldehyde Oxidase, Nitrate Reductase and Sulphite Oxidase.

Molybdenum is required for Aldehyde Oxidase break down formaldehyde and many other aldehydes which we absorb from the clothes we wear, furniture we own, chipboard, carpets, glues, perfumes, etc. These are inhaled and need to be eliminated, but aldehydes can also be produced internally by bacteria, parasites, fungi, yeast, etc. Molybdenum has been shown to prevent Breast and Gastrointestinal cancers.

Molybdenum protects the body from the carcinogenic effects of dietary nitrosamines (due to its incorporation into the Nitrate Reductase enzyme that prevents the conversion of nitrates to nitrosamines within the Stomach).

Molybdenum has been used in the treatment of Wilson's disease because it facilitates the excretion of excess Copper. Hence it is extremely useful in treating copper excess. Male impotence has benefited from Molybdenum supplementation. Molybdenum is blocked by lead and copper excess. Excess molybdenum can lead to gout (need 15,000mg per day to cause this).

The most important function of molybdenum is to keep copper in check. You see Mother Nature is aware of copper's Jekyll and Hyde personality. She knows that when copper becomes too plentiful that it ceases to be a nutrient and starts becoming a nuisance! So she built in a moderator to control this tendency: Molybdenum.

See the figure below to see where molybdenum fits into the puzzle of copper excess.

Now we have three problems in Western Australia. Firstly, molybdenum is very scarce and needs to be added to fertilisers. The second problem is that fluoride inhibits the absorption of molybdenum. The third problem is that when molybdenum is low, copper absorption is much higher than expected.

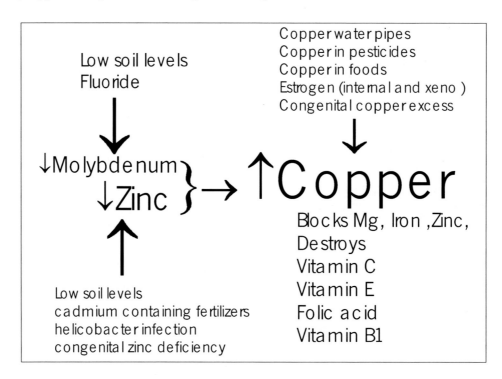

When evaluating the WHO calculation (see below) for safe copper levels in water. The assumption of 10% absorption is based on a normal molybdenum level, which acts as a natural barrier. Low Molybdenum levels (the commonest deficiency I see!!) increase absorption to 40-50%. The other assumption is that copper mainly comes in the first flow of tap water. So, the recommendation is to run the tap for 30 seconds to release any copper. Mentally imagine how much water escapes from a tap during 30 seconds and ask yourself "Are these assumptions realistic?" Overall, this means the "conservative" calculations of the total absorption of copper through water that are published by the Water Authority underestimates *actual* copper absorption under these circumstances. So "safe" levels of copper in water are no longer safe in the presence of Molybdenum deficiency.

Derivation of Guideline
The health-based guideline value of 2 mg/L (rounded up) for copper in drinking water was derived as follows:

$$2\ mg/L\ =\ \frac{0.5\ mg/kg\ body\ weight\ per\ day\ \times\ 70\ kg\ \times\ 0.1}{2\ L/day}$$

where:
- 0.5 mg/kg body weight per day is the provisional maximum tolerable daily intake for humans (WHO, 1982);
- 70 kg is the average weight of an adult;
- 0.1 is the proportion of total daily intake attributable to the consumption of water; **(i.e. 10%)**
- 2 L/day is the average amount of water consumed by an adult.

**Sources** are Wheat Germ, Oats, Brown Rice, Cottage Cheese, Eggs, Lentils, Green Peas, Split Peas, Fish, Kidneys, Spinach, Cauliflower and Brewer's Yeast.

The recommended daily allowance (RDA) of Molybdenum (for adults) is 75 - 250 mcg per day.

The therapeutic uses of molybdenum are Asthma, recurrent tinea or thrush, cancers of the gastrointestinal system, Copper excess, Mercury toxicity, Anxiety, Arthritis, and dental caries (tooth decay).

References:
1] Berg, J. W., et al. Epidemiology of gastrointestinal cancer. Proc Natl Cancer Congr. 7:459-463, 1973.
2] Brewer, G. J. Treatment of Wilson's disease with ammonium tetrathiomolybdate; Initial therapy in 17 neurologically affected patients. Archives of Neurology. 51:545-554, 1994.
3] Brewer, G. J. Practical recommendations and new therapies for Wilson's disease. Drugs. 50:240-249, 1995.
4] Erdmann R & Jones M: Minerals: the Metabolic Miracle Workers. Century. London, UK. 110-111 1988
5] Fleisher MA Mercury detoxification Townsend Letter for Doctors and Patients 214 May 64-71 2001
6] Komada, K., et al. Effects of dietary molybdenum on esophageal carcinogenesis in rats induced by N-methyl-N-benzylnitrosamine. Cancer Res. 50:2418-2422, 1990.
7] Losee, FL et al. A study of the mineral environment of caries-resistant navy recruits. Caries Res 3:23-31, 1969.
8] Luo, X. M., et al. Molybdenum and oesophageal cancer in China. Federation Proceedings. Federation of the American Society for Experimental Biology. 46:928, 1981.
9] Luo, X. M., et al. Inhibitory effects of molybdenum on esophageal and forestomach carcinogenesis in rats. J Natl. Cancer Inst. 71:75-80, 1983.
10] Moss, M. A. Effects of Molybdenum on Pain and General Health: A Pilot Study Journal of Nutritional & Environmental Medicine. 5(1):56-61, 1995.
11] Nakadaira H et al Distribution of selenium and molybdenum and cancer mortality in Niigata, Japan. Arch Envir Health Sep 50:5 374-80 1995
12] Papaioannou R et al: Sulfite sensitivity unrecognised threat: Is molybdenum the cause? J Ortho Mol Psyhc 13 (2) 105-110 1984
13] Sardessi VM Molybdenum: an essential trace element. Nur Clin Pract Dec 8:6 277-81 1993
14] Turnlund JR et al Molybdenum absorption, excretion and retention studies with stable isotopes in young men at five intakes of dietary molybdenum Am J Clin Nutr Oct 62:4 790-6 1995
15] Wei, H. J., et al. Effect of molybdenum and tungsten on mammary carcinogenesis in Sprague-Dawley (SD) rats Chung Hua Liu Tsa Chih. 9:204-207, 1987.
16] Yang, C. S. Research on esophageal cancer in China: a review. Cancer Research. 40:2633-2644, 1980.

## Selenium is a dirty word

Selenium is an unusual element. It's conduction of electricity increases with the amount of light hitting it. It sits in the periodic table below oxygen and sulphur and next to Arsenic and Bromine. Both arsenic and bromine have had interesting medical applications over the years.

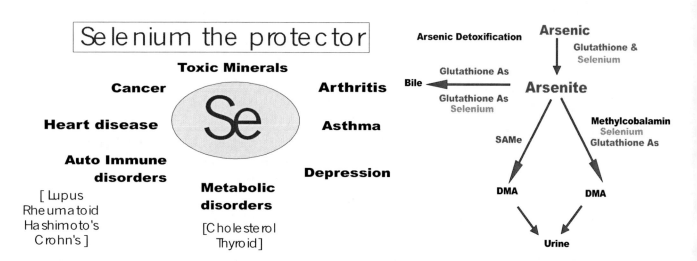

Selenium has had a chequered history in Australia. There was a time when the authorities declared that no one in Australia could possibly be selenium deficient and therefore banned selenium supplements. Then a strange thing happened. They changed their mind. Anyway, now you can buy selenium supplements as long as the tablet does not exceed 25 micrograms in quantity. Natural sources include Wheat Germ, Whole Grain Bread, Wheat Bran, Barley, Eggs, Mushrooms, Legumes, Liver, Kidneys, Rabbit, Chicken, Brazil Nuts, Peanuts, Herring, Tuna, Shellfish, Asparagus, Cabbage, Celery, Garlic, Onions, Potatoes, Radish, Tomatoes and Brewer's Yeast.

Selenium falls in the category of a metallic antioxidant. That is, a metal that prevents oxidation (rusting) and hence free radical build up. Free radicals damage the inside structure of cells like DNA. Their build up has been implicated in many major diseases including cancer. Interestingly, both low and high levels of antioxidants are associated with immune suppression.

Why is selenium so important, and why don't doctors know about this? I guess that if you found that significant cancer, heart disease, diabetes was associated with low selenium levels and this information got out, then you'd have somewhat of a panic on your hands, especially if you had previously issued an edict stating that selenium deficiency couldn't happen in Australia.

Selenium deficiency is very well hidden from doctors and the general population. Anyone mentioning it is immediately eyed suspiciously rather like an alien abductee would be. Selenium? Oh *that* conspiracy theory again! Funnily enough, all the farmers know about it (I guess they couldn't kill all of *them* could they?). So does the Agriculture department and the dieticians and the nutritionists and even some pharmacists.

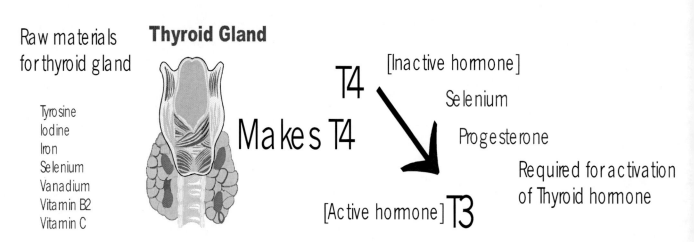

## Cancers associated with Selenium Deficiency

Lung Cancer
Leukemia
Breast Cancer
Oesophageal Cancer
Stomach Cancer.
Colon Cancer
Liver Cancer
Pancreatic Cancer
Skin Cancer
Basal Cell Carcinoma.
Squamous Cell Carcinoma
Melanoma
Bladder Cancer
Ovarian Cancer
Cervix Cancer
Uterus Cancer
Prostate Cancer

Why is selenium a dirty word? Because we find it (or can't find it) in soil. Considering the low levels of selenium in our soils (a fact known to all except the medical profession), it's difficult to know what a normal serum level of selenium should be. One way to check the tissue level is to look at the conversion of T4 (the inactive thyroid hormone) to T3 (the active level of thyroid hormone). Good levels of selenium mean that the ratio is about 2:1. That is T3 should be half of T4.

Low seleniums have been associated with several major illnesses. These are heart disease, high cholesterol, arthritis, cancer, hypothyroidism, diabetes, psoriasis and even depression. The references at the end of this article show the scope of the research and are not a complete list (only 82) by any means.

The majority of studies have looked at selenium and immunity especially resistance to infection and cancer. In this sense it concords with the general trend of antioxidants such as Vitamin C, beta-carotene, zinc, manganese and Vitamin E. These nutrients seem to improve immune function and/or low levels are associated with immunosuppression.

Selenium has a strong role in thyroid function. It is important for both thyroid hormone production and conversion of the inactive thyroid hormone (the one the doctor gives you) into the active hormone. So without selenium even Oroxine won't improve thyroid function. Selenium has been implicated in poor heart function (cardiomyopathy) and it may have this function because it is needed for co-enzyme Q10 production. Most of the medical profession are not aware that co-enzyme Q10 is step 2 of the cytochrome system, which powers every single cell in the body (except Red Blood Cells). This feature may explain why selenium is useful in angina. It simply helps the heart function more efficiently and hence because it needs less oxygen and can work better on a reduced blood flow such as in coronary artery disease.

The amino acid taurine facilitates the transport of selenium into the cells from the blood stream. This may explain why taurine has been used for palpitations and hypertension, because it increases cellular selenium and hence co-enzyme Q10.

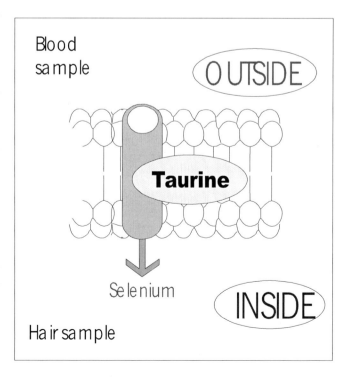

# Mitochondrial Energy Pathway

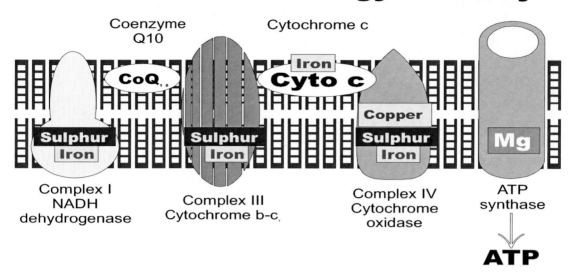

Coenzyme Q10 — CoQ₁₀

Cytochrome c — Cyto c — Iron

Sulphur Iron — Complex I NADH dehydrogenase

Sulphur Iron — Complex III Cytochrome b-c₁

Copper — Sulphur Iron — Complex IV Cytochrome oxidase

Mg — ATP synthase → ATP

Most problems with low selenium are due to poor soil levels, diet or absorption. Land-based sources of selenium such as alfalfa sprouts or wheat depend upon the levels of selenium in the soil where they are grown. Plants can grow on selenium poor soils without overt signs of deficiency. The best sources are from marine based products like shellfish, but cost and cholesterol levels in these foods often mean people may not include these in their diets. Interestingly, selenium is needed for cholesterol metabolism and is also found in these foods. Just as an egg has the cholesterol in the yolk balanced by the lecithin in the white, these foods are also balanced.

Malabsorption can occur for several reasons. Reduced stomach acid from (low zinc, helicobacter stomach infection, drugs like Losec, Zoton, Somac) and/or reduced pancreatic juice production (often as result of low stomach acid) can impair selenium absorption because selenium can be absorbed as the picolinic acid form (see article on zinc last month). Cadmium and selenium can compete for absorption and there is a suspicion that cadmium may substitute for selenium in soils treated with super phosphates. This could create a toxic product high in cadmium and low in antioxidants.

Alcohol and smoking can deplete selenium levels. Vitamin C supplements can interfere with the absorption of sodium selenite drops (one form of selenium supplement).

**Selenium, the immune system and cancer:**

1] Batist, G., et al. Selenium induced cytotoxicity of human leukemia cells: interaction with reduced glutathione. Cancer Research. 46(11):5482-5485, 1986.

2] Buljevac, M., et al. Serum selenium concentration in patients with liver cirrhosis and hepatocellular carcinoma. Acta Med Croatica. 1(50):11-14, 1996.

3] Burke, E. R. Selenium: low levels linked to liver cancer. Muscular Development. 36(11):34, 1999.

4] Burke, E. R. Selenium could lower risk of prostate cancer. All Natural Muscular Development. 35(12):56, 1998.

5] Burnley, P. G. J., et al. Serologic precursors of cancer: Serum micronutrients and the subsequent risk of pancreatic cancer. American Journal of Clinical Nutrition. 49:895-900, 1989

6] Broghamer, W. L., et al. Relationship between serum selenium levels and patients with carcinoma. Cancer. 37:1384, 1976.

7] Cheng, K. K., et al. Nutrition and oesophageal cancer. Cancer Causes and Control. 7:33-40, 1996.

8] Clark, L. The epidemiology of selenium and cancer. Federation Proceedings. 44:2584-2589, 1985.

9] Clark, L. C., et al. Plasma selenium and skin neoplasms: A case control study. Nutr Cancer. 6:13, 1985.

10] Clark, L. C., et al. Decreased incidence of prostate cancer with selenium supplementation: results of double-blind cancer prevention trial. Br J Urol. 81:730-734, 1998.

11] Clark, L. C., et al. Effects of selenium supplementation for cancer prevention in patients with carcinoma of the skin. A randomised controlled trial. Nutritional Prevention of Cancer Study Group. JAMA. 276:1957-1963, 1996.

12] Combs, G. F., et al. Can dietary selenium modify cancer risk? Nutr. Rev. 43:325-331, 1985.

13] Coldsitz, G. A. Selenium and cancer prevention: promising results indicate further trials required. The Journal of the American Medical Association. 276(24):1984, 1996.

14] Combs, G. F Jr., et al. Reduction of cancer mortality and incidence by selenium supplementation. Med Klin. 92(Supplement 3):42-45, 1997.

15] Contreras, V. National cancer institute spotlights nutrients: prestigious panel focuses on substances found in plants. Journal of Longevity. #48, 1999.

16] Davis, C. D., et al. The chemical form of selenium influences 3,2'-dimethyl-4- National Research Council: Diet and Health.

17] Fex, G., et al. Low plasma selenium as a risk factor for cancer death in middle-age men. Nutr Cancer. 10:221-229, 1987.

18] Hocman, G. Chemoprevention of cancer: Selenium. Int J Biochem. 20(2):123-132, 1988.

19] Ip, C. Selenium inhibition of chemical carcinogenesis. Federation Proceedings. 44:25373-2578, 1985.

20] Ip, C. Interaction of vitamin C and selenium supplementation in the modification of mammary carcinogenesis in rats. J N C I. 77:299, 1986.

21] Kandaswami, C., et al. Differential inhibition of proliferation of human squamous cell carcinoma, gliosarcoma and embryonic fibroblast-lung cells in culture by plant flavonoids. Anticancer Drugs. 3(5):525-530, 1992.

22] Kiremidjian-Schumacher, L., et al. Supplementation with selenium and human immune cell functions; II, Effect on cytotoxic lymphocytes and natural killer cells. Biol Trace Elem Res. 41:115-127, 1994.

23] Kiremidjian-Schumacher, L., et al. Selenium and immune responses. Environmental Res. 42:277-303, 1987.

24] Knekt, P., et al. Serum selenium and subsequent risk of cancer among Finnish men and women. Journal of the National Cancer Institute. 82:864-868, 1990.

25] Kobayashi, M., et al. Inhibitory effect of dietary selenium on carcinogenesis in rat glandular stomach induced by N-Methyl-N'-nitro-N-nitro. Cancer Research. 46:2266-2270, 1986.

26] Ksrnjavi, H., et al. Selenium in serum as a possible parameter for assessment of breast disease. Breast Cancer Research and Treatment. 16:57-61, 1990.

27] Menkes, M. S., et al. Serum beta-carotene, vitamins A and E, selenium and the risk of lung cancer. New England Journal of Medicine. 315:1250, 1986.

28] Mervyn, L. Thorsons Complete Guide to Vitamins and Minerals (2nd Edition). Thorsons Publishing Group, Wellingborough, England. 1989:79.

29] McConnell, K. P., et al. The relationship between dietary selenium and breast cancer. Journal of Surgical Oncology. 15(1):67-70, 1980.

30] Moss, Ralph W. Cancer Therapy: the Independent Consumer's Guide to Non-Toxic Treatment & Prevention. Equinox Press, Brooklyn, New York, USA. 1992:109-114.

31] Moss, Ralph W. Cancer Therapy: the Independent Consumer's Guide to Non-Toxic Treatment & Prevention. Equinox Press, Brooklyn, New York, USA. 1992:109-114.

32] Nelson, R. L. Is the changing patterns of colorectal cancer caused by selenium deficiency?. Dis Colon Rectum. 459-461, 1984.

33] Nelson, R. L., et al. Serum selenium and colonic neoplastic risk. Diseases of the Colon and Rectum. 38:1306-1310, 1995.

34] Rajcok, P. Selenium: the trace element for the next millennium. Mother Nature's Health Journal Biweekly Newsletter. 2(18), 1999.

35] Redman, C., et al. Involvement of polyamines in selenomethionine induced apoptosis and mitotic alterations in human tumour cells. Carcinogenesis. 18(6):1195-1202, 1997.

36] Redman, C., et al. Inhibitory effect of selenomethionine on the growth of three selected human tumour cell lines. Cancer Letters. 125(1-2):103-110, 1998.

37] Redman, C., et al. Involvement of polyamines in selenomethionine induced apoptosis and mitotic alterations in human tumour cells. Carcinogenesis. 18(6):1195-1202, 1997.

38] Roy, M. Supplementation with selenium and human immune cell functions; I, Effect on lymphocyte proliferation and interleukin 2 receptor expression. Biol Trace Elem Res. 41:103-114, 1994.

39] Salonen, J. T., et al. Association between serum selenium and the risk of cancer. American Journal of Epidemiology. 120:342, 1984.

40] Salonen, J. T., et al. Risk of cancer in relation to serum concentrations of selenium and vitamins A and E: matched case control analysis of prospective data. British Medical Journal. 290:417-420, 1985.

41] Scheer, J. F. 12 key antioxidants: may their 'force' be with you. Better Nutrition. 61(1):58-60, 1999.

42] Schrauzer, G. N., et al. Effects of temporary selenium supplementation on the genesis of spontaneous mammary tumours in inbred female C3H/St mice. Carcinogenesis. 1:199, 1980.

43] Schrauzer, G. N. Selenium and cancer: A review. Bioinorganic Chemistry. 5:275-281, 1976.

44] Schrauzer, G. N., et al. Cancer mortality correlation studies III: Statistical associations with dietary selenium intakes. Bioinorganic Chemistry. 7:23-34, 1977.

45] Sundstrom, H., et al. Serum selenium in patients with ovarian cancer during and after therapy. Carcinogenesis. 5(6):731-734, 1984.

46] White, E. L., et al. Screening of potential cancer preventing chemicals for induction of glutathione in rat liver cells. Oncol Rep. 5(2):507-512, 1998.

47] Yoshizawa, K., et.al. Study of prediagnostic selenium level in toenails and the risk of advanced prostate cancer. J Natl Cancer Inst. 90:1219-24, 1998.

48] Yu, S. Y., et al. A preliminary report on the intervention trials of primary liver cancer in high-risk populations with nutritional supplementation of selenium in China. Biological Trace Element Research. 29:289-294, 1991.

49] Yu, S. Y., et al. Protective role of selenium against hepatitis B virus and primary liver cancer in Qidong. Biol Tr Elem Res. 56(1):117-124, 1997.

50] Yu, S-Y, et al. Intervention trial in selenium for the prevention of lung cancer among tin miners in Yunnan, China. Biological Trace Element Research. 24:105-108, 1990.

51] Yu, S. Y., et al. Protective role of selenium against hepatitis B virus and primary liver cancer in Qidong. Biol Tr Elem Res. 56(1):117-124, 1997.

## Selenium and Heart disease:

52] Addis, P. B., et al. Atherogenic and anti-atherogenic factors in the human diet. Biochem Soc Symp. 61:259-271, 1995.

53] Beaglehole, R., et al. Decreased blood selenium and risk of myocardial infarction. Int J Epid. 19:918-922, 1990.

54] Kok, F. J., et al. Decreased selenium levels in acute myocardial infarction. JAMA. 261:1161-1164, 1989.

55] Korpela, H., et al. Effect of selenium supplementation after acute myocardial infarction. Res Commun Chem Pathol Pharmacol. 65:249-252, 1989.

56] Moore, J. A., et al. Selenium concentrations in plasma of patients with arteriographically defined coronary atherosclerosis. Clin Chem. 30:1171. 1984.

57] Oster, O., et al. The serum selenium concentration of patients with acute myocardial infarction. Annals of Clinical Research. 18:36, 1986.

58] Schiavon, R., et al. Selenium enhances prostacyclin production by cultured epithelial cells: Possible explanation for increased bleeding times in volunteers taking selenium as a dietary supplement. Thrombosis Research. 34:389, 1984.

59] Schone, N. W., et al. Effects of selenium deficiency on aggregation and thromboxane formation in rat platelet. Federation Proceedings. 43:477, 1984.

60] Salonen, J. T. Association between cardiovascular death and myocardial infarction and serum selenium in a matched-pair longitudinal study. The Lancet. 2:175-179, 1982.

61] Salonen, J. T. Association between cardiovascular death and myocardial infarction and serum selenium in a matched-pair longitudinal study. The Lancet. 2:175-179, 1982.

62] Stansbury, J. Sidestep heart disease. Nutrition Science News. March 1999.

63] Suadicani, P., et al. Serum selenium concentration and risk of ischemic heart disease in a prospective cohort study of 3000 males. Atherosclerosis. 96:33-42, 1992.

**Selenium and Diabetes:**

64] Battell, M. L., et al. Sodium selenate corrects glucose tolerance and heart function in STZ diabetic rats. Mol Cell Biochem. 179(1-2):27-34, 1998.

65] Mukherjee, B., et al. Anbazhagan S, Roy A, Ghosh R, Chatterjee M. Novel implications of the potential role of selenium on antioxidant status in streptozotocin-induced diabetic mice. Biomed Pharmacother. 52(2):89-95, 1998.

66] Pryor, K. Nutritional approaches to optimal blood glucose and insulin levels: key factors in longevity and resistance to diabetes and other degenerative diseases. Vitamin Research News. April 2000.

**Selenium and arthritis:**

67] Aeseth, J., et al. Trace elements in serum and urine of patients with rheumatoid arthritis. Scand J Rheumatol. 7:237-240, 1978.

68] Honkanen V., et al. Serum zinc, copper and selenium in rheumatoid arthritis. J Trace Elem Electrolytes Health Dis. 5(4):261-263, 1991.

69] Kose, K., et al. Plasma selenium levels in rheumatoid arthritis. Biological Trace Element Research. 53:51-56, 1996.

70] Munthe, E., et al. Treatment of rheumatoid arthritis with selenium and vitamin E. Scandinavian Journal of Rheumatology. 53(Suppl.):103, 1984.

71] Peretz, A., et al. Adjuvant treatment of recent onset rheumatoid arthritis by selenium supplementation: preliminary observations [letter]. Br J Rheumatol. 31(4):281-282, 1992.

72] Tarp, U., et al. Low selenium level in severe rheumatoid arthritis. Scandinavian Journal of Rheumatology. 14:97-101, 1985.

73] Tarp, U. et al. Selenium treatment in rheumatoid arthritis. Scandinavian Journal of Rheumatology. 14:364-368, 1985.

74] Tarp, U. Selenium in rheumatoid arthritis. A review. Analyst. 120(3):877-881, 1995.

*Selenium in Psychiatry:*

75] Benton, D., et al. Selenium supplementation improves mood in a double-blind trial. Psychopharmacology. 102(4): 549- 550, 1990.

76] Benton, D., et al. The impact of selenium supplementation on mood. Biological Psychiatry. 29(11):1092-1098, 1991.

Clausen, J., et al. Selenium in chronic neurological diseases - multiple sclerosis and Batten's Disease. Biol Trace Elem Res. 15:179-203, 1988.

77] Foster, H. D. Schizophrenia and esophageal cancer: Comments on similarities in their spatial distributions. Journal of Orthomolecular Medicine. 5(3):129-134, 1990.

78] Foster, H. D. The geography of schizophrenia: Possible links with selenium and calcium deficiencies, inadequate exposure to sunlight and industrialization. Journal of Orthomolecular Medicine. 3(3):135-140, 1988.

79] Shamberger, R. J. Selenium and the antioxidant defense system. Journal of Advancement in Medicine. 5(1):7-19, 1992.

**Selenium and Skin:**

80] Juhlin, L., et al. Blood glutathione peroxidase levels in skin diseases: Effect of selenium and vitamin E treatment. Acta Dermat Vener (Stockholm). 62:211-214, 1982.

81] Michaelsson, G., et al. Selenium in whole blood and plasma is decreased in patients with moderate and severe psoriasis. Acta Dermatology Venereology (Stockholm). 69:29-34, 1989.

82] White A et al. Role of lipoxygenase products in the pathogenesis and therapy of psoriasis and other dermatoses. Arch. Dermatol. 119:541-547, 1983.

Manganese is an underrated nutrient mineral. It is one of the three transitional elements I treat with great respect. The other two are iron and copper. This is because these three minerals have narrow therapeutic ranges. Their absence or blockade causes problems and certainly high levels (or retention) of these minerals will also cause problems. Manganese's place in the mineral tetrahedra is with the minerals that affect *cognitive* function. Interestingly, three of these minerals appear as consecutive elements in the transition series of the periodic table. Total body manganese is about 20 mg with high levels in kidneys, liver and bone. It is excreted in the bile, like copper.

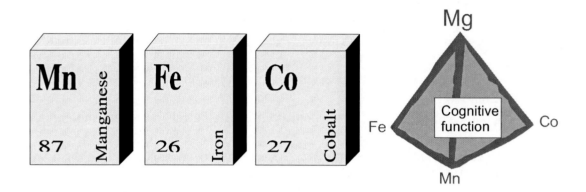

### Brain function and manganese.

Studies identifying problems with both low and high levels of manganese confirm the importance of this mineral with respect to the nervous system. Low levels are associated with epilepsy, poor memory, muscle twitching, dizziness and Schizophrenia. High levels are associated with severe brain dysfunction with some writers even blaming high manganese levels for "mad cow disease". In particular, Manganese excess can cause aggressiveness, apathy dementia, hallucinations, Schizophrenia and speech impairment.

One of the reasons for these symptoms is due to the role of Manganese in the adrenergic neurotransmitter pathways. In the conversion of tyrosine to adrenaline, Manganese turns up twice as shown by the asterixes (see below).

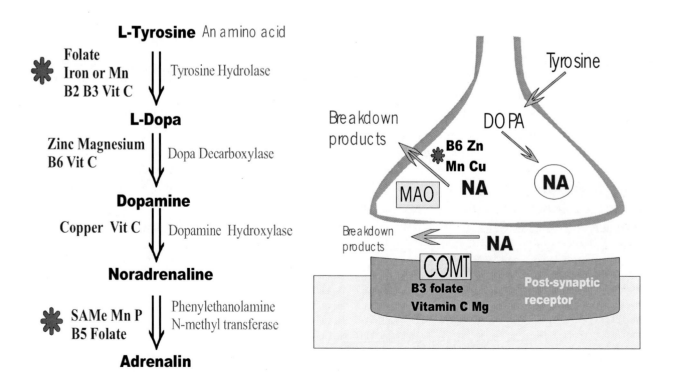

In the terminal bulb of a noradrenergic neuron (see figure above) Manganese is important for the efficient breakdown of noradrenaline.

The balance of the neurotransmitters Dopa and Noradrenaline is important in the prevention of hallucinations and Schizophrenia. It turns out that Manganese, Copper, Vitamin B3 and Vitamin C must all be in balance for this system to function normally.

## Manganese and glucose regulation.

Manganese turns up in the glycolytic pathway in an enzyme called enolase, where it can substitute for magnesium. Some authors suggest that Manganese may actually be more important in glycolysis than previously thought. Manganese is also important for the production of insulin, and it is worthwhile checking blood levels for deficiency in Diabetes.

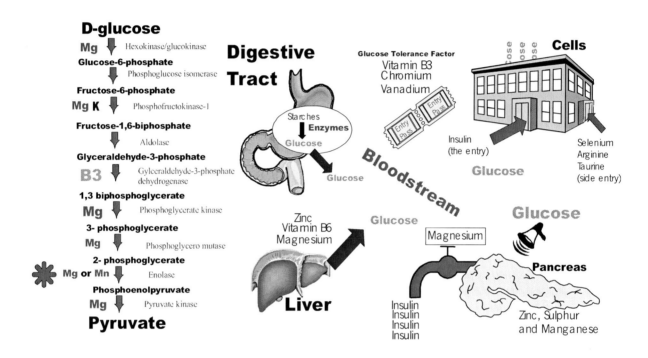

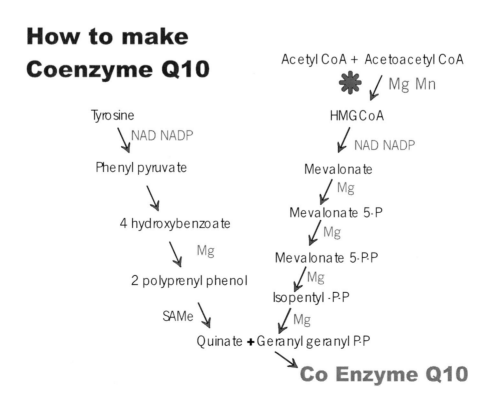

Manganese and energy.
In addition to its role in glycolysis, Manganese is important for the production of Coenzyme Q10 as shown below.

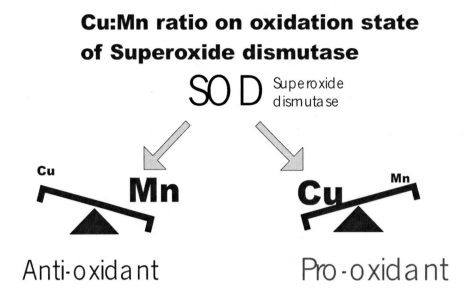

## Cu:Mn ratio on oxidation state of Superoxide dismutase

SOD Superoxide dismutase

Cu / Mn — Anti-oxidant

Cu / Mn — Pro-oxidant

In *mitochondrial* Superoxide dismutase (SOD), Manganese and copper must be in balance. Imbalances will affect the way SOD handles free radicals. Copper overload drives the enzyme to a pro-oxidant state, while Copper deficiency will create an anti-oxidant state.

Manganese and allergy.
Manganese deficiency can cause skin rashes and eczema. This may be due to its importance in the breakdown of histamine. In fact the balance of copper, zinc, molybdenum and manganese significantly affects histamine metabolism (see pathways below)

## Histamine Metabolism

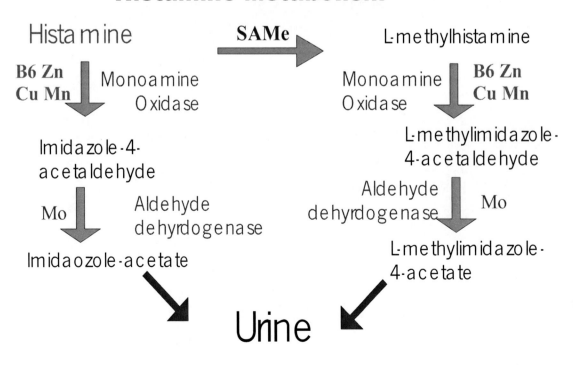

Histamine

**B6 Zn Cu Mn** ↓ Monoamine Oxidase

Imidazole-4-acetaldehyde

**Mo** ↓ Aldehyde dehyrdogenase

Imidaozole-acetate

**SAMe** → L-methylhistamine

Monoamine Oxidase ↓ **B6 Zn Cu Mn**

L-methylimidazole-4-acetaldehyde

Aldehyde dehyrdogenase ↓ **Mo**

L-methylimidazole-4-acetate

Urine

## Manganese and bone/cartilage production.
Numerous studies link manganese deficiency to joint and bone problems. This due to a combination of important functions including cartilage repair, joint lubrication and bone production.

## Manganese and cholesterol.
Manganese is important for the correct breakdown of LDL by the liver. Patients with high cholesterol may well turn out to be manganese deficient.

There is no RDA for manganese, but intakes of 2 to 15 mg would be appropriate in areas where refined foods abound.

**Manganese References:**

1] Amdur M.O., et al.  The need for manganese in bone development by the rat. Proc Soc Exp Biol Med. 59:254-55, 1945

2] Aston B.A. Manganese & Man. J. Orthomol. Psych. 9,4, 1980

3] Baly D., et al. Effect of manganese deficiency on insulin binding, glucose transport & metabolism in rat adipocytes. J Nutr. 120:1075-1079, 1990

4] Banta et al Elevated manganese levels associated with dementia and extrapyramidal signs. Neurology 27:213-216 1977

5] Bentley O.G. & Philips P.H. The Effect of Low Manganese Rations upon Dairy Cattle. J. Dairy Sci. 34:396-403, 1951

6] Bolas B.D. & Portsmouth G.B. Effect os CO2 on the Availability of Manganese in Soil Producing Manganese Deficiency. Nature. 162:737, 1948

7] Burger O.J. & Hauge S.M. Relation of Manganese to the Carotene and Vitamin Contents of Growing Crop Plants. Soil Sci. 72:303-13, 1951

8] Carl E.G., et al. Association of low blood manganese concentrations with epilepsy. Neurology. 336:1584-1587, 1986

9] Caskey C.D. & Norris L.C. Further Studies on the Role of Manganese in Poultry Nutrition. Poult. Sci. 17:433, 1938

10] Chandra S.V. Neurological Consequences of Manganese Imbalance. Neurobiology of The Trace Elements,Vol.2. Dreosti, I.E., Smith R.M., Eds. Humana Press. N.J. 1983

11] Cotzias G.C. Manganese in Health and Disease. Physiol. Rev. 38:503-31, 1958

12] Cotzias G.C., et al. Slow turnover of manganese in active rheumatoid arthritis 7 acceleration by prednisone. J Clin Invest. 47:992, 1968

13] Cranton E.M. Update on hair element analysis in clinical medicine. J Holistic Med. 7(2):120-134, 1985

14] Davis et al Longitudinal changes of manganese-dependent superoxide dismutase and other indexes of manganese and iron status in women Am J Clin Nutr 55:747-752 1992

15] Davidsson et al Manganese retention in man: a method fro estimating manganese absorption in man. Am J Clin Nutr  49:170-179 1989

16] Dexter D.T., et al. Increased nigral iron content & alterations in other metal ions occuring in brain in Parkinson's disease. J. Neurochem. 52(6):1830-6, 1989

17] Doisy C.A.Jr. Micronutrient Cntrol on Biosynthesis of Clotting Proteins & Cholesterol. Trace substances in environmental health, VI. Hemphill, D.D., et al : Eds. Univ. Mo. Press. Columbia, Mo. 1973

18] Donaldson J., McGregor D., et al. Manganese neurotoxicity: a model for free radical medicated neurodegeneration. Can.J.Physiology & Pharmacol. 60:1398-1405, 1982

19] Donaldson J. & Barbeau A. Possible clues to the etiology of human brain disorders. in S.Gabay et al, Eds. Metal Ions in Neurology & Psychiatry. N.Y. Alan R. Liss, 259-85, 1985

20] Dupont C.L. & Tanaka Y. Blood manganese levels in children with convulsive disorder. Biochem Med. 33(2):246-55, 1985

21] Failla M.L. Hormonal regulation of manganese. Manganese in Metabolism & enzyme function. Schrammk V.L.,Wedler F.C.,Eds. Academic Press. N.Y., 1986

22] Florence T.M. & Stauber J.L. Neurotoxicity of manganese. Letter. Lancet. 1:363, 1988

23] Freeland-Graves J.H.  Manganese: An essential nutrient for humans. Nutrition Today. Nov./Dec. 13-19, 1988

24] Freeland-Graves J.H. & Lin P-H. Plasma uptake of manganese as affected by oral loads of manganese, calcium, milk, phosphorus, copper, & zinc. J Am Coll Nutr. 10(1):38-43, 1991

25] Gallup W.D. & Norris L.C. The Effect of a Deficiency of Manganese in the Diet of the Hen. Poult. Sci. 18:83-88, 1939

26] Greger JL Dietary standards for manganese: overlap between nutritional and toxicological studies. J Nutr 128:368S-371S 1998.

27] Guillard O., et al. Manganese concentration in the hair of greying ("salt & pepper" men reconsidered. Clin Chem. 31(7):1251, 1985

28] Hill R.M., et al. Manganese Deficiency in Rats with Relation to Ataxia and Loss of Equilibrium. J. Nutr. 53:359-371, 1950

29] Hunnisett A., et al. A new functional test of manganese status. J Nutr Med. 1:209-15, 1990

30] Hurley L.S., et al. Influence of manganese on susceptibility of rats to convulsions. Am J Physiol. 204:493-496, 1963

31] Hurley L.S. & Keen C.L. Manganese. In E. Underwood & W. Mertz, Eds. Trace Elements in Human Health & Animal Nutrition. N.Y., Academic Press. 185-223, 1987

32] Keen C.L., et al. Whole blood manganese as an indicator of body manganese. N Engl J Med. 308:1230, 1983

33] Keen C.L. & Zidenberg-Cherr S. Manganese. In: Present Knowledge in Nutrition (6th Edition). Brown M.L. (editor). International Life Sciences Institute, Washington DC, USA. 279-286, 1990

34] Keen C.L. & Lonnerdal B. Manganese Toxicity in Man & Experimental Animals. Manganese in Metabolism & enzyme Function. Schramm, V.L., Wedler F.C., Eds. Academic Press. N.Y. 1986

35] Keller J.N., et al. Mitochondrial manganese superoxide dismutase prevents neural apoptosis & reduces ischemic brain injury: supression of peroxynitrite production, lipid peroxidation, & mitochondrial dysfunction. J. Neurosci Jan. 18:2,687-97, 1998

36] Kies C., et al. Manganese availability for humans, effect of selected dietary factors. Nutritional Bioavailability of Manganese. Kies C., Ed Am Chem Soc Wash, D.C. 1987

37] Leach R.M.,Jr. Metabolism & Function of Manganese. Trace elements in Human Health & Disease. Vol.III. Prasea, A.S.,Ed. Academic Press, N.Y.,1976

38] Leach R.M., Jr., et al. Studies on the role of manganese in bone formation. II. Effect upon chondroitin sulfate synthesis in chick epiphyseal cartilage. Arch Biochem Biophys. 133:22-28, 1969

39] Leach R.M., Jr. Mn (II) and glycosyltransferases essential for skeletal development. In: Manganese in Metabolism and Enzyme Function. Schramm B.L & Wedler F.W. (editors). Academic Press, New York, NY, USA. 981-91, 1986

40] Lindegard B. Aluminium & Alzheimer's disease. Letter. Lancet. 1:267-68, 1989

41] Liu A.C., et al. Influence of manganese deficiency on the characteristics of proteoglycans of avain epiphyseal growth plate cartilage. Poultry Science. 73:663-669, 1994

42] Löhnis M.P. Manganese Toxicity in Field and Market Garden Crops. Plant and Soil. 3:193-221, 1951

43] Matsuda A., et al. Quantifying manganese in lymphocytes to assess manganese nutritional status. Clin Chem. 35(9):1939-41, 1989

44] Meissner D. [Manganese and arteriosclerosis.] Z Gesamte Inn Med. 41(4):114-115, 1986

45] Mena I. Manganese. In F Bronner,J.W. Coburn, Eds. Disorders of Mineral Metabolism. I . Trace Minerals. N.Y., Academic Press, 233-70, 1981

46] Mena I., et al. Chronic manganese poisoning. Clinical picture & manganese turnover. Neurology. 17:128-36, 1967

47] Miller E.J. Chemistry, structure & function of collagen. In L Manaker, Ed. Biologic Basis of Wound Healing. N.Y., Harper & Row. 164-9, 1975

48] Nickolova, V et al Effect of Manganese on essential trace element metabolism. Tissue concentrations and excretion of manganese, iron, copper cobalt and zinc. Trace Elem Med 10:141-147 1993

49] Papavasilou P.S., et al. Seizure disorders and trace metals: Manganese tissue levels in treated epileptics. Neurology . 29:1466, 1979

50] Pasquier C., et al. Manganese containing superoxide dismutase deficiency in polymorphonuclear lymphocytes in rheumatoid arthritis. Inflammation. 8:27-32, 1984

51] Pfeiffer,C & Bacchi,D Copper,zinc, manganese, niacin and pyridoxine in the schizophrenias. J Appl Nutr 27(223):9-39 1975

52] Pfeiffer C.C. & LaMola S. Zinc & manganese in the schizophrenias. J Orthomol. Psychiatry. 12:215-34, 1983

53] Plumlee M.P., et al. The Effects of Manganese Deficiency upon the Growth, Development and Reproduction of Swine. J. Animal Sci. 15:352-67, 1956

54] Raloff J. Reasons for boning up on manganese. Science News. Sept. 199, 1986

55] Reginster et al Trace elements and postmenopauseal osteoporosis: a preliminary study of decreased serum manganese Med Sci Res 16:337-338 1988

56] Rosa G.D., et al. Regulation of superoxide dismutase activity by dietary manganese. Journal of Nutrition. 110(4):795-804, 1980

57] Rossander-Hulten L., et al. Competitive inhibition of iron absorption by manganese & zinc in humans. Am J Clin Nutr. 54:152-6, 1991

58] Rubinstein A.H. Manganese-induced hypoglycemia. The Lancet. 2:1348-1351, 1962

59] Rubenstein A.H., et al. Hypoglycemia induced by manganese. Nature. 194:188-9, 1962

60] Sampson P. Low manganese levels may trigger epilepsy. Journal of the American Medical Association. 238:1805, 1977

61] Sanchez-Morito N., et al. Magnesium-manganese interactions caused by magnesium deficiency in rats. J. Am Coll Nutr. 18(5),475-480, 1999

62] Schuler P., et al. Manganese Poisoning: Environmental and Medical Study at a Chilean Mine. Indus. Med. & Surg. 26:167-73, 1957

63] Shils M.E. & McCollum E.V. Further Studies on the Symptoms of Manganese Deficiency in the Rat and Mouse. J. Nutr. 26:1-19, 1943

64] Smialowicz R.J., et al. Manganese chloride enhances natural cell-mediated immune effector cell function: Effects on macrophages. Immunopharmacol. 9:1-11, 1985

65] Somers I.J. & Shive J.W. The Iron-Manganese Relation in Plant Metabolism. Plant Physiol. 17: 582-602, 1942

66] Strause L. & Saltmar P. Role of manganese in bone metabolism. Nutritional Bioavailability of Manganese. Kies C., Ed. Am.

Chem. Soc. Wash., D.C. 1987

67] Sziraki I., et al. Implications for atypical antioxidative properties of manganese in iron-induced brain lipid peroxidation and copper-dependent low density lipoprotein conjugation. Neurotoxicology. 20(2-3):455-466, 1999

68] Tanaka Y. Low manganese level may trigger epilepsy. JAMA. 238:1805, 1977

69] Thome J., et al. Increased concentrations of manganese superoxide dismutase in serum of alcohol dependent patients. Alaohol alcohol. Jan. 32:1,65-9, 1997

70] Thompson S.G. The Cure of Deficiencies of Iron and Manganese. Ann. Report East Malling Research Station for 1944, 119-23, 1945

71] Thomson A.B.R., et al. Interrelation of intestinal transport system for manganese and iron. J Labs Clin Med. 73:6422, 1971

72] Van Koetsveld E.E. The Manganese and Copper Contents of Hair as an indication of the feeding condition of cattle regarding Manganese & Copper. Tijdschr. Dieregeneesk. 83:229, 1958

73] Watts D.L. The nutritional relationships of manganese. J. Orthomol. Med. 5(4):219-22, 1990

74] Watts D.L. The nutritional relationships of magnesium. J. Orthomol. Med. 3(4):197-201, 1988

75] Weiner W.J., et al. Effects of chlorpromazine on central nervous system concentrations of manganese, iron, & copper. Life Sci. 20, 1971

76] Weiner W.J. et al. Regional brain manganese levels in an animal model of tardive dyskinesia. in W.E. Fann et al, Eds. Tardive dyskinesia: Research & Treatment. N.Y.,SP Medical & Scientific Books,159-163, 1980

77] Weldie G.W. & Pound G.S. Manganese Nutrition of N. Tabacum L. in Relation to the Multiplication of Tobacco Mosaic Virus. Virology. 5:92-109, 1958

78] Wilgus H.S., et al. Factors affecting manganese utilization in the chicken. Journal of Nutrition. 18:35, 1939

79] Wimhurst J.M., et al. Comparison of the ability of Mg and Mn to activate the key enzymes of glycolysis. FEBS Letters. 27:321-326, 1972

80] Yase Y. Environmental contribution of the amyotrophic lateral sclerosis process. in G. Serratrice et al, Eds. Neuromuscular Diseases. N.Y., Raven Press, 335-39, 1984

81] Yase Y. The pathogenesis of amyotrophic lateral sclerosis. Lancet. 2:292-96, 1972

82] Zayed J., et al. Environmental factors in the etiology of Parkinson's disease. Can J Neurol Sci. 17(3):286-91, 1990

**The functions of Iron can be categorised as follows.**

Immune system.
Energy.
Neurotransmitters.
Steroidal Hormones.
Thyroid function
Apoptosis
Haemoglobin & Myoglobin
Liver function

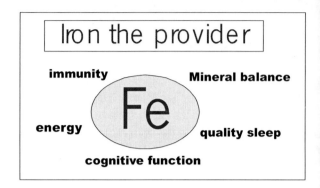

## Introduction.

In order to fully understand iron, there are four "myths" that need to be cleared up. The first is that only iron deficiency anaemia causes symptoms. Readers may care to note that many references talk about iron deficiency as a disease condition in itself. They are not referring to the anaemia, which ensues months or years after iron deficiency has affected the patient.

The second myth is that iron is primarily used in making red cells. Most iron is stored in cells *other* than red blood cells. Iron is stored in muscle, liver and brain and the ratio of these stores to the marrow store is about 3 million to one. Said in another way, for every haematopoietic cell with iron, there are 3 million other cells that need iron. Said another way; by the time a patient has iron deficiency anaemia; the patient has been suffering an age of the purgatory of health that iron deficiency causes. Said in another way: the haemoglobin is the *least* sensitive measurement of iron stores.

The third myth is that heavy periods cause iron deficiency. Three references cited which claim the opposite. And in my own practice, Menorrhagia settled after iron infusion in the majority of my patients who did not have an intrauterine structural cause. I have to concur with the investigators.

The last myth is that giving megadoses of ferrous gluconate has to be better than smaller doses of a more efficient iron supplement. Large doses of industrial strength iron will block the absorption of zinc. The reason is that the extra unabsorbed iron binds picolinate. That is why these dinosaur supplements cause nausea and constipation. Iron picolinate is the way to get around this problem. Severe iron deficiency in the face of copper overload is best treated by intravenous iron infusion. Iron injections stain, can be painful and be ineffective.

## Immune system.

Iron deficiency and blockade result in immune defects. One of the mechanisms of this is the lack of peroxide and hypochlorate in the Neutrophils. Iron is required for the function of myeloperoxidase which helps kill ingested organism that white cells engulf. When iron is low or blocked, the organism cannot be killed effectively. Iron and copper are used by white cells to "carve up" bacteria, because they are proxidant minerals. Although useful, they need to be kept under lock and key and released only when needed! See the section "lock up your cations".

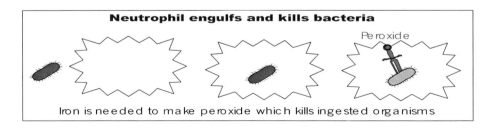

**Figure 1. Neutrophil function and iron**

## Iron and energy

Iron is required in the Krebs cycle as depicted in figure 2.

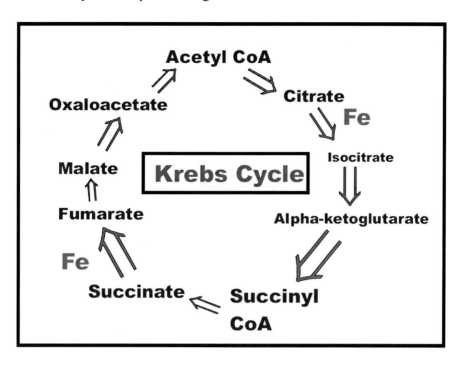

**Figure 2. Iron in the Krebs cycle**

# Mitochondrial Energy Pathway

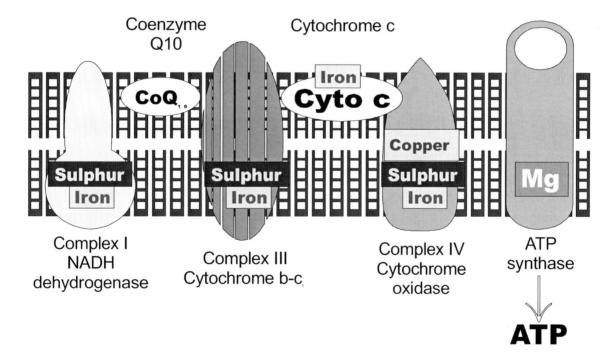

Figure 3 shows where Iron is required in the cytochromes that convert electrons to ATP.

**Figure 3. Iron in the electron transport chain**

Iron is required in the conversion of lysine to carnitine. Carnitine shovels fatty acids into mitochondria. Muscles rely heavily on carnitine for correct function. For optimum energy, the best ratio of iron to copper is 10:1.

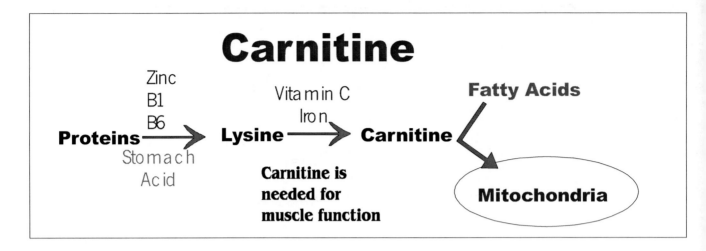

**Figure 4. Production of carnitine**

**Iron and Neurotransmitters**

Iron is a cofactor in the rate limiting steps of Adrenaline and Melatonin production. Optimal levels within the CNS are required. Blood test will underestimate CNS levels. Normal is not good enough, optimal is better. Figure 5 shows these crucial steps.

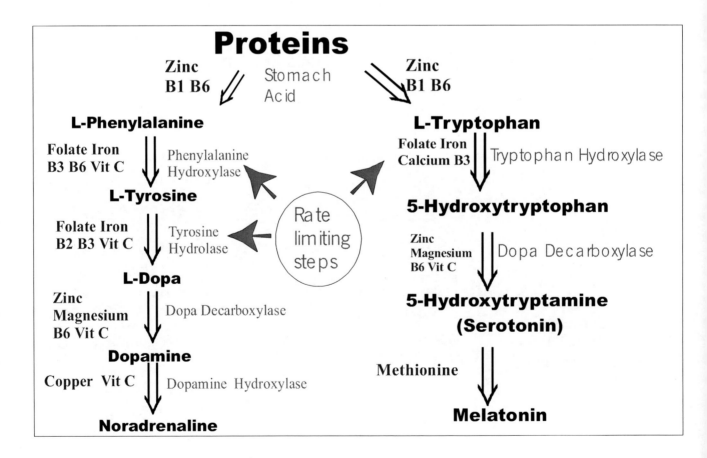

**Figure 5. Iron and neurotransmitters**

**Production of Steroidal hormones**

The figure 6 shows the importance of iron in the steroid hormone pathway.

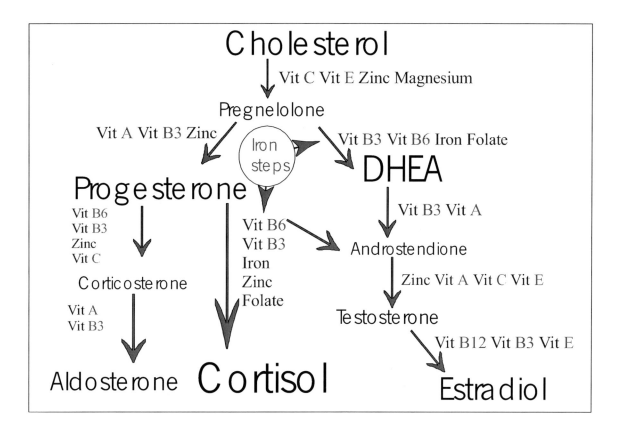

**Figure 6. Iron and steroidal hormones**

**Iron and thyroid hormone**

The figure 7 shows the effect of iron on the initial steps of thyroxine synthesis

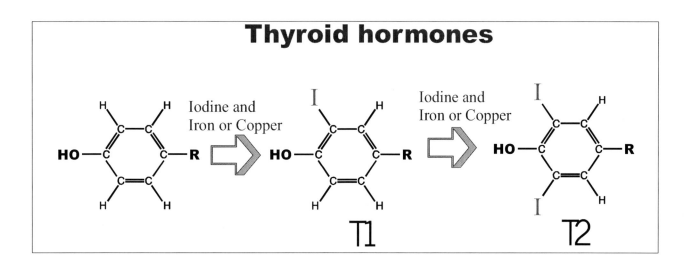

**Figure 7. Iron in the first processes of iodinisation of thyronine**

## Apoptosis

In the apoptosis mechanism, cytochrome C must be abundant enough to leave the mitochondria and stimulate the correct mechanism. Iron is the central ion in cytochrome C. Figure 8 shows the passage of cytochrome C out of the mitochondria in its quest to activate apoptosis.

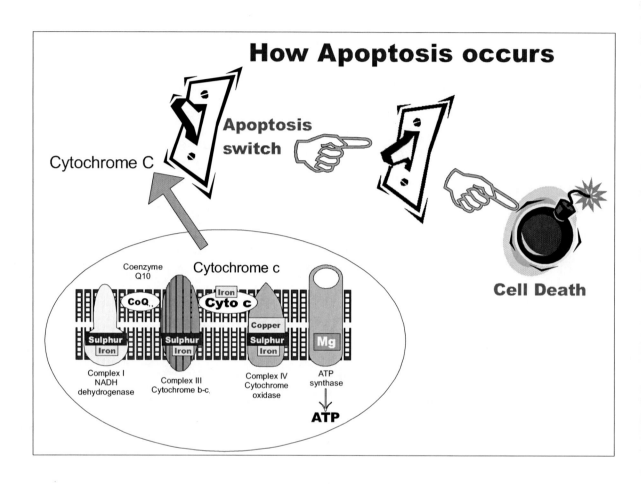

**Figure 8. Iron, cytochrome C and apoptosis**

## Haemoglobin & Myoglobin

The ability to retain oxygen in tissues is dependent upon the levels of Haemoglobin (oxygen carrier in red cells) and myoglobin (oxygen carried in red muscle). The amount of body iron in red cells compared to the other body tissues is outweighed by a factor of 3 million to one. Pity this fact isn't stressed in medical school.

## Liver Function

Iron is a component of most cytochromes. Iron also turns up as a cofactor for 2 Krebs cycle enzymes. Iron dependent enzymes include aldehyde oxidase, cytochrome oxidase, cytochrome P450, monamine oxidase, NAD dehydrogenase, succinate dehydrogenase, tyrosine hydroxylase and xanthine oxidase.

References
1] Arvidsson, B., et al. Iron prophylaxis in menorrhagia. Acta Obstet Gynecol. Scandinavia. 60:157-160, 1981.
2] Bates CJ Vitamins, Iron and physical work Lancet 2:313-14 1989
3] Beutler E et al Iron therapy in chronically fatigued non-anaemic women: A double-blind study Ann Intern Med 52:378-394 1960
4] Beisel WR Single nutrients and immunity Am J Clin Nutr 35:417-68 1982
5] Dallman et al Iron deficiency and the immune response Am J Clin Nutr 46:329-334 1987
6] Dhur et al Iron status, immune capacity and resistance to infections Comparative Biochemistry and Physiology

94A:11-19 1989

7] Dillman E et al <u>Hypothermia in iron deficiency due to altered triiodothyronine metabolism</u> Am J Physiol 239 1980

8] Edgerton VR et al <u>Iron deficiency anaemia and its effect on worker productivity and activity patterns</u> Br Med J 2:1546-1549 1979

9] Fairbanks, V.F. <u>Clinical disorders of iron metabolism</u> 2nd Ed Grune & Stratton. 1971

10] Fielding J et al <u>Iron deficiency without anaemia</u> Lancet 2 1965

11] Halberg L. <u>Search for nutritional confounding factors in the relationship between iron deficiency and brain function.</u> Am J Clin Nutr 50:598-606 1989

12] Hambidge KM et al <u>Acute effects of iron therapy on zinc status during pregnancy.</u> Obstet Gynecol 70(4): 593-6 1987

13] Heinrich, H.C. <u>Iron deficiency without anaemia.</u> Lancet 1968

14] Helman AD Darnton Hill I . <u>Vitamin & iron status in new vegetarians</u> Am J Clin Nutr 45(4): 785-9 1987

15] Herscko et al <u>Iron and infection</u> Br Med J 296:660-664 1988

16] Kuleschora EA Riabova NV <u>Effect of iron deficiency of the body on the work capacity of women engaged in mental work.</u> Ter Arkh 61(1): 92-95

17] Leiber RL <u>Behavioural and biochemical correlates of iron deficiency</u> J Am Diet Assoc 77:398-404 1977

18] Lewis, G. J. <u>Do women with menorrhagia need iron?</u> British Medical Journal. 284:1158, 1982.

19] Lozoff B Brittenham GH <u>Behavioural aspects of iron deficiency.</u> Proc Hematol New York 14:23-53 1986

20] MacDougall, L.G. <u>The immune response in iron deficient children: Impaired cellular defence mechanisms with altered humoral components.</u> J Paediatrics 86 1975

21] O'Brien et al <u>Prenatal iron supplements impair zinc absorption in pregnant Peruvian women</u> J Nutr 130 22251-5 2000

22] O'Keefe, S. T., et al. <u>Iron status and restless legs syndrome in the elderly.</u> Age and Ageing. 23(5):200-203, 1994.

23] Oppenheimer SJ <u>Iron and infection: the clinical evidence</u> Acta Paed Scand Sci 361:53-62 1989

Oski, F. <u>Iron deficiency in infancy and childhood.</u> The New England Journal of Medicine. 329:190-193, 1993.

24] Parks YA Wharton BA <u>Iron deficiency and the brain.</u> Acta Paed Scand Suppl 361:71-77 1984

25] Pollet E <u>Cognitive effects of iron deficiency anaemia</u> Lancet 1:158 1985

26] Pollet E et al <u>Iron deficiency & behavioural development in infants and pre-school children.</u> Am J Clin Nutr 43(4): 555-65 1989

27] Rosen, G. M., et al. <u>Iron deficiency among incarcerated juvenile delinquents.</u> J Adolesc Health Care 6:419-23, 1985.

28] Rushton DH et al <u>Ferritin and fertility</u> Letter Lancet 337: 155415 1991

29] Scrimshaw NS <u>Functional consequences of iron deficiency in human populations</u> J Nutr Sci Vitaminol 30:47-63 1984

30] Sherman AR <u>Influence of iron and immunity and disease resistance</u> Ann NY Acad Sci 587: 140-146 1990

31] Taymor, M. L., et al. <u>The etiological role of chronic iron deficiency in production of menorrhagia.</u> JAMA. 187:323-327, 1964.Sandstrom B et al <u>Oral iron dietary ligands and zinc absorption</u> J Nutr 115: 411-4 1985

32] Tucker DM et al <u>Iron status and brain function: serum ferritin levels associated with asymmetrics of cortical electro-physiology and cognitive performance.</u> Am J Clin Nutr 39(1):105-113 1984

33] Wallenberg HSC et al <u>Effect of oral iron supplements during pregnancy on maternal and foetal iron status.</u> J Perinatal Med 12(1):7-12 1984

34] Webb, T. E., et al. <u>Behavioural status of young adolescents with iron deficiency anaemia.</u> J. Special Ed. 8(2):153-156, 1974.

35] Youdim, M. B., et al. <u>Putative biological mechanisms of the effect of iron deficiency on brain biochemistry and behaviour.</u> American Journal of Clinical Nutrition. 50(3 Supplement):607-15, 1990.

# Are you copping too much Copper?

In all the time I have been looking at copper, I have only found a handful of patients with copper deficiency. However, I have found **hundreds** of people with excessive copper. What sort of problems did these people have? They fell into 5 categories. Hormone imbalance, joint pains, chronic fatigue, anxiety/depression or cancer.

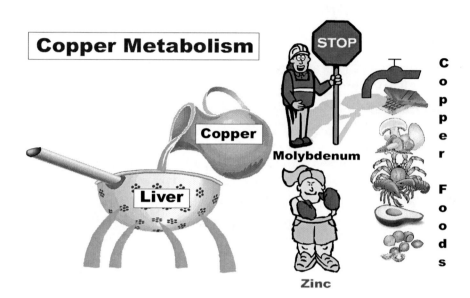

The distribution of copper in the body by tissue is as follows: Bones (44%), Muscles (25%), Liver (10%), Brain (9%), Blood (6%), Kidneys (3%), Heart (2%) and Lungs (1%). The problem with copper is that it one of the few minerals that can be absorbed from the gullet and stomach when in the ionic form. But that's OK you say because we only get in it food when its chelated. Yes, that was until we started to use copper pipes for water supplies. But wait, we have a defence system called metallothionine in the upper gut to protect us from ionic copper. That's if you have enough zinc and cysteine to supply the production of Metallothionine.

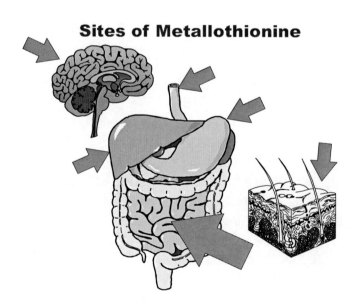

But clearly, just being on a high copper diet could not cause the results I see. We know quite a bit about copper from human and animal studies. Copper accumulates in the mother (serum copper rises 2-3 times prepregnancy levels) and unborn child during gestation. Stockpiling occurs mostly in the liver. Neonatal liver copper may be 5- 10 times that of an adult. The reason is that zinc is required for growth of the baby and also provides the topical protection against infections for babies until their immune systems mature. It is secreted into breast milk at the expense of the mother's

149

stores. The problem is that zinc and copper antagonise each other. The answer for most mammals is to stockpile the neoneate with truckloads of copper and give zinc in the breast milk. As long as the baby feeds and weans properly the two metals even themselves out. As long as the baby hasn't inherited any Xenoestrogens that floated across the placenta. Well, that's in a perfect world of course. No environmental Xenoestrogens, lots of zinc in the mother and 2-3 years of breast feeding.

From the diagram, you can see the dynamics of copper metabolism. Copper ingestion is very easy, but there are two minerals, which limit copper absorption. These are Zinc and Molybdenum. Think of these as sentinels. What copper gets past them can always get out through the bile via the liver. However, the Xenoestrogens block the body's ability to excrete copper. Therefore Xenoestrogen exposure on a background of low zinc or low molybdenum eventually leads to copper overload because of *copper retention*. Hair sample coppers match liver biopsy levels and hence are meaningful.

Copper has several functions. It is needed for neurotransmitter production (L-Dopa and noradrenaline); Cytochrome C oxidase: and the enzyme that breaks down Vitamin C. It is important for lactase (the enzyme you need for digesting milk); and it is needed to make collagen and elastin (the fibres that gives strength and elasticity to tissues). Normally, we have several substances that protect us against the absorption of copper. These are zinc, Vitamin C, manganese and molybdenum. If copper tends to accumulate then we have cysteine, glutamine, histidine and threonine to chelate (bind to) and remove it from the body. If it accumulates in the tissues, then DHEA helps to prevent copper induced lipid peroxidation (fat breakdown that releases free radicals). It is important to keep it in balance with iron (10:1 iron:copper ).

What about the work of Dr John R Lee linking estrogens to copper excess? Copper accumulation has been linked to both prescribed estrogens (HRT and the pill) and ingested xenoestrogens (false Estrogen or Estrogen mimickers). Where do false estrogens come from? There are 4 main sources. The first are pesticides like DDT, DDE and the modern equivalents. These behave as estrogens in the body and are accumulated permanently in fat cells at 70,000 times background levels. The second group are the petroleum products. Two hours in city traffic per week will incur enough of these to have an estrogenic effect. The next group are the plastics such as PVC's. Plastic wraps, plastic drink bottles, microwave containers, motor car seats and trims. We all have exposure to these. The last group are the hormones. There are two main categories. Prescribed hormones and those that come in the food chain. The food chain group has two main subtypes. These come from the poultry industry and antibiotics. Seventy five percent of the antibiotics used in Australia are *not* prescribed by doctors. They are used for animals, but they are not prescribed by Vets. They are used by farmers to enhance the growth rate of animals grown for commerce.
So, when we add up all the internal and external estrogens, this can create confusion for the body. One of the effects is the accumulation of copper. In fact a high copper to zinc ratio found in hair analysis is very suggestive that there are false estrogens in the patient.

Copper interferes with zinc, magnesium, vitamin C, folic acid, vitamin B1 and vitamin E. For example one can have adequate zinc levels, but appear to be zinc deficient because of the high copper level. I had one patient who said that after intravenous vitamin C, there was no vitamin C detectable in her urine. She turned out to have a very high copper level, which caused the instantaneous oxidation of the vitamin C in her body. So a combination of low zinc, low vitamin C in the diet coupled with xenoestrogens and copper piping could cause a serious escalation of tissue copper levels.

There are two quite disturbing implications of this finding. The first is that many of the patients that present to doctors may be suffering from a manifestation of copper excess. The second is that because copper interferes with tissue function, this will not show up on any blood test, X-ray, ultrasound etc.

An interesting phenomenon occurs when copper is high, the patient may have cravings for foods that have high copper to zinc ratios such as mushrooms, lobster, crab, pecans, hazelnuts, sunflower seeds, chocolate, dried peaches, canned prawns, walnuts, cod, almonds, brazil nuts, sesame seeds, French fries, brewer's yeast, oysters and liver.

So what can go wrong when the copper accumulates? Imagine a body where zinc and magnesium didn't work and none of your vitamin C lasted more than a few minutes. This is the summary of the effects of copper excess. Previous articles have discussed the functions of zinc, magnesium and Vitamin C, so refer back to these for more detailed information. The most affected systems are immunity, hormones, joints and brain function. High copper predisposes people to viral, fungal and yeast infections. Vitamin C can help to remove copper from the body and hence may explain some of its immunostimulant activity.

Imagine such a person getting glandular fever. The chances of chronic fatigue syndrome would be extremely high. The chances of developing depression and anxiety would be extremely high. The likelihood would be that this person would be female and would give birth to a zinc deficient child who would eventually accumulate copper themselves. This combination of low zinc high copper could manifest as the fashionable diagnosis of ADD/ADHD. What would that child crave? French fries and chocolate.

Does this sound like an epidemic to anyone? How many paediatricians or psychiatrists perform hair analysis? How many are likely to pick up this abnormality? Would the governmental agencies want parents to find out about this? Would the pharmaceutical companies like parents to find out about this? If copper excess can lead to cancer, would pharmaceutical companies that make chemotherapy drugs want people to know about this? Hair analysis has been used extensively in the USA to investigate criminal behaviour and delinquency. Guess what types of abnormalities seem to crop up regularly? Yes, you guessed it; excessive metal accumulation or nutrient metal imbalance.

The way to rectify the problem is to take a combination of zinc, molybdenum and a chelating agent, which can remove the backlog of stored xenoestrogens. Reducing the copper: zinc ratio foods also help. High copper to zinc ratio foods are Chocolate, Crab, Haddock, Pecans, Almonds Sesame Seeds, bakers yeast, mushrooms, Avocado, Liver, Walnuts, Bran flakes, Peanut paste, prawns, Trout, Brazil nuts, Sunflower seeds, and Grapes.

Sources of copper. Bee Pollen, Buckwheat, Oats, Wheat Bran, Wheat Germ, Butter, Eggs, Apples, Apricot Kernels, Bananas, Olives, Oranges, Peaches, Prunes, Raisins, Mushrooms Burdock, Chickweed, Cocoa, Dandelion Greens, Echinacea, Eyebright, Goldenseal Parsley, Barley, Lentils, Soya Beans, Split Peas, Chicken, Liver, Pork, Almonds, Brazil Nuts, cashew Nuts, Chestnuts, Hazelnuts, Macadamia Nuts, Peanuts, Pecan Nuts, Pistachio Nuts, Coconut, Walnuts, Pine Nuts, Sunflower Oil, Chocolate, Molasses, Tomato Puree, Crab, Lobster, Oysters, Salmon, Kelp Sunflower Seeds Avocado, Green Beans, Beetroot, Broccoli, Fennel, Garlic, Radish, Brewer's Yeast.

Copper References:
1] Aggett P.J., Fairweather-Tait. Adaptation to High and Low Copper Intakes: Its relevance to Estimated Safe and adequate daily dietary intakes. Am J Clin Nut.67:1061S-63, 1998
2] Allcroft R. & Uvarov O. Parenteral Administration of Copper Compounds to Cattle with Special Reference to Copper Glycine (Copper Amino-acetate). Vet. Rec. 71: 797-810, 1959
3] Aminoff M.J. Pharmacologic management of Parkinsonism and other movement disorders. In: Katzung, B. G. (editor), Basic & Clinical Pharmacology (sixth edition). Prentice-Hall International, London. 419-431,1995
4] Arnon D.I. & Stout P.R. The Essentiality of Certain Elements in Minute Quantity for Plants, with Special Reference to Copper. Plant Physiol. 14: 371-5, 1939
5] Barber R.S. et al. Further Studies on Antibiotic and Copper Supplements for Fattening Pigs. Brit. J. Nutr. 11: 70-79, 1957
6] Baumslag N., et al. Trace metal Content of maternal and neonate hair. Arch Environ Health. 29, 1974
7] Baxter J.H. & Wyk J.S. Van A Bone Disorder Associated with Copper Deficiency. Bull. Johns Hopk. Hosp. 93: 1-23, 1953
8] Bennets H.W., et al. Studies on Copper Deficiency in Cattle: the Fatal Termination (Falling Disease). Aust. Vet. J. 18: 50-63, 1942
9] Beshgetoor L. & Hambridge M. Clinical conditions altering copper metabolism in humans. Am J Clin Nutr. 67: 1017S-21S, 1998
10] Boccuzzi G., et al. Protective effect of dehydroepiandrosterone against copper-induced lipid peroxidation in

the rat. Free Radical Biology & Medicine. 22(7): 1289-1294, 1997

11] Bremner I. Manifestations of Copper excess. Am J Clin Nutr. 67 1069S-73, 1998

12] Bremner K.C. & Keath R.K. The Effect of Copper Deficiency on Trichostrongylosis in Dairy Calves. Aust. Vet. J. 35: 389-95, 1959

13] Brewer G. J. Treatment of Wilson's disease with ammonium tetrathiomolybdate; Initial therapy in 17 neurologically affected patients. Archives of Neurology. 51:545-554, 1994

14] Brewer et al. Treatment of metastatic cancer with tetrathiomolybdate, an anticopper, antiangiogenic agent. Phase I study. Clin Cancer Res. 6(1): 1-10, 2000

15] Cartwright G.E. Copper metabolism in Human Subjects. Copper Metabolism, Eds. McElroy W.D. & Glass B. (Johns Hopkins Press, Baltimore) 1950

16] Cartiwright G.E., et al. Studies on Copper Metabolism. XVII. Further Observations on the Anemia of Copper Deficiency of Swine. Blood. 9: 143-53, 1956

17] Cartiwright G.E., et al. The Role of Copper in Erythropoiesis. Biosynthesis of Hemoglobin. Conference on Hemoglobin. Part II, May 1957 (Division of Med. Sci., Nat. Res. Council, U.S.A.) 1958

18] Cartwright et al. Copper metabolism in normal subjects. J Clin Nut. 14, 1964

19] Casdorph R., Walker M. Toxic Metal Syndrome: How Metal poisoning can affect your brain. Avery Press. 1995

20] Cervantes C., Gutierrez-Corona F. Copper resistance mechanisms in bacteria and fungi. FEMS Microbiol Rev. 14:121–37, 1994

21] Chandra R.H., Newberne A.M. Nutrition Immunity and Infections. Plenum Press. 1977

22] Chuong et al. Zinc and copper levels in premenstrual syndrome. Fertility & Sterility. 62 313-20, 1994

23] Cunningham I.J. & Hogan K.G. The Influence of Diet on the Copper and Molybdenum Contents of Hair, Hoof and Wool. N.Z.J. Agric. Res. 1: 841-6, 1958

24] Dabrowska E., Jablonska-Kaszewska I., Lukasiak J., et al. Serum iron and copper and their relations to hepatocellular carcinoma in porphyria cutanea tarda and hemochromatosis patients—case report. Biofactors. (Netherlands) 11(1-2) p131-4, 2000

25] Dameron et al. Mechanisms for protection against copper toxicity. AM J Clin Nut. 67 1091S-1097S, 1998

26] Daniels A.L., Wright O.E. Iron and copper retention in Young Children. J of Nutrition. 8, 1934

27] Davis G.K. The Influence of Copper on the Metabolism of Phosphorus and Molybdenum. A Symposium on Copper Metabolism, Ed. McElroy W.D. & Glass B. (Johns Hopkins Press, Baltimore) 1950

28] Deeming S.B., Weber C.W. Hair analysis of Trace Minerals in Human Subjects as Influenced by Age, Sex, and Oral Contraceptive Use. Am J of Clin Nutrition. 23, 1970

29] Dick A.T. Studies on the Assimilation and Storage of Copper in Crossbred Sheep. Aust. J. Agric. Res. 5: 511-44, 1954

30] Dutt B. & Mills C.F. Reproductive Failure in Rats Due to Copper Deficiency. J. Comp. Path. 70: 120-5, 1960

31] Eck P. Insight into copper elimination. Ph oenix AZ Eck Institute reference sheet. 1991

32] Eck P. Introduction to copper toxicity. Phoenix AZ Eck Institute reference sheet. 1989

33] Epstein et al. Hair copper in primary biliary cirrhosis. Am J Clin Nutr. 33: 965-967

34] Fearn J.T. & Habel J.D. Parenteral Copper Therapy for Sheep in South Australia. Aust. Vet. J. 37: 224-6, 1961

35] Ferrigno D., Buccheri G., Camilla T. Serum copper and zinc content in non-small cell lung cancer: abnormalities and clinical correlates. Monaldi Arch Chest Dis (Italy), Jun. 54(3) p204-8, 1999

36] Finley E. B., et al. Influence of ascorbic acid supplementation on copper status in young adult men. American Journal of Clinical Nutrition. 47:96-101, 1988

37] Finley et al. Influences of ascorbic acid supplementtion on copper status in young adult men. Am J Clin Nut. 37, 1983

38] Fitzgerald D. Safety guidelines for copper in water. Am J Clin Nut. 67 1098S-1120S, 1998

39] Flesch P. The Role of Copper in Mammalian Pigmentation. Proc. Soc. Exp. Biol. 70: 79-83, 1949

40] Friedrich J. Stop the pain: natural remedies for migraines. Nutrition Science News. June, 1999

41] Gallagher C.H. The Pathology and Biochemistry of Copper Deficiency. Aust. Vet. J. 33: 311-17, 1957

42] Gallagher C.H., et al. The Biochemistry of Copper Deficiency. I. The Enzymological Disturbances, Blood Chemistry and Excretion of Amino Acids. Proc. Roy Soc.,Series B. 145: 134-50, 1956

43] Gallagher C.H. et al. The Biochemistry of Copper Deficiency. II Synthetic Processes. Proc. Roy. Soc., Series B. 145: 195-205, 1956

44] Greaves J.E. & Anderson A. Influence of Soil and Variety on the Copper Content of Grains. J. Nutr. 11: 111-17, 1936

45] Gubler C.G., et al. Studies on Copper Metabolism. XX. Enzyme Activities and Iron Metabolism in Copper and Iron Deficiencies. J. Biol. Chem. 224: 533, 1957

46] Harrison D. P. Copper as a factor in the dietary precipitation of migraine. Headache. 26(5): 248-250, 1986.

47] Howell J.S. The Effect of Copper Acetate in p-Diethylaminoazobenzene Carcinogenesis in the Rat. Brit. J. Cancer. 12: 594-608, 1958

48] Howell J., McC. & Davison A.N. Copper and Cytochrome Oxidase in Swayback. Biochem. J. 72: 365-8, 1959

49] Jacob et al. Hair as a biopsy material. V. Hair metal as an index of hepatic metal in rats: copper and zinc. Am J Clin Nutr. 31: 477-480

50] Joshi N.V. & Joshi S.G. Effect of Copper Sulphate on Rice in Bombay State. Science & Culture (India) 18: 9607, 1952 (Chemical Abstracts. 47: 4538)

51] Karcioglu et al. Zinc and copper in Medicine. Springfield Charles C Thomas Pub. 1980

52] Klevey L.M. Hair as a biopsy material II. Assesment of copper nutriture. Am J Clin Nutr. 23, 1970

53] Klevay L.M. The role of copper and zinc in cholesterol metabolism. Advances in Nutritional research Draper Plenum Pub. 1971

54] Knobeloch L., Schubert C., Hayes, Clark J., Fitzgerald C., Fraundorff A. Gastrointestinal upsets and new copper plumbing-is there a connection? W.M.J. Jan. 97:1, 49-53, 1998

55] Koch M. Laugh with health. Mastertech Publishing. 1996

56] Kivirikko K., et al. Abnormalities in copper metabolism and disturbances in the synthesis of collagen and elastin. Med Biol. 60:45-48, 1982

57] Levenson C. Mechanisms of copper conservation in organs. Am J Clin Nut. 67 978S-981S, 1998

58] Lizotte L. The woman with too much copper. Total health. 19: 49, 1997

59] Lucas R.E. The Effect of Copper Fertilization on Carotene, Ascorbic Acid, Protein & Copper Contents of Plants Grown on Organic Soils. Soil Sci. 65: 461-9, 1948

60] Malter R. Copper toxicity: Psychological implications for children, adolescences and adults. Hoffman estates A Malter institute for natural development reference sheet. 1984

61] Marinov B, Tsachev K, Doganov N, et al. [The copper concentration in the blood serum of women with ovarian tumors (a preliminary report)]Akush Ginekol (Sofiia) (Bulgaria). 39(2) p36-7, 2000

62] Marston H.R. Cobalt, Copper and Molybdenum in the Nutrition of Plants and Animals. Physiol. Rev. 32: 66-121, 1952

63] Martin J.M. Overdosing on copper? Alive. 62:43-44, 1985

64] Mason K.E. A conspectus of research on copper metabolism and requirements of man. J Nutr. 109, 1979

65] Matrone G. Interrelationships of Iron and Copper in the Nutrition and Metabolism of Animals. Fed. Proc. 19: 659-65, 1960

66] McKenzie J.M. Alteration of the zinc anc copper concentration of hair. Am J Clin Nutr. 31: 470-476

67] Linder M.C.& Hazegh-Azam M. Copper biochemistry and molecular biology. Am J Clin Nutr.63: 797S-811S

68] Milde D., Novak O., Stu ka V., et al. Serum levels of selenium, manganese, copper, and iron in colorectal cancer patients. Biol Trace Elem Res (United States), Feb.79(2) p107-14, 2001

69] Mills C.F. Comparative Studies of Copper, Molybdenum and Sulphur Metabolism in the Ruminant and the Rat. Proc. Nutr. Soc. 19: 162-9, 1960

70] Morgan D.E., et al. The Effect of Copper Glycine Injections on the Live Weight Gains of Sucking Beef

Calves. Anim. Prod. 4: 303-7, 1962

71] Nakakoshi T. Copper and hepatocellular carcinoma. Radiology (United States), Jan. 214(1) p304-6, 2000

72] Narasaka S. Studies in the Biochemistry of Copper. XX. Thyroid as a Factor in the Regulation of Blood Copper Level. Jap. J. Med. Sci. 4: 33-36, 1938

73] Neelakantan V. & Mehta B.V. Copper Status of Soils in Western India. Soil Sci. 91: 251-6, 1961

74] Nolan K.R. Copper toxicity syndrome. J Orthomol Psych. 12:270-282, 1983

75] O'Dell B.L. Biochemistry of Copper. The Medical Clinics of North America 60. Saunders Press. 1960

76] Osiecki Henry The Nutrient Bible. Bio Concepts Publishing. 1998

77] Owen C.A. Copper deficiency and toxicity: Acquired and inherited in plants, animals and man. Park Ridge NJ Noyes Pub. 1981

78] Pfeiffer C. Mental and Elemental Nutrients. Keats New Canaan. 1975

79] Pirrie R. Serum Copper and its Relationship to Serum Iron in Patients with Neoplastic Disease. J Clin. Path. 5: 190-3, 1952

80] Polukhina I.N.& Masljanaja H.K. Influence of Nitrogen and Copper on the Anatomical Structure of Oat Stems in Relation to the Resistance of Oats on Peat Soils. (English translation), Izv. Timir. Sol. Shokh Akad., No.1, 205-8, 1961

81] Pratt W.B. Elevated hair copper in idiopathic scoliosis and of normal individuals. Clin Chem. 24 ,1978

82] Ramaswamy M.S. Copper in Ceylon Teas. Tea Quart. 31: 76-80, 1960

83] Reavley Nicola The New encyclopaedia of Vitamins, Minerals, Supplements and Herbs. Bookman Press. 1998

84] Robertson H.A. & Broome A.W.J. Factors Influencing the Blood Copper Level of Sheep: the Effect of change in Basal Metabolic Activity. J. Sci. Fd. Agric. (Supp. Issue), 8, s. 82-s. 87, 1957

85] Roelofsen H., Wolters H., Van Luyn M.J., et al. Copper-induced apical trafficking of ATP7B in polarized hepatoma cells provides a mechanism for biliary copper excretion. Gastroenterology (United States), Sep. 119(3) : 782-93, 2000

86] Sandstead H H. Copper bioavailability and requirements. American Journal of Clinical Nutrition. 35:809-814, 1982

87] Schultze M.O. The Effect of Deficiencies in Copper and Iron on the Cytochrome Oxidase of Rat Tissues. J. Biol. Chem. 129: 729-37, 1939

88] Shore D., et al. CSF copper concentrations in chronic schizophrenia. American Journal of Psychiatry. 140:754-757, 1983

89] Sidhu K. S., et al. Need to revise the national drinking water regulation for copper. Regul Toxicol Pharmacol. 22(1): 95-100, 1995

90] Solioz M. et al Copper pumping ATPases: common concepts in bacteria and man. FEBS Lett. 346:44–7, 1994

91] Stine J.B., et al. Copper and Cheddar Flavour. Dairy World, Chicago. 32: 10-14, 1953 (Chemical Abstracts, 48,900)

92] Sugimoto Y., et al Cations inhibit specifically type 1 5 alpha-reductase found in human skin. J Invest Dermatol. 104(5): 775-778, 1995

93] Takamiya K. Anti-tumour Activities of Copper Chelates. Nature. 185: 190-1, 1960

94] Timberlake C.F. Complex Formation between Copper and some Organic Acids, Phenols and Phenolic Acids Occurring in Fruit. J. Chem. Soc. 2795-8, 1959

95] Turnlund et al. Copper absorption, excretion and retention by young men consuming low dietary copper determined by using stable isotope 65Cu. AM J Clin Nut. 67: 1219-1225, 1998

96] Van Campen D.R. Zinc interference with copper absorption in rats. Journal of Nutrition. 91:473, 1967

97] Van den Berg G.J., et al. Dietary ascorbic acid lowers the concentration of soluble copper in the small intestinal lumen of rats. Br J Nutr. 71(5): 701-707, 1994

98] Van Koetsveld E.E. The Manganese and Copper contents of hair as an indication of the feeding condition of cattle regarding manganese and copper. Tijdschr. Dieregeneesk. 83: 229, 1958

99] Vir et al. Serum and hair concentrations of copper during pregnancy. Am J Clin Nutr. 34: 2382-2388, 1981

There are several features of iron metabolism that can be affected by copper. Iron levels are like a bank account; they depend on how much you put in, how much you take out and how often you put in and take out.

**INPUT**

Firstly, iron sources may not be plentiful in the diet. Below is a list of such sources with the corresponding amounts. It is believed that concurrent vitamin C will enhance iron absorption.

<u>**Sources Of Iron:**</u>

| Food | Amount | Iron (mg) | Food | Amount | Iron (mg) |
|---|---|---|---|---|---|
| Branflakes | 1 cup | 10.8 | Hamburger Patty | 1 serve | 2.4 |
| Lambs Liver (Fried) | 100g | 8.2 | Pearl Barley (Boiled) | 1 cup | 2.1 |
| Spinach (Cooked) | 1 cup | 6.4 | Cashews (Salted) | 1/2 cup | 2 |
| Apricots (Dried) | 1 cup (Halves) | 6.1 | Lamb | 100g | 2 |
| Chickpeas (Boiled) | 1 cup | 4.7 | Bulgur (Boiled) | 1 cup | 1.7 |
| All Bran | 1/2 cup | 4.5 | Raisins | 1/2 cup | 1.7 |
| Oysters (Fried) | 6 Oysters | 4.4 | Sausages (Grilled) | 2 (thick,10cm in length) | 1.3 |
| Salmon (Canned) | 1 can | 3.8 | Liverwurst | 1 slice | 1.2 |
| Oats | 1/2 cup | 3.7 | Wholegrain Bread | 1 slice | 1.1 |
| Beef (Cooked) | 3/4 cup (Diced) | 2.6 | Wholewheat Pita Bread | 1 (small) | 0.8 |
| Almonds | 1/2 cup | 2.6 | Pate | 1 tbsp | 0.7 |
| Tuna (Canned) | 1 can | 2.5 | Baked Beans | 1 cup | 0.7 |

## How Picolinate binds zinc

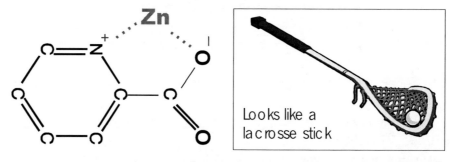

Looks like a lacrosse stick

Also absorbed in this way are Selenium Manganese Molybdenum Boron Chromium and Vanadium

**ABSORPTION**

Secondly, iron needs to be charged with a two-plus charge to be absorbed. This requires stomach acid. Unfortunately stomach acid requires the presence of Zinc, Vitamin B1 and vitamin B6. Calcium and Magnesium also need stomach acid to absorb them. When the stomach makes acid for digestion a second message is sent to the pancreas gland to release picolinate into the intestine. This special molecule acts like a lacrosse stick to pick up ions like zinc, selenium, molybdenum, chromium, manganese and vanadium. The irony is that if you don't absorb zinc, you don't make stomach acid and if you don't make acid, you don't absorb zinc (and the iron).

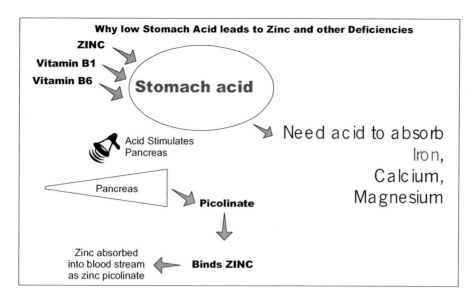

The next step is that iron must traverse the intestinal wall to get to bloodstream. Copper in the intestinal wall will affect this transfer.

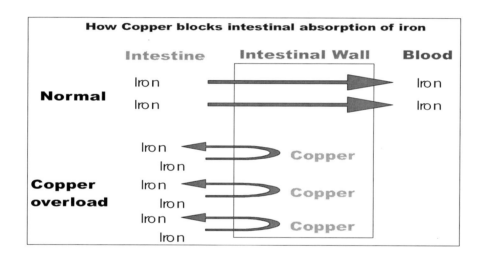

**LOSS**

Iron may be lost if there is blood loss.

Nose bleeds
Stomach ulcers
Haemorrhoids
Menstrual Fluid

## STORAGE

Lastly, the efficiency of iron storage is dependent on the presence of the mineral molybdenum. If you could imagine iron as eggs in the palm of your hand, there would be a limit to how many you could hold. Molybdenum allows efficient iron storage rather like the egg cartons.

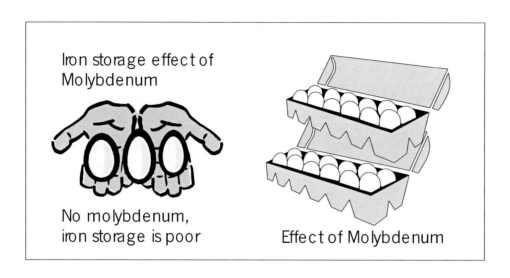

Iron storage effect of Molybdenum

No molybdenum, iron storage is poor

Effect of Molybdenum

The following tissue mineral analyses show the typical pattern for iron deficiency. High copper levels and low molybdenum's are the common finding in most of my patients.

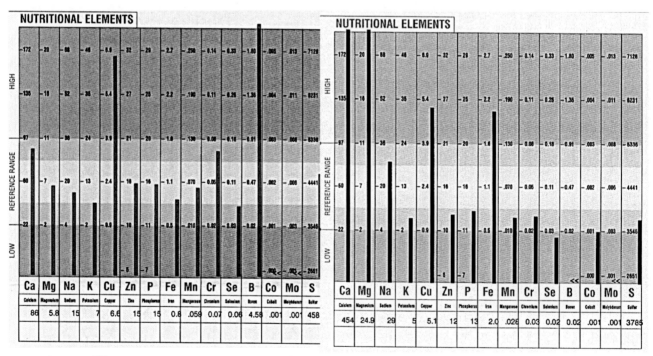

| | Ca | Mg | Na | K | Cu | Zn | P | Fe | Mn | Cr | Se | B | Co | Mo | S |
|---|---|---|---|---|---|---|---|---|---|---|---|---|---|---|---|
| | Calcium | Magnesium | Sodium | Potassium | Copper | Zinc | Phosphorus | Iron | Manganese | Chromium | Selenium | Boron | Cobalt | Molybdenum | Sulfur |
| | 86 | 5.8 | 15 | 7 | 6.6 | 15 | 15 | 0.8 | .059 | 0.07 | 0.06 | 4.58 | .001 | .001 | 458 |

| | Ca | Mg | Na | K | Cu | Zn | P | Fe | Mn | Cr | Se | B | Co | Mo | S |
|---|---|---|---|---|---|---|---|---|---|---|---|---|---|---|---|
| | Calcium | Magnesium | Sodium | Potassium | Copper | Zinc | Phosphorus | Iron | Manganese | Chromium | Selenium | Boron | Cobalt | Molybdenum | Sulfur |
| | 454 | 24.9 | 29 | 5 | 5.1 | 12 | 13 | 2.0 | .028 | 0.03 | 0.02 | 0.02 | .001 | .001 | 3785 |

# Why copper excess causes fatigue.

In previous articles I have mentioned the unwanted effect of having too much copper. This is a problem within the tissues and not in the blood. Naïve doctors who think that a normal blood test for copper disproves this should go back to basic cell physiology books and realise that blood tests for intracellular minerals are not representative of tissue levels.

**Copper causes fatigue for several reasons.**
a] Iron deficiency and/or tissue iron blockade
b] Magnesium deficiency and/or tissue blockade
c] Carnitine deficiency leading to weak muscles
d] Hypoglycaemia
e] Poor sleep pattern
f] Depression
g] Tissue blockade of thyroid hormone

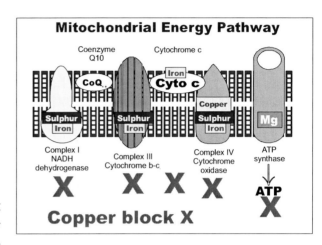

Let's take iron deficiency first.
Copper excess is probably the commonest cause of persistent iron deficiency. It causes gastritis, hypochlorhydria (low stomach acid) and blocks the transfer of iron across the intestinal wall.
Once iron is in the cells, copper blocks the effect of iron. This is most notable in the mitochondria. See the figure about Mitochondrial energy pathway and see that copper blocks most of the steps.

Carnitine is a vitamin, which is required for the metabolism of fatty acids. Tissues which need this type of metabolism cannot function properly. The most important tissue is the muscle. Copper blocks the production of carnitine as shown in the figure below.

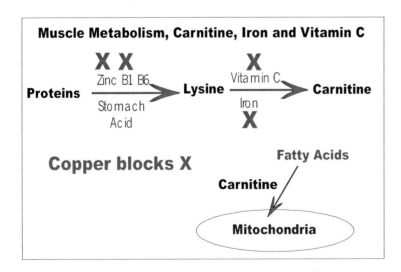

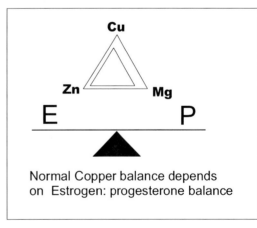

Copper leads to hypoglycaemia because of several mechanisms. Firstly it affects digestion and may impair the absorption of sugars. Secondly it causes an inappropriate rise in Insulin, which causes the blood sugar to drop. Thirdly it affects liver function and gluconeogenesis. This is where the liver makes glucose during the fasting state. The effect on insulin is part of the Syndrome X spectrum. Its relationship to Estrogen dominance is shown below. Two hormones, Estrogen and progesterone affect normal copper metabolism and balance. If total estrogens (endogenous and foreign) are high then copper is retained. This causes the Insulin level to rise and the DHEA level to fall.

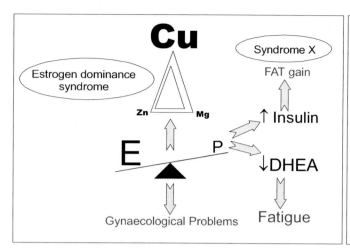

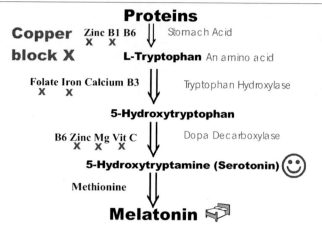

Poor sleep pattern and depression are direct results of copper blocking serotonin and melatonin production. Lastly, the effect upon thyroid function.

***Warning, after reading this section you will know more about thyroid function than any Endocrinologist in this state.***

Normal thyroid function involves the release of TSH (thyroid stimulating hormone) from the pituitary. This requires Vitamin E and Vitamin A. TSH stimulates the thyroid to release T4 (thyroxine). To make T4, the thyroid needs to get tyrosine. We get this from proteins, but we need good digestion to extract this amino acid (and Zinc, B1, B6). Then the thyroid needs Selenium, Vanadium, Vitamin C, Vitamin B2 and Iodine to make T4. To activate T4 to T3 we need Progesterone and Selenium. The effect by Copper is to destroy Vitamin E and C, promote the back conversion from T3 to T4 and block T3 in the cells. Does this show up on a blood test? No. Do the doctors believe the blood test or the patient? You guessed it.

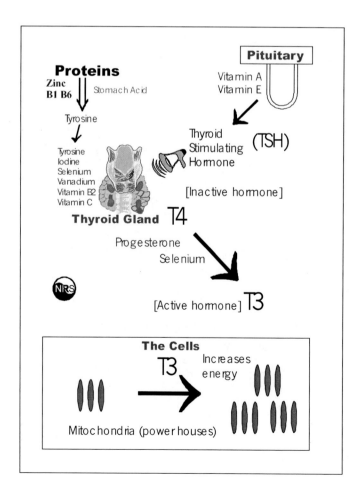

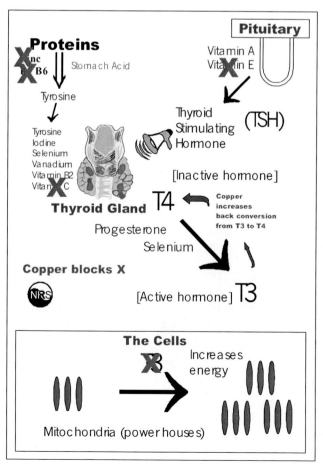

Those with high coppers find that they feel better taking supplements like Zinc, Magnesium, Vitamin C and Vitamin E. They are trying to match the disruptive effect of copper with the nutrients that copper blocks or destroy. The analogy is a railway bridge. The burden of copper is met by propping up the bridge with extra nutrients. Unfortunately, a life event such as a stress, infection, anaesthetic, pregnancy, etc depletes Zinc, Magnesium and Vitamin C and may sabotage this attempt to deal with copper in this manner. The best solution, of course, is to get rid of the copper.

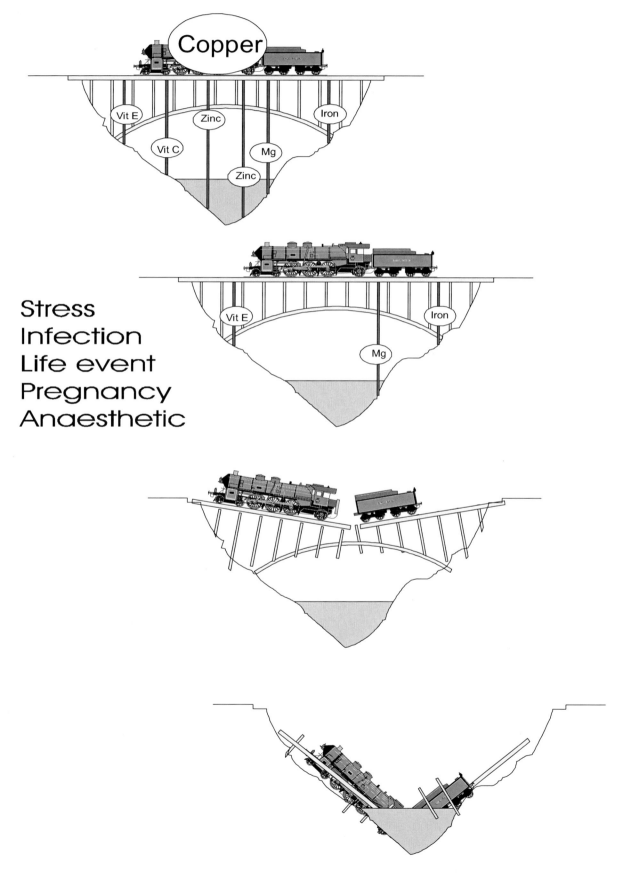

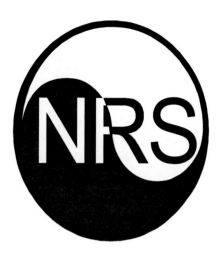

# Nutrient Charts

**How to read the Nutrient Charts**

The figure below shows what parts the graphics represent. With the specific tissue symptoms, not all patients get all the symptoms. Some symptoms may be potential problems which arise the longer the deficiency progresses.

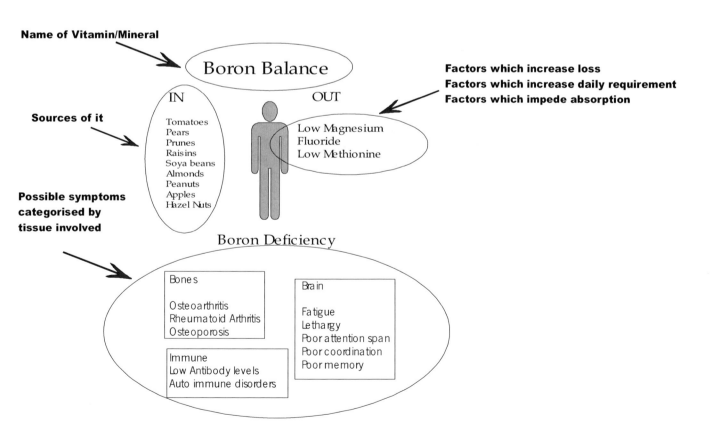

**Name of Vitamin/Mineral**

Boron Balance

**Factors which increase loss**
**Factors which increase daily requirement**
**Factors which impede absorption**

IN

OUT

**Sources of it**

Tomatoes
Pears
Prunes
Raisins
Soya beans
Almonds
Peanuts
Apples
Hazel Nuts

Low Magnesium
Fluoride
Low Methionine

**Possible symptoms categorised by tissue involved**

Boron Deficiency

Bones

Osteoarthritis
Rheumatoid Arthritis
Osteoporosis

Brain

Fatigue
Lethargy
Poor attention span
Poor coordination
Poor memory

Immune
Low Antibody levels
Auto immune disorders

# Vitamin A Balance

## IN

Apricots
Carrots
fish liver oils
Cod
Salmon
Halibut
green leafy vege
kohlrabi
liver
mint
egg yolk

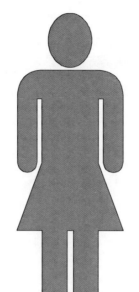

## OUT

Alcohol
diabetes
diarrhoea
gall bladder problems
pancreas problems
smoking
stress

# Vitamin A Deficiency

Serum Vitamin A < 1.0 micromol/L

Senses

Poor taste
Poor smell

Metabolic
Low cortisol
Weight loss

Bone
Poor bone growth

Immune System

Colds
Ear infections
Gastroenteritis
Thrush
Boils
Sinusitis
Delayed healing
Prolonged infections

Skin & Hair

Acne
Corneal ulcers
Sebaceous cysts
Dry eyes
Dry hair
Flaky skin

Eyes

Night blindness
Conjunctivitis
Corneal ulcers
Poor tear production

# Thiamin (Vit B1) Balance

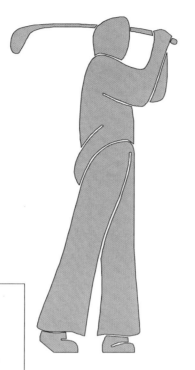

## IN
Legumes
Liver
Nuts
Pork
Wheat Germ
Whole grains
Yeast

**Needs Mg
to activate it**

## OUT
Alcohol
Coffee
Diuretics
Diarrhoea
Exercise
Pregnancy
Stress
Surgery

Destroyed
by Copper
Aluminium

## Thiamin Deficiency

Serum Thiamin < 11 nmol/L
or Red Cell Thiamin < 190 nmol/L

Brain

Poor sleep
Poor Memory
Poor balance
Nervous exhaustion
Depression
Problem with eye movements

Skin

Sweating
Burning feet

Gut
Nausea
Constipation
Abdominal pains

Muscle & Bone

Backache
Muscle weakness
Fatigue

Nerves

Numbness
Burning feet
Muscle weakness

Blood stream

Unstable blood pressure
Fluid retention

Heart

Palpitations
Fast heart rate
Shortness of breath
Enlarged heart

# Vitamin B2 Balance

## IN

Avocados
Beans
Currants
Eggs
Milk/dairy
organ meats
Sprouts
wholegrain cereals
yeast
broccoli

## OUT

Alchohol
Coffee
Diabetes
Fever
OCP
Smoking
Stress
Surgery
Thyroid disease

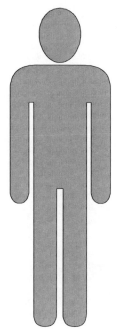

Affected by
Cadmium
Boron
Copper

## Vitamin B2 Deficiency

Eyes

Blood shot eyes
Blurred vision
Conjuctivitis
Eye fatigue
Photophobia
Cataracts

Not measurable in Aust

Nerves & Muscle

Excessive feeling of cold and pain
Weakness

Oral Cavity

Sore red lips
Sore tongue
Sore mouth
Cracks and sores on lips
Geographic tongue

Blood

Anaemia

Skin
Hair loss
Greasy scaling
Sore mouth
Seborrheic Dermatitis
Facial oiliness
Dry skin

# Vitamin B3 Balance

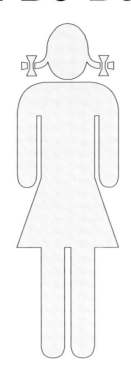

## IN

Almonds
Chicken
Legumes
Eggs
Mackerel
Meat
Peanuts
Salmon
Sardines
Sunflower seeds
yeast

## OUT

Alcohol
Coffee
Diarrhoea
Diabetes
Fever
High Cholesterol
Smoking
Ulcerative colitis

NAD & NADP affected by Aluminium

# Vitamin B3 Deficiency

Brain

Anxiety
Confusion
Depression
Fatigue
Insomnia
Headaches

Not measurable in Aust

Gut
Anorexia
Nausea
Diarrhoea
Indigestion
Vomiting

Oral Cavity

Canker sores in mouth
Sore red tongue
Sore mouth

Skin

Scaly Dermatitis

Nerves & Muscle

Fatigue
Weakness

# Vitamin B5 Balance

## IN

Avocado
Baker's yeast
Beans
brains
egg yolk
green vege
liver
lobsters
milk
mushrooms
oranges
royal jelly
sweet potato
whole grain

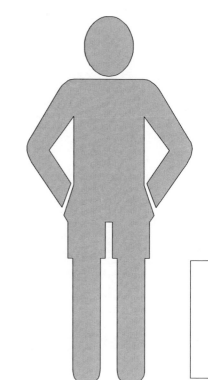

## OUT

Alcohol
Coffee
pregnancy
stress

Coenzyme A
affected by
copper

# Vitamin B5 Deficiency

Brain

Depression
Fatigue
Hyperirritability
Insomnia
Nervousness
Poor co-ordination

Not Measurable in Aust

Blood & Vessels

Low BP
Anaemia

Metabolic

Raised Cholesterol

Muscle & Joints

Fatigue
Muscle spasm
Muscle cramps

Nerves

Altered feeling in hands/feet
Tender heels

Skin & Hair

Hair loss
Dermatitis

Immune System

Increased infection

# Vitamin B6 Balance

## IN

Brewer's yeast
Cereal
Chicken
Egg yolk
Legumes
Mackerel
Oatmeal
Offal
Peanuts
Salmon
Tuna
Walnuts

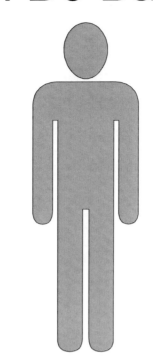

## OUT

Diabetes
coffee
tea
alcohol
pregnancy
coeliac disease

**needs Zinc and B2 to activate it**

Affected by Copper

# Vitamin B6 Deficiency

Serum < 25 nmol/L

Brain

Depression
Fatigue
Irritability
Insomnia
Poor balance
Confusion

Blood

Anaemia
Fluid retention

Kidney

Stones

Skin
Pimples
Sore mouth
Dermatitis
Facial oiliness

Muscle

Fatigue
Weakness
Carpal Tunnel Syn

Heart & Blood vessels

Abnormal ECG
Hardening of arteries

Gut

Abdominal pain
Anorexia
Nausea

# Folate Balance

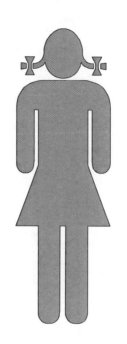

## IN

Beans
Eggs
Green leafy Vege
Lentils
Organ meats
Yeast

## OUT

Alcohol
Antibiotics
Coeliac disease
Diarrhoea
Pregnancy
Gastric Surgery

Destroyed
by Copper

# Folate Deficiency

Serum Folate < 2.2 ng/ml
Red Cell Folate < 200 ng/mL

Blood

Anaemia

Brain

Poor sleep
Poor Memory
Irritability
Apathy
Headaches
Depression
Mental sluggishness

Skin
Cracks on lips
Skin irritation

Gut

Constipation
Red tongue
Cracks on the lips

Bone & Joint

Rheumatoid arthritis
osteoporosis

Nerves & Muscle

Restless legs
Weakness

# Vitamin B12 Balance

## IN

Brain
Clams
Egg yolk
Herring
Kidney
Liver
Meat
Milk
Oysters
Salmon
Sardines

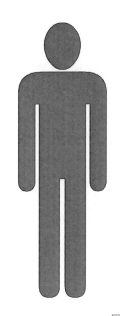

## OUT

Bacterial overgrowth
Diabetes
Coeliac disease
Alcohol
Smoking
Ulcerative colitis
Crohn's disease
Pregnancy
Gastric Surgery
Helicobacter

Coenzyme B12
blocked by copper
lead and mercury

# Vitamin B12 Deficiency

Vitamin B12 < 200 pg/ml

Joints

Bursitis

Blood

Anaemia

Mental

Paranoia
Schizophrenia
Temper outbursts
Dementia
Negative thinking
Psychosis
Violence

Skin
Brown areas over joints

Brain

Mood swings
Dizziness
Poor Memory
Irritability
Depression
Restlessness

Nerves& Muscle
Tingling in the nerves
Restlessness
Weakness

Gut

Sore tongue
Pale smooth tongue
Nausea
Diarrhoea

# Vitamin C Balance

**IN**

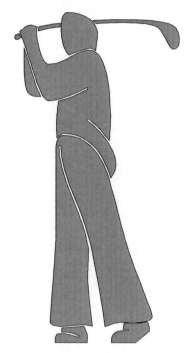

Black currant
Broccoli
citrus fruit
guava
parsley
Peppers
Pineapple
potatoes
raw cabbage
rosehips
Strawberries

**OUT**

Allergies
Antibiotics
cancer
infection
pregnancy
OCP
smoking
stress
surgery

Destroyed
by Copper
Aluminium

## Vitamin C Deficiency

Metabolic
Iron deficiency
Raised Cholesterol

< 4.0 mg/L
or
< 40 µmol/L

Bone

Soft bones

Brain

Abnormal function
Depression
Malaise
Listlessness

Lung

Asthma

Muscle & Joints

Painful joints
Weakness

Immune System

Increased infection
Prolonged infection
Poor healing

Blood vessels

Easy bruising
Raised BP
Fluid retention

Skin & Hair

Coiled hair
Bruising
Rough skin
Bleeding gums
Scurvy

# Vitamin D Balance

## IN

Sunlight
Fish liver oils
Egg yolk
milk
sprouted seeds

## OUT

Alcohol
Crohn's disease
lactation
pregnancy
ulcerative colitis

**Needs Boron to activate it**

# Vitamin D Deficiency

$< 50$ nmol/L

### Bone

Bone pain
Arthritis
Osteoporosis

### Gastrointestinal

Burning in mouth & throat
Diarrhoea

### Brain

Insomnia
Short sightedness
Nervousness
?Multiple Sclerosis

### Immune system

Frequent infections
Prolonged infections
Auto-immune disorders?

### Metabolic

Low Calcium
Glucose intolerance

# Vitamin E Balance

## IN

Almonds
beef
corn
egg yolk
nuts
safflower
sunflower
wheat germ

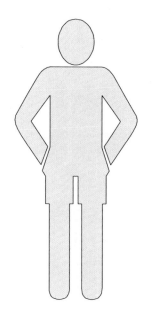

## OUT

Alcohol
coeliac disease
diabetes
lactation
liver disease
gall bladder disease
pregnancy

# Vitamin E Deficiency

Serum Vitamin E  <  18μmol/L

Destroyed
by Copper
Aluminium
Arsenic

Senses

Poor taste
Poor smell

Blood

Fluid retention
Anaemia
Sticky platelets

Metabolic

Raised Cholesterol

Immune System

Colds
Ear infections
Gastroenteritis
Thrush
Boils
Sinusitis
Delayed healing
Prolonged infections

Nerve & Muscle

Loss of reflexes
Loss position sense
Poor balance
Muscle wasting

Liver & Gall Bladder

Chronic live disease
Gall bladder cirrhosis

# Boron Balance

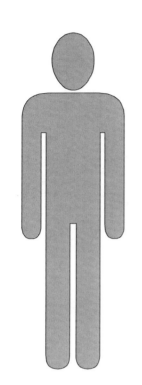

## IN

Tomatoes
Pears
Prunes
Raisins
Soya beans
Almonds
Peanuts
Apples
Hazel Nuts

## OUT

Low Magnesium
Fluoride
Low Methionine

Blocked by
Copper
Arsenic

## Boron Deficiency

Bones

Osteo Arthritis
Rheumatoid Arthritis
Osteoporosis

Brain

Fatigue
Lethargy
Poor attention span
Poor coordination
Poor memory

Immune
Low Antibody levels
Auto immune disorders

# Calcium Balance

## IN

Almonds
dairy products
egg yolk
green leafy vege
molasses
sardines
soyabeans

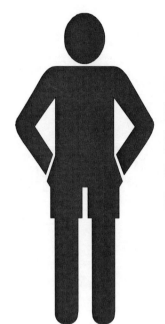

## OUT

High phosphate intake
high protein intake
lack of exercise
magnesium deficiency
pregnancy

Blocked
by Lead

# Calcium Deficiency

Corrected Serum calcium < 2.15 mmol/L
Ionised calcium < 1.14 mmol/L

Heart & Blood Vessels

Palpitations
Irregular heart rate
Raised BP

Nerves

Numbness
tingling

Muscle & Bone

Muscle spasm
Cramps
Tetany
Soft bones
Soft teeth

Skin & Nails

Brittle nails
Eczema

Brain

Agitation
Cognitive impairment
Depression
Hyperactivity
Insomnia

# Chromium Balance

## IN
Asparagus
cheese
egg yolk
grape juice
liver
lobster&prawns
molasses
mushrooms
nuts
oysters
pepper
prunes
raisins
wheat
yeast

## OUT

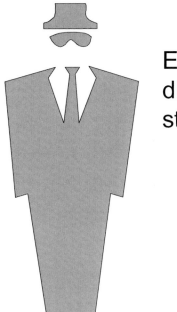

Excess refined foods
diabetes
strenuous exercise

Blocked
by Lead

# Chromium Deficiency

Deficiency if < 6 nmol/L

Brain

Anxiety
Poor balance
Fatigue

Heart & Vessels
Atherosclerosis
Heart disease

Metabolism

Raised sugar
Raised insulin levels
Impaired glucose tolerance
Raised cholesterol

Nerves

Loss of feeling in hands/feet

# Copper Balance

## IN

Almonds
beans
crab
lamb
mushrooms
oysters
pecans
perch
pork
prunes
sunflower seeds
wholegrain

## OUT

Alcohol
pregnancy
excessive sugar intake

# Copper Deficiency

Plasma Copper < 11µmol/L

| | | |
|---|---|---|
| **Hair**<br><br>Hair loss<br>Grey hair | **Lung**<br><br>Emphysema<br>Chest infections | **Metabolic**<br><br>Raised Cholesterol<br>Raised uric acid |

| | | |
|---|---|---|
| **Blood**<br>Anaemia<br>Low White cell count | **Brain**<br><br>Depression<br>Hyperaccusis<br>Loss of white matter<br>Reduced dopamine<br>Reduced noradrenaline<br>Reduced enkephalin<br>Poor coordination | **Immune System**<br><br>Colds<br>Ear infections<br>Gastroenteritis<br>Thrush<br>Boils<br>Sinusitis<br>Delayed healing<br>Prolonged infections |

**Infertility**

Spontaneous abortion
Still births

# Copper Balance

## IN

Almonds
beans
crab
lamb
mushrooms
oysters
pecans
perch
pork
prunes
sunflower seeds
tap water
whole grains

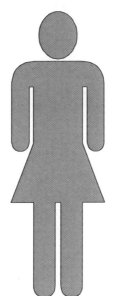

## OUT

Vitamin C
Zinc
Molybdenum
Cysteine
Glutamine
Histidine
Threonine

## Copper Excess

### Brain

Headaches

**Pattern 1:**
Anxiety "worrier"
Agitation
Depression
Insomnia

**Pattern 2:**
Constantly needs
reassurance
"Emotional"
"Hypochondria"

**Pattern 3:**
Surly
Aggressive
Pushy
Beligerent

### Hair

Hair loss
Grey hair
Early greying

### Joints
Arthritis

### Blood
Anaemia
Iron deficiency

### Metabolic

Fatigue
Osteoporosis
Raised Cholesterol
Syndrome X
Hypoglycaemia
Hormone imbalance
Thyroid dysfunction

### Liver
Fatty Liver
Impaired liver function
Sluggish bile
Gallstones

### Gastric Tract
Gastritis
Constipation
Salicylate Intolerance

### Immune System

Viral infections
Fungal infections
Delayed healing
Prolonged infections

### Skin
Flushing
Red skin
Allergies
Rashes
Easy bruising

# Iron Balance

## IN

Apricots
Clams
Beef
Liver
Oysters
Parsley
Pine nuts
Soya beans
Sunflower seeds
Pumpkin seeds
Wheat germ
Yeast

## OUT

Menstrual Fluid
Pregnancy
Faeces
Hemorrhoids
Stomach Ulcers
Blood Noses
Recurrent bruising
Molybdenum deficiency

## Iron Deficiency

Ferritin $< 30\,\mu\,mol/L$

Blocked
by Copper
Mercury
Lead

Marrow

Anaemia

Gynaecological
Heavy Periods

Immune System

Sinusitis
Ear infections
Colds
Thrush
Chronic Herpes
Mouth ulcers

Lung

Breathing difficulties

Skin

Generalised itching
Cracked corners of the mouth
Sore tongue
Brittle nails
Thrush
Hair loss
Mouth ulcers
Pimples/acne

Brain

Disrupted sleep
Dizziness
Headaches
Fatigue
Depression
Restless legs

Muscle

Fatigue on exertion
Restless legs

# Magnesium Balance

## IN
Almonds
Cashews
Cocoa
Mineral Water
Molasses
Parsnips
~~Soyabeans~~
Wholegrain Cereals
Tap water *

\* Low levels of magnesium
in ground water in Perth

## OUT
Sweating
Urine (increased by
Alcohol and coffee)
Stress
The pill
HRT
Pregnancy
Diuretics,
ACE inhibitors
Beta blockers

Blocked by
Cadmium
High Copper

# Magnesium Deficiency

Plasma Magnesium < 0.7 mmol/L or Red Cell Magnesium < 2.3 mmol/L
or Red Cell Magnesium < 6.0 µ mol/gHb

## Heart
Palpitations
Rapid Pulse
Spasm of Arteries
Cold hands/feet
Fluid retention
Shortness of breath
Exertional Chest Pain

## Mouth & Gullet
Mouth ulcers
Sore tongue
Gullent spasm
Swallowing problem

## Abdomen
Intestinal cramp
Uterine cramp
Painful periods
Biliary colic
Constipation

Urinary frequency
Nocturia
Bladder spasm
Kidney stones

## Sleep
Unrefreshed Sleep
Insomnia

## Brain
Anxiety
Agitation
Irritability
Dizziness
Headaches
Depression
Seizures
Poor Concentration

### Ear
Tinnitus
Vertigo

## Lung
Persistent dry cough
Post Viral Cough
Exertional wheeze
Asthma
cold/Flu induced Asthma

## Nerves
Reduced pain threshold
Chronic pain
Tremor of hands
Carpal tunnel syndrome
Sensitivity to sound

## Metabolic
Low Temperature
Unstable Blood Sugar
Fatigue
Osteoporosis

## Blood Vessels
Raised BP
Unstable BP

## Muscle
Muscle pain
Easy fatigue
Twitching
Leg Cramps
Muscle weakness
Uterine cramp
Intestinal cramp
Blurred vision

# Manganese Balance

## IN
Almonds
beans
coconuts
corn
kelp
liver
olives
pecans
pineapple
fruit juice
sunflower seeds
walnuts

## OUT

Diabetes
pregnancy

Blocked
by Lead
copper

# Manganese Deficiency

Deficiency if < 0.11μmol/l

Brain

Poor balance
Dizziness
Seizures
Poor concentration
Poor cognitive function

Joints
Arthritis

Hearing

Loss of hearing
Tinnitis

Heart & Vessels

Atherosclerosis

Metabolism

Fatigue
Glucose intolerance
Raised cholesterol
Diabetes

Skin

Dermatitis
Reduced growth hair & nails

# Molybdenum Balance

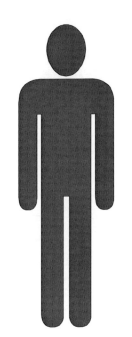

## IN

Beans &peas
butter
kidney
lamb
legumes & lentils
lima beans
liver
oats
pork
soyabeans
sunflower seeds
wheat germ

## OUT

High protein diets
Fluoride in water
Low Zinc
High Copper

Blocked
by Lead
Copper

## Molybdenum Deficiency

| | | | |
|---|---|---|---|
| Lung<br><br>Asthma | Immune<br><br>Fungal infections<br>Yeast infections<br>GIT cancers<br>Breast cancer | **Brain**<br>Anxiety<br>Irritability<br>Insomnia | Heart<br><br>Rapid heart rate |

Blood

Anaemia

Metabolic

Fatigue
Weight gain
Copper Excess
Zinc Deficiency

Gut

Digestive problems
Gullet cancer
Stomach cancer
Nausea
Vomiting
Colon cancer.

Nerves

Night blindness
Headache

Joints

Gout

Allergy

Increased sensitivity to sulphites
Sensitivity to sulphur foods

# Selenium Balance

## IN

Alfalfa
brazil nuts& cashews
crab
eggs
fish
garlic
human breast milk
liver
mackeral
oysters
peanuts
tuna
wholegrain
yeast

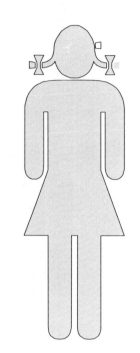

## OUT

alcohol
pregnancy
smoking
vitamin C deficiency

Blocked by
Mercury
Arsenic Cadmium
Aluminium

## Selenium Deficiency

$<0.6 \ \mu mol/L$

Heart
Heart disease
Cardiomyopathy

Lung

Asthma

Joints

Arthritis

Brain
Depression

Immune system

Increased infections
Autoimmune diseases
Cancer

Metabolism

Low thyroid
Raised cholesterol
Diabetes

# Zinc Balance

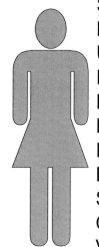

## IN

* Zinc deficient soils create zinc deficient cows

Milk *
Beef *
Liver *
Herring
Oysters
Sunflower seeds
Pumpkin seeds
Ginger
Whole grains
Yeast

## OUT

Sweating
Menstrual Fluid
Urine (increased by Food Colouring 102)
Pregnancy
Breast feeding
Faeces
Diuretics, ACE Inhibitors
Stress & Anaesthetics
OCP & HRT
Vitamin B6 deficiency

NRS

Blocked by
Mercury
Cadmium
High Copper

# Zinc Deficiency

Plasma Zinc < 11 µmol/L or
Red Cell Zinc < 200 µmol/L

### Skin

Dermatitis
Dry Skin
Eczema
Warts
Psoriasis
Pimples
Hair loss
Tinea
Thrush
Stretch Marks

### Low Stomach Acid
Salicylate Intolerance

### Allergy
Hay fever
Runny nose
Itchy skin

### Joints
Joint pain
Joint stiffness

### Sexual Function
Loss of libido
Infertility
Missed periods

### Metabolic
Raised Cholesterol
Low Sugar 3 hours after meals
Alcohol intolerance

### Hair & Nails
Brittle nails
Hair Loss
Early Greying

### Brain

Disrupted sleep
Poor Memory
Moodiness
Depression
Poor coping with stress
Temper outbursts

### Immune System
Frequent sore throats
Colds & Sinusitis
Ear infections
Gastroenteritis
Thrush
Boils/pimples
Delayed healing
Prolonged infections
Conjunctivitis
Low White cell count

### Lung

Asthma
Bronchitis
Pneumonia
Chest infections

### Children
Hyper activity
Fidgeting
Pre-dinner tantrums

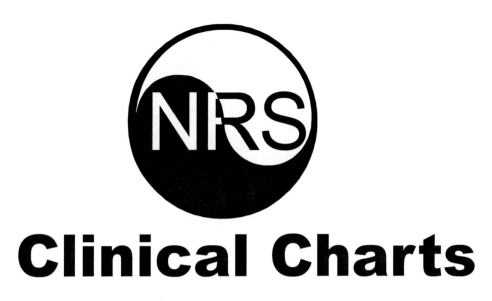

# Clinical Charts

**How to read the Clinical Problem Charts**

The figure below shows a typical clinical problem. Think of the rows as a shopping list that tissues that manage joints would like the body to supply. Conversely think of the columns as a list of things which the tissue does not want too much of.

Some symptoms will occur even if levels are normal, if there is an antagonist to the nutrient (so-called anti-nutrients). With regards to the B-Vitamins, both low levels and failure to be activated equate to the same tissue problem. Biochemistry occurs in the tissues, not the blood; so don't rely on blood for your answers.

**Nutrients needed for arthritis prevention**

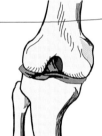

# Say arthritis is the clinical problem

Basic Anti-nutrient List

| | Copper block | Cadmium Block | Mercury Block | Arsenic Block | Lead Block | Aluminium Block | Antimony Block |
|---|---|---|---|---|---|---|---|
| Magnesium | X | X | | | | | |
| Boron | X | | | X | | | |
| Zinc | X | X | X | X | | X | X |
| Molybdenum | X | | | | X | | |
| Selenium | X | X | X | X | | X | X |
| Calcium | | | | | X | | |
| Manganese | X | | | | X | | |
| Vitamin D | | | | X | | | |
| Vitamin C | X | | | | | X | |

Basic Nutrient list

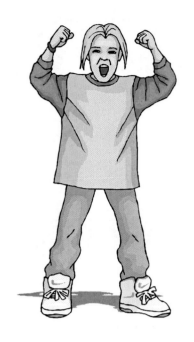

## Proteins

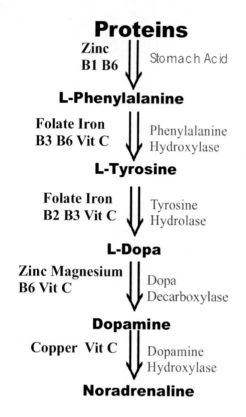

Zinc
B1 B6 — Stomach Acid

**L-Phenylalanine**

Folate Iron
B3 B6 Vit C — Phenylalanine Hydroxylase

**L-Tyrosine**

Folate Iron
B2 B3 Vit C — Tyrosine Hydrolase

**L-Dopa**

Zinc Magnesium
B6 Vit C — Dopa Decarboxylase

**Dopamine**

Copper  Vit C — Dopamine Hydroxylase

**Noradrenaline**

# Nutrients important for prevention of ADD ADHD

| | Copper block | Cadmium Block | Mercury Block | Arsenic Block | Lead Block | Aluminium Block | Antimony Block |
|---|---|---|---|---|---|---|---|
| Vitamin C | X | | | | | X | X |
| Iron | X | | X | | X | | |
| Zinc | X | X | X | | | X | X |
| Magnesium | X | X | | | | | |
| Folate | X | | | | | | |
| B2 & B3 | | | | | | | |
| B1 & B6 | X | | | | | X | |

185

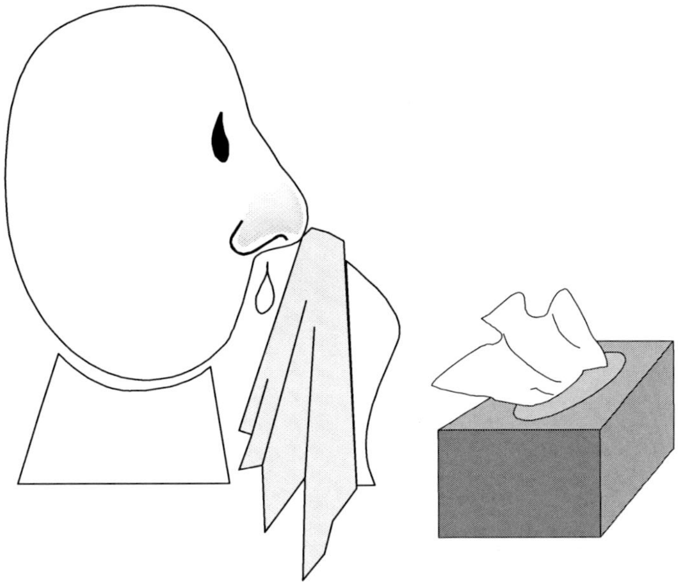

# Nutrients needed for allergy prevention

| | Copper block | Cadmium Block | Mercury Block | Arsenic Block | Lead Block | Aluminium Block | Antimony Block |
|---|---|---|---|---|---|---|---|
| Zinc | X | X | | | | X | X |
| Molybdenum | X | | | | X | | |
| Selenium | | X | X | X | | X | X |
| Vitamin C | X | | | | | X | |
| Vitamin E | X | | | X | | X | |

## Factors involved with Allergies

1. Low Zinc
2. High Copper
3. Low Zinc:Copper ratio
4. Low Molybdenum
5. Low Vitamin C
6. Digestive problems
7. Helicobacter stomach infection
8. Candida overgrowth
9. Hormone imbalance

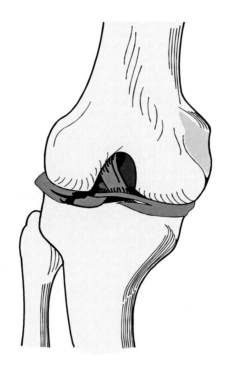

# Nutrients needed for arthritis prevention

|  | Copper block | Cadmium Block | Mercury Block | Arsenic Block | Lead Block | Aluminium Block | Antimony Block |
|---|---|---|---|---|---|---|---|
| Magnesium | X | X |  |  |  |  |  |
| Boron | X |  |  |  |  |  |  |
| Zinc | X | X | X | X |  | X | X |
| Molybdenum | X |  |  |  | X |  |  |
| Selenium | X | X | X | X |  | X | X |
| Calcium |  |  |  |  | X |  |  |
| Manganese | X |  |  |  | X |  |  |
| Vitamin D |  |  |  |  |  |  |  |
| Vitamin C | X |  |  |  |  | X |  |

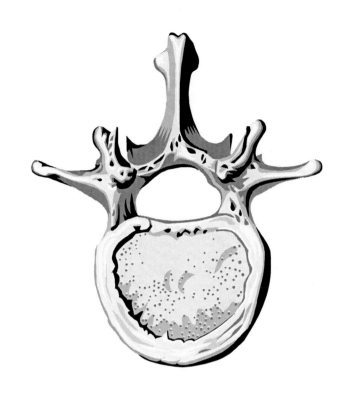

# Nutrients needed for correct bone density

| | Copper block | Cadmium Block | Mercury Block | Arsenic Block | Lead Block | Aluminium Block | Antimony Block |
|---|---|---|---|---|---|---|---|
| Magnesium | X | X | | | | | |
| Boron | X | | | | | | |
| Zinc | X | X | X | X | | X | X |
| Potasssium | | | | | | X | |
| Molybdenum | X | | X | X | X | X | |
| Calcium | | | | | X | | |
| Manganese | X | | | | X | | |
| Phosphorus | | | | | | X | |
| Vitamin D | | | | | | | |
| Vitamin C | X | | | | | X | |
| Parathyroid hormone | | | | | | | |
| Progesterone | | | | | | | |

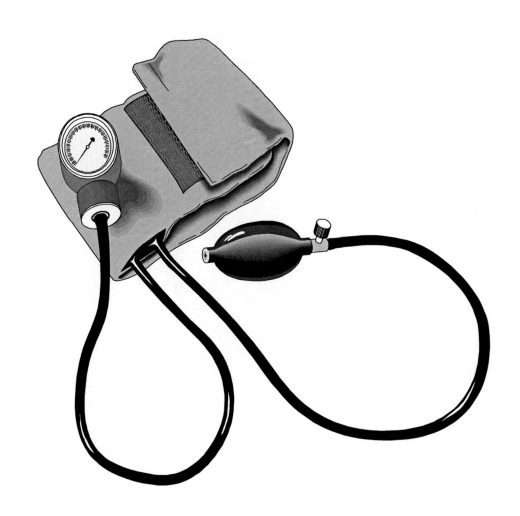

# Nutrients needed for correct Blood pressure control

| | Copper block | Cadmium Block | Mercury Block | Arsenic Block | Lead Block | Aluminium Block | Antimony Block |
|---|---|---|---|---|---|---|---|
| Magnesium | X | X | | | | | |
| Potassium | | | | | | | |
| Calcium | | | | | X | | |
| Selenium | | X | X | X | | X | X |
| Vitamin A | | | | | | | |
| Vitamin D | | | | | | | |
| Vitamin C | X | | | | | | |

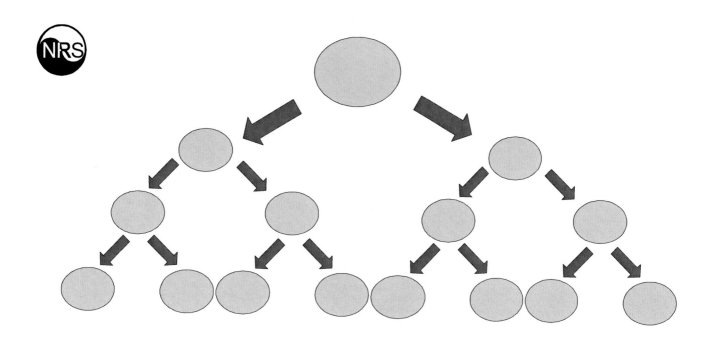

# Nutrients needed for cancer prevention

|  | Copper block | Cadmium Block | Mercury Block | Arsenic Block | Lead Block | Aluminium Block | Antimony Block |
|---|---|---|---|---|---|---|---|
| Magnesium | X | X | | | | | |
| Zinc | X | X | X | | | X | X |
| Molybdenum | X | | | | X | | |
| Selenium | | X | X | X | | X | X |
| Iron | X | | X | | X | | |
| Vitamin D | | | | | | | |
| Vitamin C | X | | | | | X | |
| Vitamin E | X | | X | X | | X | |
| Folic acid | X | | | | | X | |
| Progesterone | | | | | | | |
| DHEA | X | | | | | | |

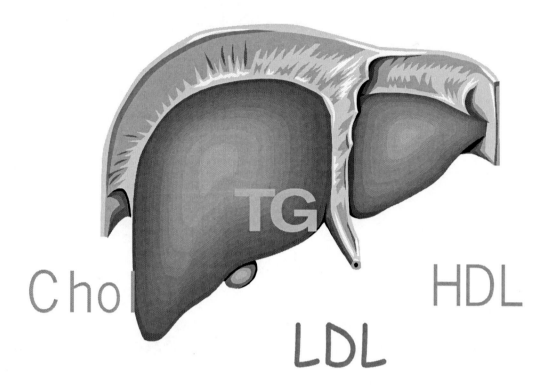

# Nutrients needed for correct Cholesterol control

| | Copper block | Cadmium Block | Mercury Block | Arsenic Block | Lead Block | Aluminium Block | Antimony Block |
|---|---|---|---|---|---|---|---|
| Manganese | X | | | | X | | |
| Chromium | | | | | X | | |
| Zinc | X | X | X | | | X | X |
| Selenium | | X | X | X | | X | X |
| Molybdenum | X | | | | X | | |
| Vitamin B3 | X | | | | | | |
| Vitamin B5 | X | | | | | | |
| Vitamin C | X | | | | | X | |
| Vitamin E | X | | | X | | X | |

# Nutrients needed for correct digestion

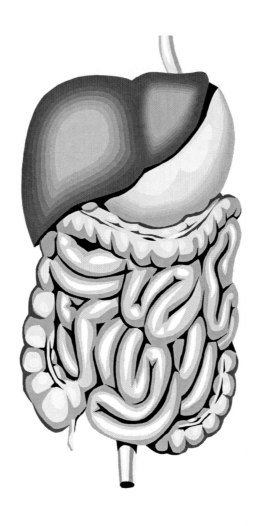

| | Copper block | Cadmium Block | Mercury Block | Arsenic Block | Lead Block | Aluminium Block |
|---|---|---|---|---|---|---|
| Zinc | X | X | X | | | X |
| Magnesium | X | X | | | | |
| Vitamin B1 | X | | | | | X |
| Vitamin B6 | X | | | | | |
| Molybdenum | X | | | | X | |
| Glutamine | | | | | | |

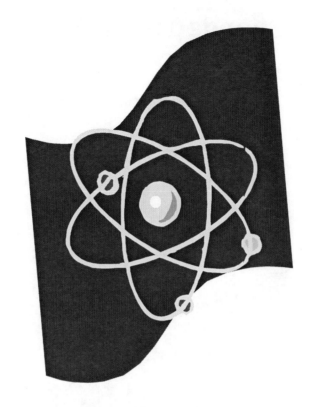

# Nutrients needed for correct Energy balance

|  | Copper block | Cadmium Block | Mercury Block | Arsenic Block | Lead Block | Aluminium Block | Antimony Block |
|---|---|---|---|---|---|---|---|
| Magnesium | X | X |  |  |  |  |  |
| Iron | X |  | X |  | X |  |  |
| Zinc | X | X | X |  |  | X | X |
| Co Enzyme Q10 | X |  | X | X |  | X |  |
| Vitamin C | X |  |  |  |  |  |  |
| B Vitamins | X |  |  |  |  | X |  |
| Carnitine | X |  | X |  | X | X | X |

193

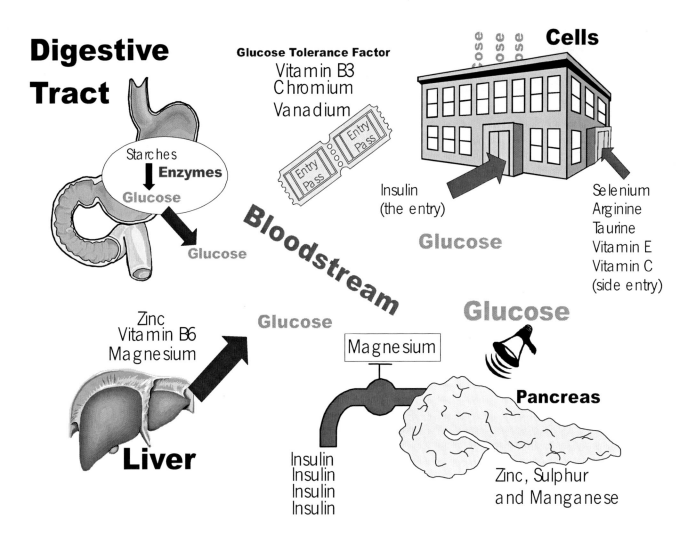

**Digestive Tract**

Starches
**Enzymes**
Glucose

Glucose

**Glucose Tolerance Factor**
Vitamin B3
Chromium
Vanadium

Entry Pass
Entry Pass

**Cells**

Glucose Glucose Glucose

Insulin
(the entry)

Glucose

Selenium
Arginine
Taurine
Vitamin E
Vitamin C
(side entry)

Zinc
Vitamin B6
Magnesium

**Bloodstream**

Glucose

**Liver**

Glucose

Magnesium

Insulin
Insulin
Insulin
Insulin

**Pancreas**

Zinc, Sulphur
and Manganese

# Nutrients needed for glucose control

| | Copper block | Cadmium Block | Mercury Block | Arsenic Block | Lead Block | Aluminium Block | Antimony Block |
|---|---|---|---|---|---|---|---|
| Zinc | X | X | X | | | X | X |
| Magnesium | X | X | | | | | |
| Selenium | | X | X | X | X | X | X |
| Manganese | X | | | | X | | |
| Sulphur | | X | X | X | X | | |
| Chromium | | | | | | | |
| Vanadium | | | | | | | |
| Vitamin C | X | | | | | | |
| Vitamin E | X | | | X | | X | |

194

# Nutrients needed for correct Heart function

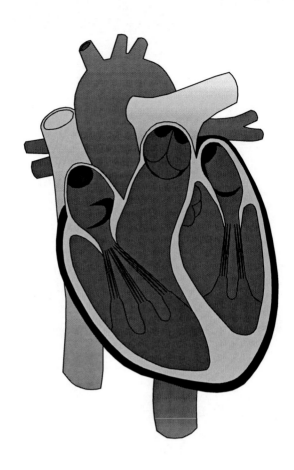

| | Copper block | Cadmium Block | Mercury Block | Arsenic Block | Lead Block | Aluminium Block |
|---|:---:|:---:|:---:|:---:|:---:|:---:|
| Magnesium | X | X | | | | |
| Iron | X | | X | | X | |
| Potassium | | | | | | X |
| Calcium | | | | | X | |
| Selenium | | X | X | X | | X |
| Co Enzyme Q10 | X | | | | | X |
| Vitamin C | X | | | | | X |
| Carnitine | X | | X | | X | X |

# Nutrients needed for lung function

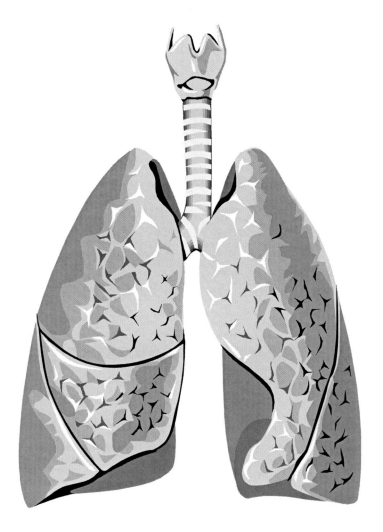

|  | Copper block | Cadmium Block | Mercury Block | Arsenic Block | Lead Block | Aluminium Block |
|---|---|---|---|---|---|---|
| Zinc | X | X | X |  |  | X |
| Magnesium | X | X |  |  |  |  |
| Vitamin C | X |  |  |  |  | X |
| Molybdenum | X |  |  |  | X |  |
| Selenium |  | X | X | X |  | X |
| Iron | X |  | X |  | X |  |
| Vitamin E | X |  |  | X |  | X |

# Nutrients needed for correct mood

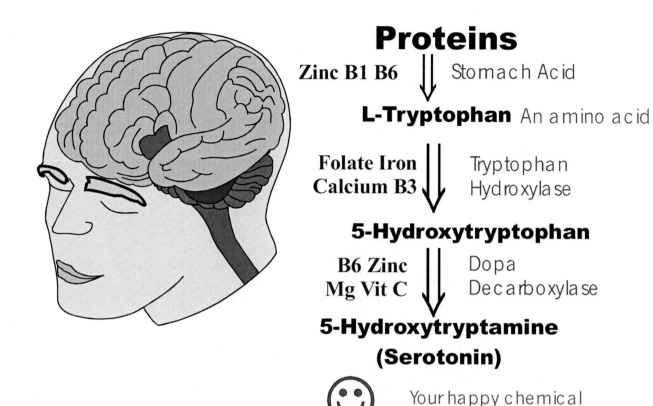

## Proteins
Zinc B1 B6 ⬇ Stomach Acid

**L-Tryptophan** An amino acid

Folate Iron
Calcium B3 ⬇ Tryptophan Hydroxylase

## 5-Hydroxytryptophan

B6 Zinc
Mg Vit C ⬇ Dopa Decarboxylase

## 5-Hydroxytryptamine (Serotonin)

☺ Your happy chemical

|  | Copper block | Cadmium Block | Mercury Block | Arsenic Block | Lead Block | Aluminium Block |
|---|---|---|---|---|---|---|
| Magnesium | X | X |  |  |  |  |
| Iron | X |  | X |  | X |  |
| Zinc | X | X | X |  |  | X |
| Calcium |  |  |  |  | X |  |
| Selenium |  | X | X | X |  | X |
| Vitamin C | X |  |  |  |  | X |
| Vitamin B1 | X |  |  |  |  | X |
| Folic acid | X |  |  |  |  |  |
| Vitamin B12 | X |  | X |  | X |  |

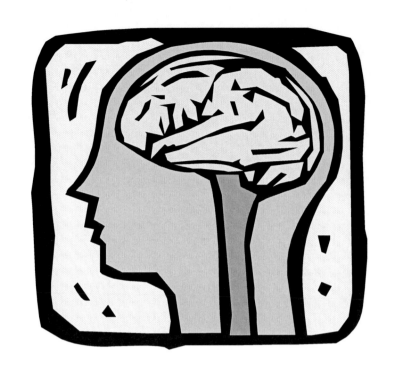

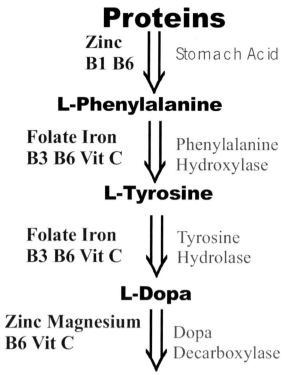

**Proteins**

Zinc
B1 B6 → Stomach Acid

**L-Phenylalanine**

Folate Iron
B3 B6 Vit C → Phenylalanine Hydroxylase

**L-Tyrosine**

Folate Iron
B3 B6 Vit C → Tyrosine Hydrolase

**L-Dopa**

Zinc Magnesium
B6 Vit C → Dopa Decarboxylase

**Dopamine**

# Nutrients important for prevention of Parkinson's disease

| | Copper block | Cadmium Block | Mercury Block | Arsenic Block | Lead Block | Aluminium Block | Antimony Block |
|---|---|---|---|---|---|---|---|
| Vitamin C | X | | | | | X | X |
| Iron | X | | X | | X | | |
| Zinc | X | X | X | | | X | X |
| Magnesium | X | X | | | | | |
| Folate | X | | | | | | |
| B2 & B3 | | | | | | | |
| B1 & B6 | X | | | | | X | |
| Melatonin | X | X | X | | X | X | X |

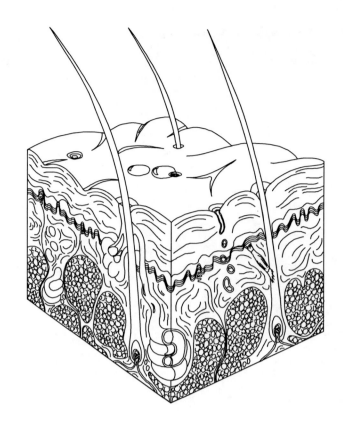

# Nutrients needed for correct skin function

| | Copper block | Cadmium Block | Mercury Block | Arsenic Block | Lead Block | Aluminium Block | Antimony Block |
|---|---|---|---|---|---|---|---|
| Zinc | X | X | X | | | X | X |
| Iron | X | | X | | | | |
| Calcium | | | | | X | | |
| Selenium | | X | X | X | | X | X |
| Sulphur | | X | X | X | X | | |
| Vitamin A | | | | | | | |
| Chromium | | | | | X | | |
| Vitamin C | X | | | | | X | |
| Vitamin B5 | | | | | | | |
| Vitamin E | X | | | X | | X | |

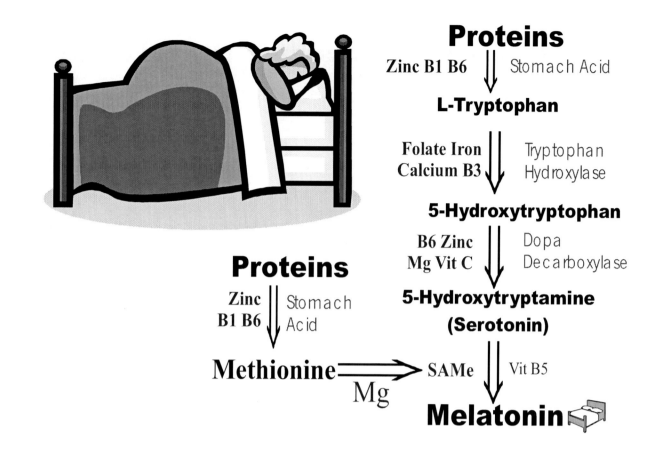

# Nutrients needed for correct sleep

| | Copper block | Cadmium Block | Mercury Block | Arsenic Block | Lead Block | Aluminium Block | Antimony Block |
|---|---|---|---|---|---|---|---|
| Magnesium | X | X | | | | | |
| Iron | X | | X | | X | | |
| Zinc | X | X | X | | | X | X |
| Calcium | | | | | X | | |
| Vitamin C | X | | | | | X | |
| Vitamin B1 | X | | | | | X | |
| Folic acid | X | | | | | | |
| Vitamin B12 | | | X | | X | | |
| Melatonin | X | X | X | | X | X | X |
| SAMe | X | X | | | | | |

# Nutrients needed for correct Thyroid function

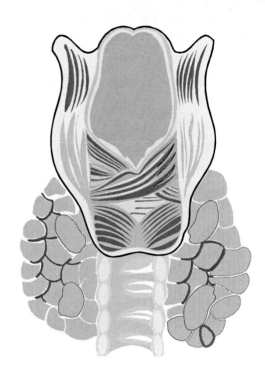

| | Copper block | Cadmium Block | Mercury Block | Arsenic Block | Lead Block | Aluminium Block | Antimony Block |
|---|---|---|---|---|---|---|---|
| Tyrosine | | | | | | | |
| Iodine | | | | | | | |
| Selenium | | X | X | X | | X | X |
| Iron | X | | X | | X | | |
| Copper | | X | | | | | |
| Vanadium | | | | | | | |
| Vitamin C | X | | | | | X | |
| B 2 | X | | | | | X | |
| Progesterone | | | | | | | |
| Vitamin A | | | | | | | |
| Vitamin E | X | | | X | | | |

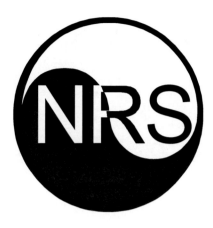

# Process Charts

About the process charts.

They are visual aids such as digestion and biochemical pathways.

## Scope of Agriculture

| Raw Materials | Production | Produce | Consumption |
|---|---|---|---|
| Oxygen<br>Nitrogen<br>Carbon<br>Minerals<br>Water | Pest control<br>→<br>Growth accelerators | 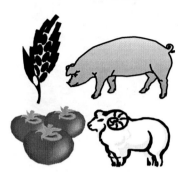 | 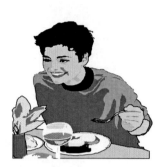 |

# Food

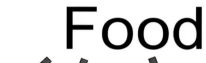

**GUT**

AA's    Mineral    Vitamins    Sugars

**Intestinal wall**

AA's    Mineral    Vitamins    Sugars

**BLOOD**

AA's    Mineral    Vitamins    Sugars

**Cell wall**

AA's    Mineral    Vitamins    Sugars

**Cells**

# Consequences of poor digestion

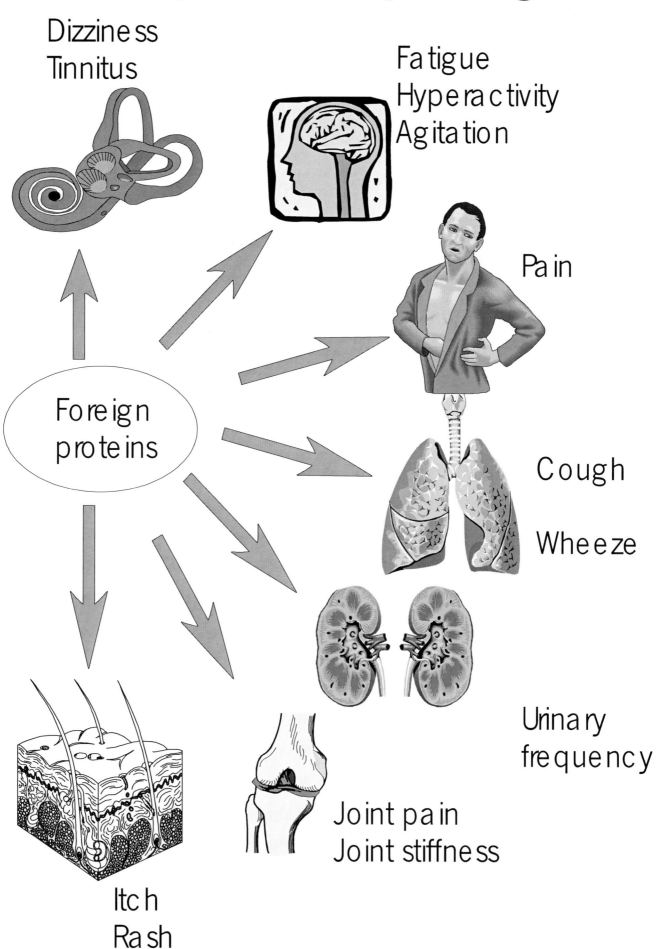

Dizziness
Tinnitus

Fatigue
Hyperactivity
Agitation

Pain

Foreign proteins

Cough

Wheeze

Urinary frequency

Itch
Rash

Joint pain
Joint stiffness

# Mitochondrial Energy Pathway

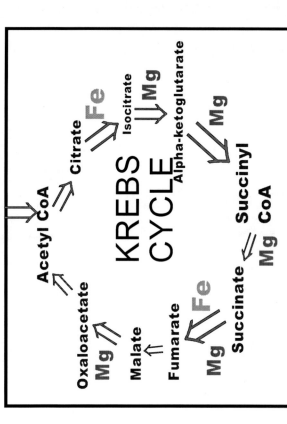

Coenzyme Q10

Cytochrome c

Cyto c

Iron

CoQ₁,₀

Copper

Sulphur
Iron

Sulphur
Iron

Sulphur
Iron

Mg

ATP synthase

**ATP**

Complex I
NADH
dehydrogenase

Complex III
Cytochrome b-c₁

Complex IV
Cytochrome oxidase

**Pyruvate**

KREBS CYCLE

Acetyl CoA

Citrate

Fe

Isocitrate

Mg

Alpha-ketoglutarate

Mg

Succinyl
Mg CoA

Succinate

Fe

Fumarate

Mg

Malate

Mg

Oxaloacetate

# D-glucose

**Mg**

Hexokinase/glucokinase

## Glucose-6-phosphate

Phosphoglucose isomerase

## Fructose-6-phosphate

**Mg K**

Phosphofructokinase-1

## Fructose-1,6-biphosphate

Aldolase

## Glyceraldehyde-3-phosphate

**B3**

Gylceraldehyde-3-phosphate dehydrogenase

## 1,3 biphosphoglycerate

**Mg**

Phosphoglycerate kinase

## 3- phosphoglycerate

**Mg**

Phosphoglycero mutase

## 2- phosphoglycerate

**Mg or Mn**

Enolase

## Phosphoenolpyruvate

**Mg**

Pyruvate kinase

# Pyruvate

# Metallic ions & Energy

# How to make Coenzyme Q10

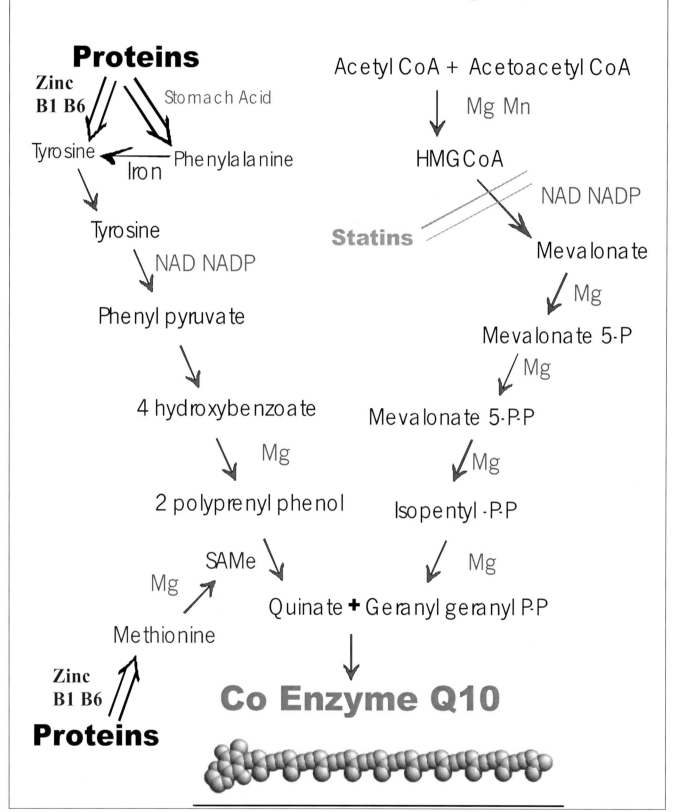

**Proteins**

Zinc
B1 B6

Stomach Acid

Tyrosine ← Phenylalanine

Iron

Tyrosine

NAD NADP

Phenyl pyruvate

4 hydroxybenzoate

Mg

2 polyprenyl phenol

SAMe

Mg

Methionine

Zinc
B1 B6

**Proteins**

Acetyl CoA + Acetoacetyl CoA

Mg Mn

HMG CoA

NAD NADP

**Statins**

Mevalonate

Mg

Mevalonate 5-P

Mg

Mevalonate 5-P-P

Mg

Isopentyl -P-P

Mg

Quinate + Geranyl geranyl P-P

**Co Enzyme Q10**

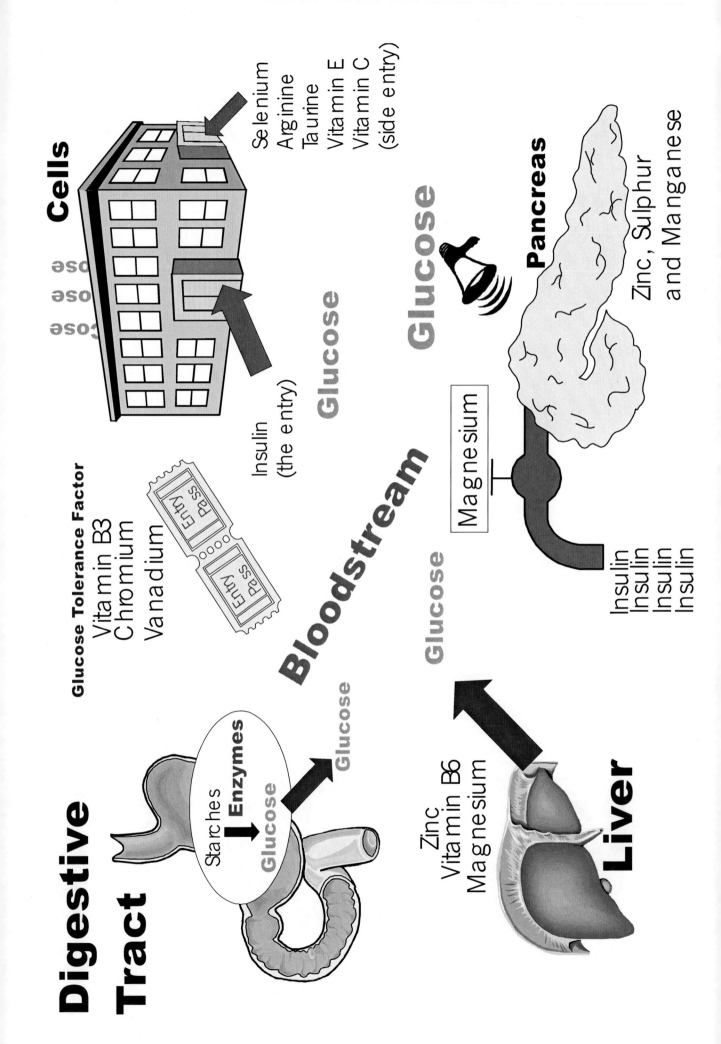

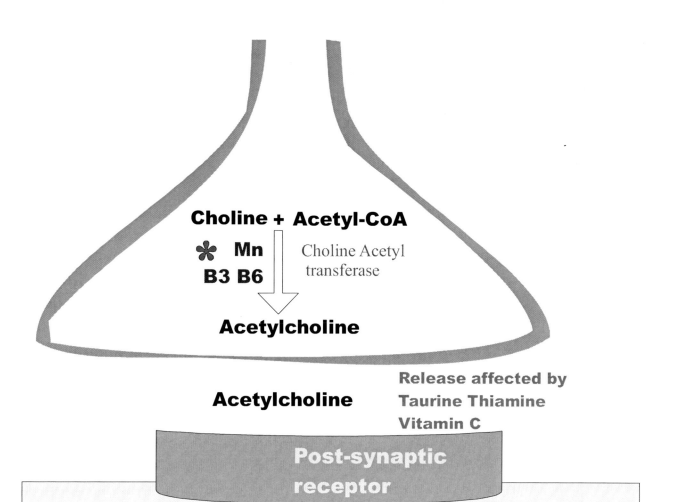

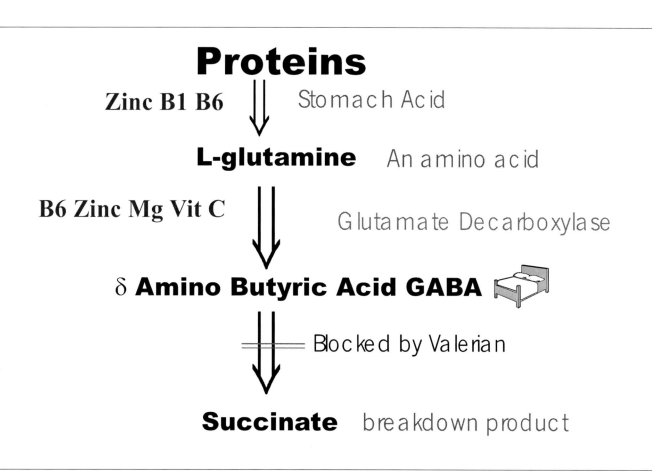

# Proteins

**Zinc**
**B1 B6**          Stomach Acid

↓↓

**L-Phenylalanine** An amino acid

**Folate Iron**          Phenylalanine
**B3 B6 Vit C**          Hydroxylase

↓↓

**L-Tyrosine** An amino acid

**Folate Iron**          Tyrosine Hydrolase
**B2 B3 Vit C**

↓↓

**L-Dopa**

**Zinc Magnesium**          Dopa Decarboxylase
**B6 Vit C**

↓↓

**Dopamine**

**Copper  Vit C**          Dopamine  Hydroxylase

↓↓

**Noradrenaline**

                              Phenylethanolamine
**SAM Mn P**          N-methyl transferase
**B5 Folate**

↓↓

**Adrenalin**

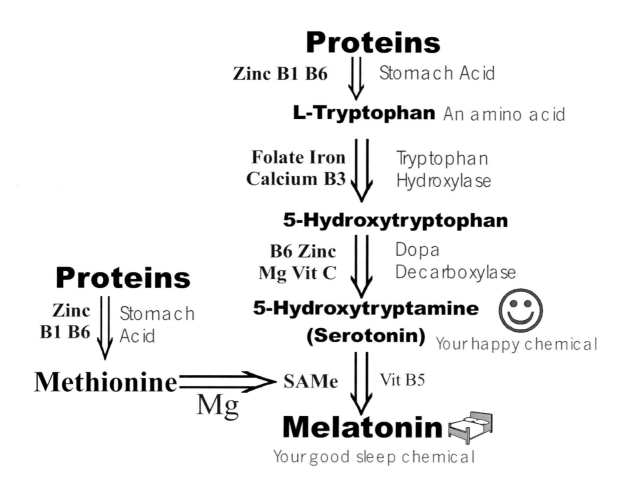

**Proteins**

Zinc B1 B6 ⇓ Stomach Acid

**L-Tryptophan** An amino acid

**Folate Iron Calcium B3** ⇓ Tryptophan Hydroxylase

**5-Hydroxytryptophan**

**B6 Zinc Mg Vit C** ⇓ Dopa Decarboxylase

**5-Hydroxytryptamine (Serotonin)** ☺ Your happy chemical

**Proteins**

Zinc B1 B6 ⇓ Stomach Acid

**Methionine** ⟹ SAMe ⇓ Vit B5

Mg

**Melatonin** 🛏 Your good sleep chemical

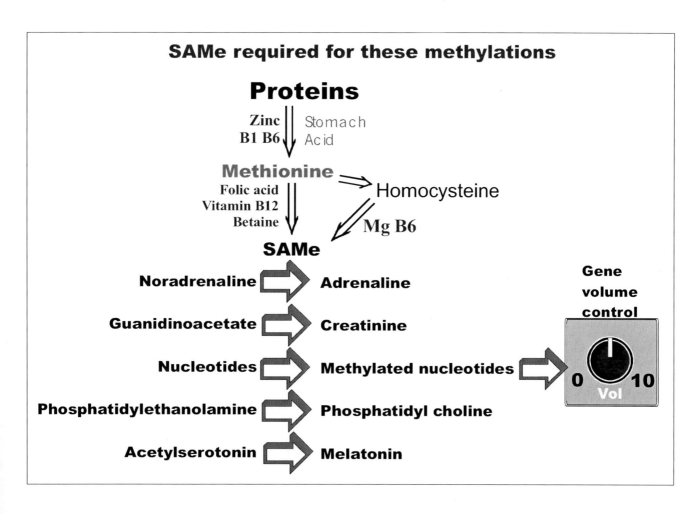

**SAMe required for these methylations**

**Proteins**

Zinc B1 B6 ⇓ Stomach Acid

**Methionine** ⟹ Homocysteine

**Folic acid Vitamin B12 Betaine** ⇓ ⟹ Mg B6

**SAMe**

Noradrenaline ⟹ **Adrenaline**

Guanidinoacetate ⟹ **Creatinine**

Nucleotides ⟹ **Methylated nucleotides** ⟹

Phosphatidylethanolamine ⟹ **Phosphatidyl choline**

Acetylserotonin ⟹ **Melatonin**

**Gene volume control**

0 | 10 Vol

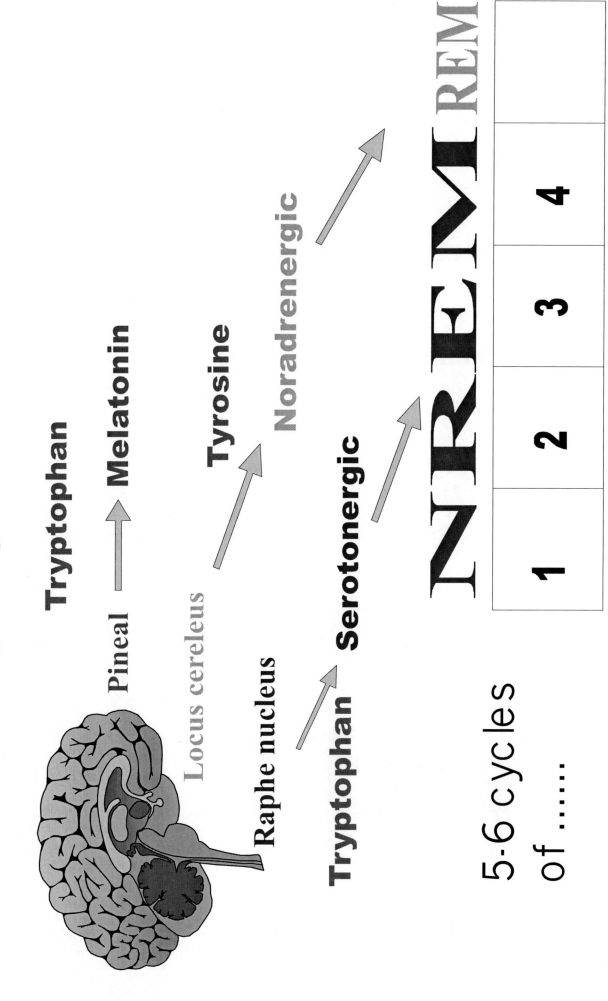

# Nutrients and antinutrients

| | Copper block | Cadmium Block | Mercury Block | Arsenic Block | Lead Block | Aluminium Block | Antimony Block |
|---|---|---|---|---|---|---|---|
| Sodium | | | | | | X | |
| Potassium | | | | | | X | |
| Magnesium | X | X | | | | | |
| Calcium | | | | | X | | |
| Iron | X | | X | | X | | |
| Zinc | X | X | X | | | X | X |
| Chromium | | | | | X | | |
| Selenium | | X | X | X | | X | X |
| Molybdenum | X | | | | X | | |
| Manganese | X | | | | X | | |
| Phosphorus | | | | | | X | |
| Vitamin B1 | X | | | | | X | |
| Vitamin C | X | | | | | X | |
| Vitamin E | X | | | X | | X | |
| Folate | X | | | | | | |
| Boron | X | | | X | | | |

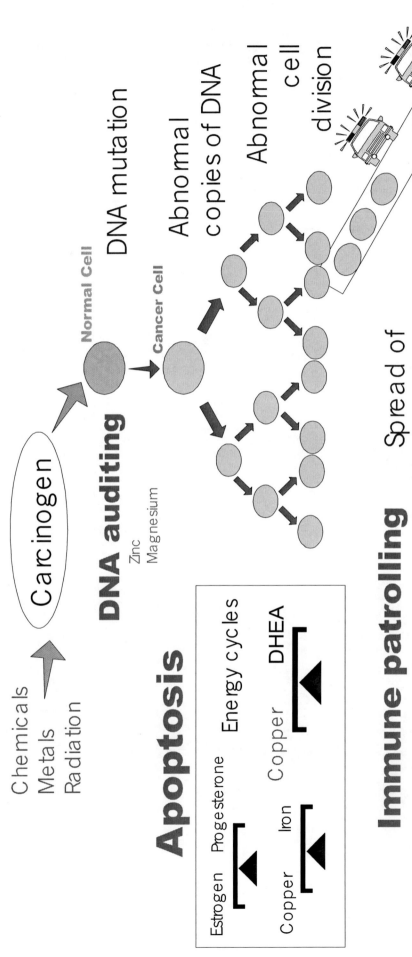
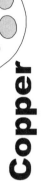

Chemicals
Metals
Radiation

Carcinogen

**Normal Cell**

DNA mutation

**DNA auditing**

Zinc
Magnesium

**Cancer Cell**

Abnormal
copies of DNA

Abnormal
cell
division

**Apoptosis**

Estrogen   Progesterone   Energy cycles

Copper   Iron

Copper   DHEA

**Immune patrolling**

Zinc        Vitamin C
Iron        Vitamin E
Selenium Vitamin D

Spread of
tumour cells

**Angiogenesis**

Encouragement
of new blood supply

**Copper**

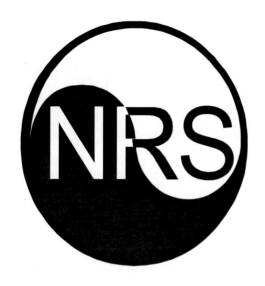

# Common Toxins Metals and Xenoestrogens

| | | | | | | | |
|---|---|---|---|---|---|---|---|
| Magnesium | X | X | | | | | |
| Calcium | | | | | X | | |
| Iron | X | | X | | X | | |
| Zinc | X | X | X | | | X | X |
| Chromium | | | | | X | | |
| Selenium | | X | X | X | | X | X |
| Molybdenum | X | | | | X | | |
| Manganese | X | | | | X | | |
| Phosphorus | | | | | | X | |
| Vitamin B1 | X | | | | | X | |
| Vitamin C | X | | | | | X | |
| Vitamin E | X | | | X | | X | |
| Folate | X | | | | | | |
| Boron | X | | | X | | | |

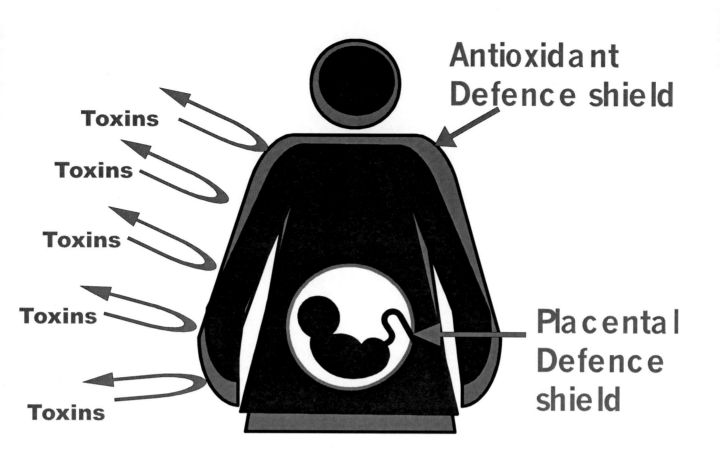

Antioxidant
Defence shield

Toxins

Toxins

Toxins

Toxins

Toxins

Placental
Defence
shield

**Defence shield down**

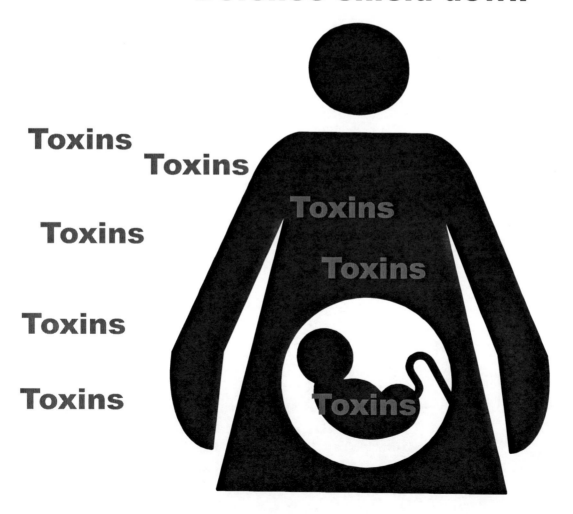

Toxins
Toxins
Toxins
Toxins
Toxins
Toxins
Toxins
Toxins

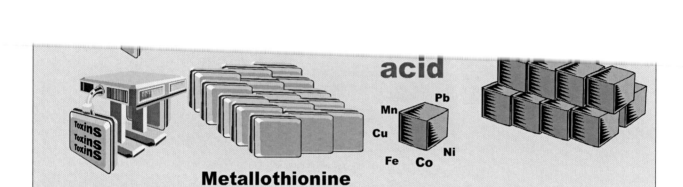

**Metallothionine**

acid

Mn  Pb
Cu
Fe  Co  Ni

# Cellular defence system

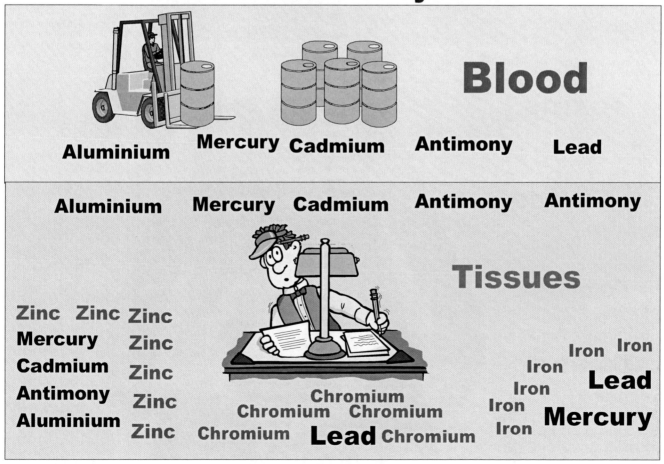

**Blood**

Aluminium    Mercury    Cadmium    Antimony    Lead

Aluminium    Mercury    Cadmium    Antimony    Antimony

**Tissues**

Zinc  Zinc  Zinc
Mercury      Zinc
Cadmium      Zinc                                        Iron  Iron
Antimony     Zinc                                    Iron
Aluminium    Zinc          Chromium              Iron    Lead
             Zinc    Chromium  Chromium    Iron
                  Chromium  Lead  Chromium    Iron    Mercury

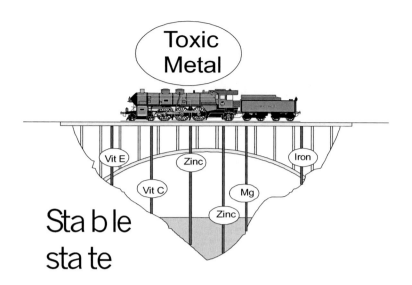

Toxic
Metal

Vit E · Zinc · Iron
Vit C · Mg
Zinc

Stable
state

Stress
Growth spurt
Vaccination
Infection
Life event
Pregnancy
Anaesthetic

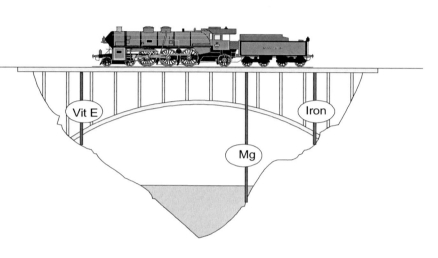

Vit E · Iron
Mg

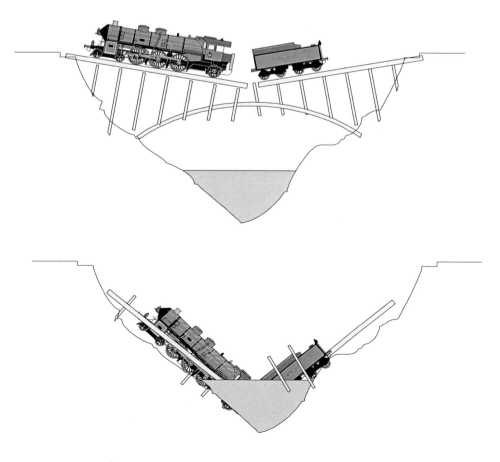

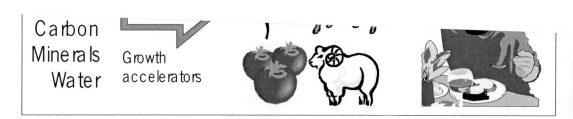

The problem all biological systems have is that members of the "zinc series" of the periodic table are interchangeable by plants and animals. That means that if a plant is faced with zinc and cadmium it will take up both because of the similarity of atomic structure.

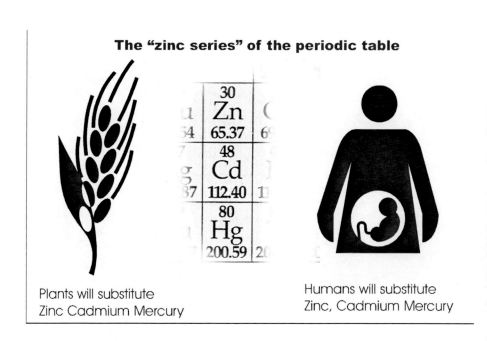

Unfortunately, our superphosphate fertilisers contain about 20mg per kg of cadmium as an unavoidable contaminant. This makes cadmium present in foods fertilised this way and is a good reason for changing to organically grown food.

Other sources of cadmium are listed below in both domestic and occupational sources.

## Sources of Cadmium

**Domestic**
Tap water
Cigarettes
Coffee, Black teas
Nuts
Refined carbohydrates
Evaporated milk
Processed meats
Organ meats
Oysters
Food grown with superphosphates fertilizers such as wheat
Industrial contamination of air and drinking water
Black rubber tyres (cars, bicycles and toys)
Pesticides
Fungicides (for tea, coffee, nuts, tobacco plants)
Paint pigments
Plastic tapes
Polyvinyl plastics (PVC's) the piping in most modern housing
Rubber carpet backing
Burned motor oil
Silver polish

**Occupational**
Cadmium alloys
Jewellery
Nickel-cadmium batteries
Process engraving
Soldering
Copper refining
Rust proofing tools
Marine hardware
Electroplating

This type of antagonism will occur at the tissue level with very small, amounts of either heavy metal. Toxicity as defined by industry is NOT relevant when describing focal tissue antagonism of zinc by cadmium and mercury. This is why any examination of zinc levels must include the Antinutrients such as Cadmium and Mercury in order to fully analyse the zinc symptoms. **Sources of mercury.**

**Domestic sources**

Body talcs and powders, Contaminated seafood, Cosmetics, Dental amalgam, Grains treated with fungicides, Fabric softeners, Fungicides used on lawns, trees & shrubs, Pesticides, Photo engraving & Wood preservatives. Vaccines (as the preservative Thiomersol). Mercurochrome

**Occupational sources**

Battery makers, Boiler makers, Dental nurses, Electroplates, Lamp makers, Mirror makers, Paint makers, Seed & Seedling handlers, Textile printers & Thermometer makers, canvas makers. Fluorescent Lights. Chlorine production.

The final point is this. Biology is the rope being tugged at by two forces (not always in opposition however). Until this changes, we will still see toxins in our community.

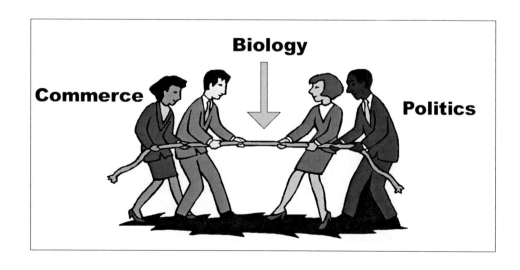

12] Atcnison [illegible]

13] Baaumslag N., et al. Trace metal content of maternal and neonate hair. Zinc, copper, iron and lead. Iron [illegible]

14] Baker E.L., et al. A nationwide survey of heavy metal absorption in children living near primary copper, lead and zinc smelter. Am J Epidemiology. 206,4, 1977

15] Bapu C., Rao P. & Sood P.P. Restoration of methylmercury inhibited adenosine triphosphatases during vitamin and monothiol therapy. J Environ Path Toxicol Oncol. 17:75-80, 1998

16] Barregard L., Sallsten G. & Jarvholm B. People with high mercury uptake from their own dental amalgam fillings. Occup Environ Med. 52:124-128, 1995

17] Barth G.,ed. The Lewis and Clark Expedition, Selections from the Journals Arranged by Topic. New York: Bedford St. Martins. 158-162, 1998

18] Batuman V., et al. Contribution of lead to hypertension with renal impairment. N.E.J.M. 309,1, 1983

19] Beattie J.H. & Peace H.S. The influence of a low-boron diet and boron supplementation on bone, major mineral and sex steroid metabolism in postmenopausal women. Brit J Nutr. 69,3, 1993

20] Bhat R.K., et al. Trace elements in hair and environmental exposure. Sci Total Environ. 22(2):169-178, 1982

21] Bigazzi P.E. Lessons from animal models: the scope of mercury-induced autoimmunity. Clin Immunol Immunopathol. 65:81-84, 1992

22] Birchall J.D. & Chappell J.S. Aluminum, chemical physiology and Alzheimer's disease. Lancet. Oct, 1988

23] Blakley B.R., Sisodia C.S. & Mukkur T.K. The effect of methylmercury, tetraethyl lead, and sodium arsenite on the humoral immunity response in mice. Toxicol Appl Pharmacol. 52:245-254, 1980

24] Blumer W. & Reich T. Leaded gasoline-a cause of cancer. Environmental International. 3:456-471, 1980

25] Bonhomme C., et al. Mercury poisoning by vacuum-cleaner aerosol. Lancet. 347:115, 1996

26] Boogaard P.J., et al. Effects of exposure to elemental mercury on nervous system and the kidneys in workers producing natural gas. Arch Environ Health. 5:108-115, 1996

27] Boyce B.F., et al. Hypercalcaemic osteomalacia due to aluminum toxicity. Lancet. Nov, 1982

28] Boyd N.D., et al. Mercury from dental "silver" tooth fillings impairs sheep kidney function. Am J Physiol. 261:R1010-R1014, 1991

29] Capel I.D., et al. Assessment of zinc status by the zinc tolerance test in various groups of patients. Clin Biochem. 15(2):257-260, 1982

30] Cavalleri A. & Gobba F. Reversible color vision loss in occupational exposure to metallic mercury. Environ Res. 77:173-177, 1998

31] Chang L.W. Neurotoxic effects of mercury. A review. Environ Res. 14:329-373, 1977

32] Cheraskin E. & Ringsdorf W.M. The distribution of lead in human hair. J Of Med Assoc of Alabama. April, 1979

33] Cheraskin E. & Ringsdorf W.M. Prevalence of possible lead toxicity as determined by hair analysis. J Orthomol Psych. 8,2. Am J Ind Med. 2,1,5-14, 1981

34] Cianciola M.E., et al. Epidemiologic assessment of measures used to indicate low-level exposure to mercury vapor. J Toxicol Environ Health. 52:19-33, 1997

35] Cimino J.A. & Demopoulos H.B. Introduction: Determinants of cancer relevant to prevention, in the war on cancer. J Environ. Path. & Toxi.3:1-10, 1980

36] Clarke N.E., Clarke C.N. & Mosher R.E. The "in vivo" disolution of metastatic calcium: An approach to athero-sclerosis. Am J Med Sci. 229:142-149, 1955

37] Clarke A.N. & Wilson D.J. Preparation of hair for lead analysis. Arch Environ Hlth. 28, 1974

38] Clarkson T.W., Amin-Zaki L. & Al-Tikriti S.K. An outbreak of methylmercury poisoning due to consumption of contaminated grain. Fed Proc. 35:2395-2399, 1976

39] Clarkson T.W., et al. Mercury. In: Clarkson T.W., Friber L., Nordberg G.F., Sager P.R.,eds. Biological Monitoring of Toxic Metals. New York: Plenum Press; 199-246, 1988

40] Coccini T., et al. Low-level exposure to methylmercury modifies muscarinic cholinergic receptor binding characteristics in rat brain and lymphocytes: physiologic implication and new opportunities in biological monitoring. Environ Health Perspect. 108:29-33, 2000

41] Collipp P.J., et al. Hair zinc levels in infants. Clin Pediatr. 22(7):512-513, 1983

42] Cooper G.P. & Manalis R.S. Influence of heavy metals on synaptic transmission: a review. Neurotoxicology. 4:69-83, 1983

43] Cornett C.R., Markesbery W.R. & Ehmann W.D. Imbalances of trace elements related to oxidative damage in Alzheimer's disease brain. Neurotoxicology. 19:339-346, 1998

44] Crapper-McLaughlin D.R. Aluminum toxicity in senile dementia: Implications for treatment. Read before the Fall Conference, American Academy of Medical Preventics, Las Vegas, NV, Nov 8, 1981

45] Cranton E.M., et al. Standardization and interpretation of human hair for elemental concentrations. J Holistic Med. 4:10-20, 1982

46] Crinnion W.J. Unpublished research. Healing Naturally. Kirkland, WA. 1999

47] David O., et al. Lead and hyperactivity, behavioral response to chelation: A pilot study. Am J Psychiatry. 133:1155-1158, 1976

48] De Souza Queiroz M.L., et al. Abnormal antioxidant system in erythrocytes of mercury exposed workers. Human & Exp Toxicol. 17:225-230, 1998

49] Del Maestro R.F. An approach to free radicals in medicine and biology. Acta Physiol Scand. 492(suppl):153-168, 1980

50] Diamond G. & Zalups R.K. Understanding renal toxicity of heavy metals. Toxicol Pathol. 26:92-103, 1998

51] Dieter M.P., et al. Immunological and biochemical responses in mice treated with mercuric chloride. Toxicol Appl Pharmacol. 68:218-228, 1983

52] Dirks M.J., et al. Mercury excretion and intravenous ascorbic acid. ArchEnviron Health. 49:49-52, 1994

53] Dix Y. Metabolism of polycyclic aromatic hydrocarbon derivatives to ultimate carcinogens during lipid peroxidation. Science. 221:77, 1983

54] Dormandy T.L. Free-radical reaction in biological systems. Ann R Coll Surg Engl. 62:188-194, 1980

55] Dormandy T.L. Free-radical oxidation and antioxidants. Lancet. i:647-650, 1978

56] Druet P., et al. Immune type glomerulonephritis induced by HgC12 in Brown-Norway rat. Ann Immunol (Inst Pasteur). 129C:777-792, 1978

57] Durham H.D., Minotti S. & Caporicci E. Sensitivity of platelet microtubles to disassembly by methylmercury. J Toxicol Enviro Health. 48:57-69, 1997

58] Ely J.T., et al. Urine mercury in micromercurialism: a bimodal distribution and its diagnostic implications. Unpublished.

59] Ely D.L., et al. Aerometric and hair trace metal content in learning-disabled children. Environ Res. 25(2):325-339, 1981

60] Emerick R.J. & Kayongo-Male H. Silicon facilitation of copper utilization in the rat. J Nutr Biochem. 1, 1990

61] Enestrom S. & Hultman P. Immune-mediate glomerular nephritis induced by mercuric chloride in mice. Experientia. 40:1234-1240, 1984

63] Enestrom S. & Hultman P. Dose-response studies in murine mercury-induced autoimmunity and immune-complex disease. Toxicol Appl Pharmacol. 113:199-208, 1992

64] Engqvist A., Colmsjo A. & Skare I. Speciation of mercury excreted in feces from individuals with amalgam fillings. Arch Environ Health. 53:205-213, 1998

65] Erickson, et al. Tissue mineral levels in victims of Sudden Infant Dealth Syndrome 1. Toxic metals – lead and cadmium. Ped Res. 17, 10, 1083

66] Falconer M.M., et al. The molecular basis of microtuble stability in neurons. Neurotoxicology. 15:109-122, 1994

67] Fiedler N., et al. Neuropsychological and stress evaluation of residential mercury exposure. Enviro Health Perspect. 107:343-347, 1999

68] Florence T.M., Lilley S.G. & Stauber J.L. Skin absorption of lead. Lancet. Jul. 16, 1988

69] Foli M.R., Hennigan C. & Errera J. A comparison of five toxic metals among rural and urban children. Environ Pollut Ser A Ecol Biol. 29:261-270, 1982

70] Fukuda Y., et al. An analysis of subjective complaints in a population living in a methylmercury-polluted area. Environ Res. 81:100-107, 1999

71] Galster W.A. Mercury in Alaskan Estimo mothers and infants. Environ Health Perspect. 15:135-140, 1976

72] Ganther H.E. Selenium: relation to decreased toxicity of methylmercury in diets containing tuna. Science. 175:1122, 1972

73] Ganther H.E. Modification of methylmercury toxicity and metabolism by selenium and vitamin E: possible mechanisms. Environ Health Perspect. 25:71-76, 1978

74] Garrett P.J., et al. Aluminum encephalopathy: Clinical and immunological features. Quart J Med. 69, 258, 1988

75] Gibson R.S. & Gage L. Changes in hair arsenic levels in breast and bottle fed infants during the first year of infancy. Sci Total Environ. 26:33-40, 1982

76] Goldberg R.L., Kaplan S.R. & Fuller G.C. Effect of heavy metals on human rheumatoid synovial cell proliferation and collagen synthesis. Biochem Pharmacol. 32:2763-2766, 1983

77] Grandjean P., et al. Methylmercury neurotoxicity in Amazonian children downstream from gold mining. Environ Health Perspect. 107:587-591, 1999

78] Grandjean P., et al. Relation of a seafood diet to mercury, selenium, arsenic and polychlorinated biphenyl and other organochlorine concentrations in human milk. Environ Res. 71:29-38, 1995

79] Giaziano J.H., Lolacono N.J. & Meyer P. Dose-response study of oral 2,3-dimercaptosuccinic acid in children with elevated

90] Harrison W., Yurachek J. & Benson C. The deter........

Clin Chim Acta. 23(1):83-91, 1969

91] Herrstrom P., et al. Dental amalgam, low-dose exposure to mercury, and urinary proteins in young Swedish men. Arch Environ Health. 50:103-110, 1995

92] Hibberd A.R., Howard M.A. & Hunnisett A.G. Mercury from dental amalgam fillings: studies on oral chelating agents for assessing and reducing mercury burdens in humans. J Nutr Environ Med. 8:219-231, 1998

93] Homma-Takeda S., et al. Selective induction of apoptosis of renal tubular cells caused by inorganic mercury in vivo. Environ Toxicol Pharmacol. 7:179-187, 1999

94] Huel G., Boudene C. & Ibrahim M.A. Cadmium and lead content of maternal and newborn hair: Relationship to parity, birth weight and hypertension. Arch Environ Health. 35(5):221-227, 1981

95] Hunt C.D., Shuler T.R. & Mullen L.M. Concentration of boron and other elements in human foods and personal-care products. J Am Diet Assoc. 91,5,1991

96] Hurry V.J. & Gibson R.S. The zinc, copper and manganese status of children with malabsorption syndromes and in-born errors of metabolism. Biol Trace Element Res. 4:157-173, 1982

97] InSug O., et al. Mercuric compounds inhibit human monocyte function by reactive oxygen species, development of mitochondrial membrane permeability transition and loss of reductive reserve. Toxicology. 124;211-224, 1997

98] Jenkins D.W. Toxic Trace Metals in Mammalian Hair and Nails. US Environmental Protection Agency publication No. (EPA)-600/4-79-049. Environmental Monitoring Systems Laboratory. 1979

99] Jenkins D.W. Biological monitoring of toxic trace metals Vol.1. Biological monitoring and surveillance. EPA 600/3-80-089, 1980 . Clin Chem. 36,3, 1990

100] Jones R.J. The continuing hazard of lead in drinking water. Lancet. Sept 16, 1989

101] Kanematsu N., et al. Mutagenicity of cadmium, platinum and rhodium compounds in cultures mammalian cells. Gifu Shika Zasshi. 17,2, 1990

102] King N., et al. The effect of in ovo boron supplementation on bone mineralization of the vitamin D-deficient chicken embryo. Biol Trace Element Res. 31,1, 1991

103] Kissel K.P. Teens fall ill after taking, playing with mercury. The Seatle Times: January 15, 1998

104] Klevay L. Hair as a biopsy material-assessment of copper nutriture. Am J Clin Nutr. 23(8):1194-1202, 1970

105] Kolata G. New suspect in bacterial resistance: amalgam. The New York Times: April 24, 1993

106] Kopito L., et al. Chronic plumbism in children. Diagnosed by hair analysis. J.A.M.A. 209,2, 1969

107] Langworth S., Elinder C.G. & Sundqvist K.G. Minor effects of low exposure to inorganic mercury on the human immune system. Scan J Work Environ Health. 19:405-413, 1993

108] Lebel J., Mergler D. & Lucotte M. Evidence of early nervous system dysfunction in Amazonian populations exposed to low-levels of methylmercury. Neurotoxicology. 17:157-167, 1996

109] Levine S.A. & Reinhardt J.H. Biochemical-pathology initiated by free radicals, oxidant chemicals and therapeutic drugs in the etiology of chemical hypersensitivity disease. J Orthomol Psychiatr. 12(3):166-183, 1983

110] Lichtenberg H. Symptoms before and after proper amalagam removal in relation to serum-globulin reaction to metals. J orthomolec Med. 11:195-204, 1996

112] Lieb J. & Hershman D. Isaac Newton: mercury poisoning or manic depression. Lancet. 1479-1480, 1983

113] Magour S., Maser H. & Grein H. The effect of mercury and methylmercury on brain microsomal Na+, K+ ATPase after partial delipidisation with Lubrol. Pharmacol Toxicol. 60:184-186, 1987

114] Maloney S.R., Phillips C.A. & Mills A. Mercury in the hair of crematoria workers. Lancet. 352:1602, 1998

115] Marlowe M., et al. Increased lead burdens and trace mineral status in mentally retarted children. J Spec Educ. 16:87-99, 1982

116] Marlowe M., et al. Lead and mercury levels in emotionally disturbed children. J Orthomol Psychiatr. 12(4):260-267, 1983

117] Marlowe M. & Mood C. Hair aluminum concentration and nonadaptive classroom behavior. J of Advancement in Med. 1,3, 1988

118] Matte T.D., et al. Acute high-dose lead exposure from beverage contaminated by traditional Mexican pottery. Lancet. 344, 8929, 1994

119] Matthews A.D. Mercury content of commercially important fish of the Seychelles and hair mercury levels of a selected part of the population. Environ Res. 30:305-312, 1983

120] Medeiros D.M. & Borgman R.F. Blood pressure in young adults as associated with dietary habits, body conformation and hair element concentrations. Nutr Res. 2:455-466, 1982

121] Medeiros D.M, Pellum L.K. & Brown B.J. The association of selected hair minerals and anthropometric factors with blood pressure in a normotensive adult population. Nutr Research. 3:51-60, 1983

122] Medeiros D.M. & Pellum L.K. Elevation of cadmium, lead and zinc in the hair of adult black female hypertensives. Bull Environ Toxicol. 32, 1984

123] Miettinen J.K. Absorption and elimination of dietary mercury (2+) ion and methylmercury in man. In: Miller MW, Clarkson T.W., eds. Mercury, Mercurials and Mercaptans. Proceedings 4th International Conference on Environmental Toxicology. New York: Plenum Press; 1973

124] Miller O.M., Lund B.O. & Woods J.S. Reactivity of Hg(II) with superoxide: evidence for the catalytic dismutation of superoxide by Hg(II). J Biochem Toxicol. 6:293-298, 1991

125] Miura K., et al. The involvement of microtubular disruption in methylmercury-induced apoptosis in neuronal and nonneuronal cell lines. Toxicol Appl Phamacol. 160:279-288, 1999

126] Moser P.B., Krebs N.K. & Blyler E. Zinc hair concentrations and estimated zinc intakes of functionally delayed normal sized and small-for-age children. Nutr Research. 2:585-590, 1982

127] Musa-Alzudbaidi L., et al. Hair selenium content during infancy and childhood. Eur J Pediatr. 139:295-296, 1982

128] Nakatsuru S., et al. Effect of mercurials on lymphocyte functions in vitro. Toxicology. 36:297-305, 1985

129] Narang A.P.S., et al. Arsenic levels in opium eaters in India. Trace Elements in Med. 4,4, 1987

130] Ngim C.H., et al. Chronic neurobehavioral effects of elemental mercury in dentists. Br J Indust Med. 49:782-790, 1992

131] Niculescu T., et al. Relationship between the lead concentration in hair and occupational exposure. Brit J Industrial Med. 40,67, 1983

132] Ninomiya T., et al. Expansion of methylmercury poisoning outside of Minamata: an epidemiological study on chronic methylmercury poisoning outside Minamata. Environ Res. 70:47-50, 1995

133] Nolan K.R. Copper toxicity syndrome. J Orhtomol Psychiatr. 12(4):270-282, 1983

134] Nordlind K. Inhibition of lymphoid-cell DNA synthesis by metal allergens at various concentrations. Effect on short-time cultured non-adherent cell compared to non-separated cells. Int Arch Allergy Appl Immunol. 70:191-192, 1983

135] Nriagu J.O. Lead and Lead Poisoning in Antiquity. Wiley N.Y. 1983

136] Orloff K.G., et al. Human exposure to elemental mercury in a contaminated residential building. Arch Environ Health. 52:169-172, 1997

137] Ortega H.G., et al. Neuroimmunological effects of exposure to methylmercury forms in the Sprague-Dawley rat. Activation of the hypothalamic-pituitary-adrenal axis and lymphocyte responsiveness. Toxicol Indust Health. 13:57-66, 1997

138] Oskarsson A., et al. Total and inorganic mercury in breast milk and blood in relation to fish consumption and amalgam fillings in lactating women. Arch Environ Health. 51:234-241, 1996

139] Oudar P., Caillard L. & Fillon G. In vitro effects of organic and inorganic mercury on the serotonergic system. Pharmacol Toxicol. 65:245-248, 1989

140] Patterson J.E., Weissberg B. & Dennison P.J. Mercury in human breath from dental amalgam. Bull Environ Contam Toxicol. 34:459-468, 1985

141] Pearl D.P., et al. Intraneuronal aluminum accumulation in Amyotrophic Lateral Sclerosis and Parkinsonism-Dementia of Guam. Science. 217, 1982

142] Pendergrass J.C., et al. Mercury vapor inhalation inhibits binding of GTP to tubulin in rat brain: similarity to a molecular lesion in Alzheimer's disease brain. Neurotoxicity. 18:315-324, 1997

143] Pendergrass J.C. & Haley B.E. Mercury-EDTA complex specifically blocks brain beta-tubulin-GTP interactions: similarity to observations in Alzheimer's disease. In: Friberg L.T., Scrauzer G.N., eds. Status Quo and Perspectives of Amalgam and other Dental Materials. Stuttgart: Georg Thieme Verlag.98-105, 1995

144] Peters H.A. Trace minerals, chelating agents and the por-phyrias. Fed Proc. 20(3)(Part II)(suppl 10):227-234. 1961

145] Peters H.A., et al. Arsenic, chromium and copper poisoning from burning treated wood. N Engl J Med. 308(22):1360-1361, 1983

146] Peters H.A., et al. Seasonal arsenic exposure from burning treated wood. J.A.M.A. 11;25,18,2393-2396, 1984

147] Peto R., et al. Can dietary beta-carotene materially reduce human cancer rates? Nature. 290:201, 1981

148] Rajanna B. & Hobson M. Influence of mercury on uptake of dopamine and norepinephrine by rat brain synaptosomes. Toxicol Lett. 27:7-14, 1985

149] Rajanna B., et al. Effects of cadmium and mercury on Na+, K+ ATPases and the uptake of 3H-dopamine in rat brain synaptosomes. Arch Int Physiol Biochem. 98:291-296, 1990

150] Redhe O. & Pleva J. Recovery form Amyotrophic Lateral Sclerosis and from allergy after removal of dental amalgam filling. Int

12:115-118, 1975

161] Stortebecker P. Mercury Poisoning from Dental Amalgam, A Hazard to Human Brain. Stockholm. Stortebecker Foundation Research. 24, 1985

162] Szylman P., et al. Potassium-wasting nephropathy in an outbreak of chronic organic mercurial intoxication. Am J Nephrol. 15:514-520, 1995

163] Thatcher R.W., et al. Effects of low levels of cadmium and lead on cognitive functioning in children. Arch Environ Health. 37(3):159-166, 1982

164] Thimaya S. & Ganapathy S.N. Selenium in human hair in relation to age, diet, pathological condition and serum levels. Sci Total Environ. 24:41-49, 1982

165] Thompson C.M., et al. Regional brain trace-element studies in Alzheimer's disease. Neurotoxicology. 9:1-8, 1988

166] Ting K.S., et al. Chelate stability of sodium dimercaptosuccinate on the intoxication from many metals. Chinese Med J. 64:1072-1075, 1965

167] Tollefson L. & Cordle F. Methylmercury in fish: a review of residue levels, fish consumption and regulatory action in the United States. Environ Health Perspect. 68:203-208, 1986

168] Trepka M.J., et al. Factors affecting internal mercury burdens among East German children. Arch Environ Health. 52:134-138, 1997

169] Vanderhoff J.A., et al. Hair and plasma zinc levels following exclusion of biliopancreatic secretions from functioning gastrointestinal tract in humans. Dig Dis Sci. 28(4):300-305, 1983

170] Vimy M.J. & Lorsheider F.L. Intra-oral air mercury released from dental amalgams. J Dent Res. 64:1069-1071, 1985

171] Vimy M.F. & Lorsheider F.L. Serial measurements of intra-oral air mercury: estimation of daily dose from dental amalgams. J Dent Res. 64:1072-1075, 1985

172] Walker P.R., LeBlanc J. & Sikorska M. Effects of aluminum and other cations on the structure of brain and liver chromatin. Biochem. 28,9, 1989

173] Watanabe C. & Satho H. Evaluation of our understanding of methylmercury as health threat. Environ Health Res. 104:367-378, 1996

174] Watts D.L. Prevalence of lead in environment threatens children. Hlth Freedom News. Oct, 1985

175] Watts D.L. Implications of lead toxicity. TEI Newsletter. 1,2, 1985

176] Wedeen R.P., Mallik D.K. & Batuman V. Detection and treatment of occupational lead nephropathy. Arch Intern Med. 139:53-57, 1979

177] Welsh S.O. & Soares J.H. Jr. The protective effect of vitamin E and selenium against methylmercury toxicity in the Japanese quail. Nutr Rep Int. 13;43, 1976

178] Westhoff D.D., et al. Arsenic intoxication as a cause of megaloblastic anemia. Blood. 75,45,2. 241-246.

179] Willett W.C., et al. Prediagnostic serum selenium and risk of cancer. Lancet. 2(8343):130-134, 1983

180] Wilson R.L. Iron, zinc, free radicals and oxygen tissue disorders and cancer control, in Iron Metabolism. Ciba Foundn Symp 51 (new series). Amsterdam, Elsevier. 331-354, 1977

181] Yamanaka S., Tanaka H. & Nishimura M. Exposure of Japanese dental workers to mercury. Bull Tokyo Den Coll. 23:15-24, 1982

182] Yokel R.A. Hair as an indicator of excessive aluminum exposure. Clin Chem. 28,4, 1982

183] Zalups R.K. & Cernichiari E. 2,3-dimercapto-1-propanesulfonic acid (DMPS) as a rescue agent for the nephropathy induced by mercuric chloride. The Toxicologist. 10:271(Abstract only), 1990

184] Zalups R.K. & Lash L.H. Interactions between glutathione and mercury in the kidney, liver and blood. In: Chang L.W., ed. Toxicology of Metals. Boca Raton: CRC Press. 145-163, 1996

185] Zheng W., et al. Choroid plexus protects cerebrospinal fluid against toxic metals. FASEB J. 5:2188-2189, 1991

# Common sources of heavy metals

**Copper** -food, water, supplements (over 100g)

**Cadmium**- Cigarettes, food, water, household items, toys

**Lead** - water, makeup, household items, petrol, paints

**Mercury**- fish, fillings, vaccines

**Aluminium**- antiperspirants, cookware, Aluminium foil, bleached flour, regional water supplies, Antacids

**Arsenic**- water, playgrounds, termite treatments

**Berylium**- light switches, fillings, copper pipes

**Antimony**- make up, fabrics, printing ink, paints

# Occupational exposure to Antinutrients

**Copper :** Plumbers, Electricians, Petroleum industry workers Fertiliser/Pesticide exposure

**Cadmium:** Mechanics, Tyre fitters, welders, plumbers, carpet layers, jewellers, toy industry, plastics industry,

**Mercury:** Dental techs, dentists, petroleum workers gold miners, medical technologists, sugar cane workers

**Arsenic:** Gold miners, metallurgists, Landscape workers, carpenters, builders, brickies, bore drillers, concrete workers

**Lead:** Mechanics, Plumbers, welders, petroleum workers, painters, renovators, lead lighting, fishermen,

**Aluminium:** Plumbers, Ducting installers, aircraft workers, welders, miners and refinery workers

Infertility
Water retention

## 2. Mineral imbalance
Zinc deficiency
Magnesium deficiency
Copper excess
Osteoporosis

## 3. Gynaecological problems
Breast lumps
Endometriosis
Fibroids
Ovarian cysts/ Polycystic ovaries

## 4. Immune system imbalance
Autoimmune disorders
Allergies

## 5. Cancers
Breast (male & female)
Uterine ,Cervical & Ovarian
Prostate
Probably melanoma & thyroid

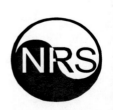

# Strangers in the night: Xenoestrogens and health.

What is Estrogen dominance? This refers to the balance of Estrogen and Progesterone. In a normal menstrual cycle (see Fig1), Estrogen is the dominant hormone up until ovulation day (usually day 14). Then progesterone is the dominant hormone until the period. Progesterone rises to increase the store of Magnesium, Zinc and Vitamin B6. It also brings down the copper, which has gradually risen to a mid-cycle peak. Overall there is no net gain of copper, if progesterone kicks in properly. If there is a lack of progesterone (see fig2), then Magnesium, Zinc and B6 tend to be low and copper tends to rise.

Another example is the oral contraceptive pill. The Estrogens in these pills do have Estrogenic effects, but the progesterone (being synthetic) tends not to have true progesterone effect (see Fig 4) . Another version of Estrogen dominance. This explains why zinc and magnesium fall and why copper rises while on the OCP.

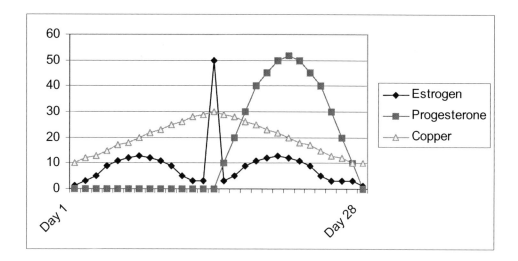

**Fig 1. Normal Cycle**

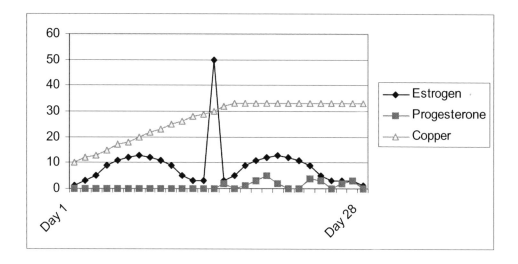

**g 2. Low Progesterone Cycle**

John R Lee's work in the 80's on Estrogen dominance was largely ignored by the medical fraternity. The suggestion has been made that they were caught up in the glossy hype generated by pharmaceutical companies pushing Estrogen therapies. His premise was that even without a uterus, the women still needed progesterone. This was never really accepted despite the expanding body of evidence that Estrogen Dominance would have been directly responsible for the woman's hysterectomy! By giving Estrogen only therapy, the doctor was perpetuating the hormone imbalance. His

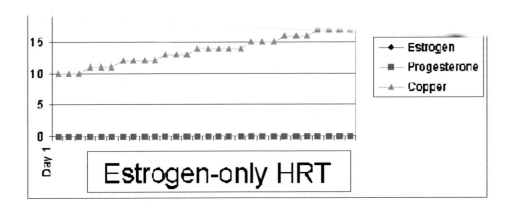

**Fig 3 Estrogen Only HRT**

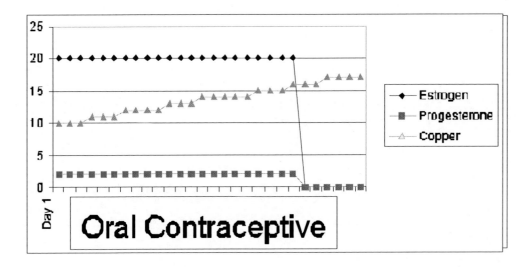

**Fig 4. Oral Contraceptive**

The effect of Xenoestrogens in the body is to shift the baseline of total Estrogen level upwards . The effect on copper is that it never returns to the starting point by day 28. Hence the connection between Xenoestrogens, Estrogen only HRT and copper excess.

# List of Estrogen Dominance Symptoms

Acceleration of aging
Agitation or Anxiety
Allergy (asthma, hives, rashes, sinus congestion)
Autoimmune disorders Lupus, Thyroiditis (Hashimoto's
Breast cancer (men and women)
Breast tenderness with period
Cervical dysplasia (abnormal pap smear)
Cold hands and feet
Copper excess
Decreased sex drive
Depression with anxiety or agitation
Dry eyes
Endometriosis
Fat gain around abdomen hips & thighs
Fatigue
Fibrocystic (lumpy breasts)
Fibroids
Foggy thinking
Gall bladder disease
Hair loss
Headaches
Hypoglycaemia (low blood sugar esp. 3-4pm)
Increased blood clotting
Infertility
Irregular menstrual periods
Irritability
Insomnia
Magnesium deficiency
Memory loss
Mood swings
Osteoporosis
Ovarian cancer
Ovarian Cysts
PMS/PMT
Polycystic ovaries
Pre-menopausal bone loss
Prostate cancer (in Men)
Sluggish metabolism
Thyroid dysfunction
Uterine cancer
Water retention, bloating
Zinc deficiency

Since that time it has become clear that many chemicals behave as Estrogens. What is also clear is that we are exposed to these *all of our lives*, not just in the womb. This group of compounds have been called the Xenoestrogens. Xeno is the Greek word for stranger, hence the comment about strangers in the night. The list is represented below. These chemicals are cumulative in some instances and increase in quantity in the body as we get older. One of the effects of Xenoestrogens is to reduce the excretion rate of copper from the body. All estrogens cause copper accumulation, xenoestrogens look like estrogens to our biochemistry and hence also cause copper retention. These patients have very high Copper levels. These Xenoestrogens (especially the pesticides) over time have progressively been classed as carcinogens. The combination of high copper (which disables iron, zinc, Vitamin C and Vitamin E) and intracellular carcinogens may explain the more unpleasant problems in his list.

## List of the Xenoestrogens

**Pesticides** (DDT, DDE, 2,4,5-T, Dieldrin, endosulfan, Cadmium, , methoxychlor, kepone, toxaphene, chloropicrin, lindane, chlordane, artrazine etc)
**Metals** Cadmium Arsenic
**Petroleum products** (PCB's, car fumes, methlybenzene, toluene, benzene, styrene, pyrene)
**Plastics** (PVC, biphenyl, nonylphenyl, octaphenyl, lunch wraps etc)

**Hormones** a. From Doctors (OCP & HRT)
    b. From Food 1) Poultry industry & 2) Antibiotics in animal feed

How would this problem manifest? Let's take a typical example. A young girl is born. She is a difficult child. Fussy eater, poor sleep pattern, lots of colds. She loves chicken and craves chocolate. She has trouble with her periods from almost the onset of menstruation. They are irregular and painful and she suffers PMT. Her doctor puts her on the oral contraceptive to suppress ovulation and this seems to quieten things down. Eventually she comes off the pill to start a family. Her periods take 6 months to resume and they are worse than ever. She has trouble conceiving because the pill has depleted her zinc levels. She is low in progesterone and loses a few pregnancies at multiples of 4 weeks (4, 8, 12 16). She eventually gets pregnant but her copper accumulates and she develops postnatal depression. Her baby is zinc deficient and probably has excess copper.
She tries for another baby but this time she can't because she's developed Endometriosis. Answer: the oral contraceptive. She starts to gain weight, starts to get depressed, then and her skin changes. Her face develops a reddish tinge. Then she develops anxiety symptoms. She is told this is anxiety/panic disorder causing her depression and is put onto antidepressants, but these don't help her tiredness. Then she finds out that she's iron deficient, but she can't raise her

... Then she's told she's got an under active thyroid and needs thyroid replacement. Still no

drain water near a toilet than the [illegible]

xenoestrogens again. Do you think that the Pharmaceutical companies who make oral contraceptives, HRT or chemotherapy stand to lose or gain if doctors were aware of these problems? No, it's probably all just a conspiracy theory with no evidence whatsoever. Or is it.....?

**References:**

1] Abraham G.E., Lubran MM. Serum and red cell magnesium levels in-patients with premenstrual tension. Am J Clin. Nut; 34(11) 2364-66 1981

2] Adlercreutz H., et al. Estrogen and Metabolite levels in Women at Risk for Breast Cancer. Cancer Res. 35:703, 1994

3] Arafah B.M. Increased Need for Thyroxine in Women with Hypothyroidism During Estrogen Therapy. N Engl J Med. 344(23):1743-1749, 2001

4] Asch R.H. & Greenblatt R. Steroidogenesis in the Post-menopausal Ovary. Clin Obstet Gynecol. 4(1): 85, 1977

5] Aufrere M.B., et al. Progesterone: An Overview and Recent Advances. J Pharmaceut Sci. 65:783, 1976

6] Backstrom T., et al. Estrogen and Progesterone in Plasma in Relation to Premenstrual Tension. J Steroid Biochem Mol Biol. 5:257-260, 1974

7] Baumslag, N et al Trace Mineral Content of Maternal and Neonatal Hair. Arch Environ Health 29 1974

8] Bell M. C., et al. Placebo-controlled trial of indole-3-carbinol in the treatment of CIN. Gynecol Oncol. 78(2):123-129, 2000

9] Beumont P.J.L., et al. Luteinizing Hormone and Progesterone Levels after Hysterectomy. Brit Med J. 836:363, 1972

10] Bloom T., Ojanotko-Harri A., Laine M., Huhtaniemi I. Metabolism of Progesterone and Testosterone in Human Parotid and Sub-mandibular Salivary Glands in Vitro. J Steroid Biochem Mol Biol. 44(1):69-76, 1993

11 Bourgain C., et al. Effects of Natural Progesterone on the Morphology of the Endometrium in Patients with Primary Ovarian Failure. Hum Reprod 5:537-543, 1990

12] Bradlow H. L., et al. Indole-3-carbinol. A novel approach to breast cancer prevention. Annals of the New York Academy of Sciences USA. 768:180-200, 1995

13 Bremner I Manifestations of Copper excess. Am J Clin Nutr 67 1069S-73 1998

14] Chang K.J., Lee T.T.Y., Linares-Cruz G., Fournier S. and de Lingieres B. Influences of Percutaneous Administration of Estradiol and Progesterone on Human Breast Epethial Cell Cycle in Vivo. Fertil Steril. 63:785-791, 1995

15] Christ J.E., et al. The Residual Ovary Syndrome. Obstet Gynecol. 46:551-556, 1975

16] Chuong C J & Dawson EB Zinc and copper levels in premenstrual syndrome. Fert. Steril 62:2, 313-20 1994

17] Ciampelli M., et al. Insulin and Polycystic Ovary Syndrome: A New Look at an Old Subject. Gynecol Endocrinol. 12(4):277-292, 1998

18] Clark G.M. and McQuire W.L. Progesterone Receptors and Human Breast Cells. Breast Cancer Res Treat. 3:157-163,1983

19] Colborn T., et al. Our Stolen Future. New York : Penguin Books, 1997

20] Corvol P., et al. Effect of Progesterone and Progestins on Water and Salt Metabolism. In Progesterone and Progestins (N.Y. Raven Press). 1983

21] Cover C. M., et al. Indole-3-carbinol and tamoxifen cooperate to arrest the cell cycle of MCF-7 human breast cancer cells. Cancer Research. 59:1244-1251, 1999

22] Cowan L.D., Gordis L., Tonascia J.A. and Jones G.S. Breast Cancer Incidence in Women with a History of Progesterone Deficiency. Am J Epidemiol. 114:209-217, 1981

23] Dalton K. The Aetiology of Premenstrual Syndrome is with the Progesterone Receptors. Med Hyp. 31:321-327, 1987

24] Dalton K. Premenstrual Syndrome and Progesterone Therapy. 2d ed. London: Heinemann. 1984

25] Dalton K. Progesterone Suppositories and Pessaries in the Treatment of Menstrual Migraine. Headache.12(4):151-159, 1973

26] Davis D.L., Bradlow H.L., Wolff M., Woodruff T., Hoel D.G. and Anton-Culver H. Medical Hypothesis: Xenohormones as Preventable Causes of Breast Cancer. Env Health Persoectuves. 101:372-377, 1993

27] Dannerstein L., Spencer-Gardner C., Brown J.B., Smith M.A. and Burrows G.D. Premenstrual Tension- Hormone Profiles. J Psychosomat Obstet Gynaec. 3:37-51, 1984

28] Del Giudice M.E., et al. Insulin and Related Factors in Premenopausal Breast Cancer Risk. Breast Cancer Res Treat. 47(2):111-120, 1998

29] Denouble Bnerstein L., et al. Progesterone and the Premenstrual Syndrome: A Double Blind Crossover Trial. Brit Med J. 290:1017-1021, 1985

30] Ducrey B., et al. Inhibition of 5 alpha-reductase and aromatase by the ellagitannins oenothein A and oenothein B from Epilobium species. Planta Medica. 63(2):111-114, 1997

31] Ellison P.T. Measurements of Salivary Progesterone. Ann NY Acad Sci. 694:161-176, 1993

32] Ellison P.T., Lipson S.F., O'Rourke M.T., Bentley G.R., Harrigan A.M., Painter-Brick C. and Vizthum V.J. Population Variation in Ovarian Function. (Letter). The Lancet. 342(8868):433-434, 1993

33] Facchinetti F et al Magnesium prophylaxis of menstrual migraine: effects on intracellular magnesium. Headache, 31:5, 298-301 1991

34] Facchinetti F et al Oral magnesium successfully relieves premenstrual mood changes. Obstet Gynecol, August; 78:2,177-81 1991

35] Foidart J.-M., et al. Estradiol and Progesterone Regulate the Proliferation of Human Breast Epithelial Cells. Fertil Steril. 69:963-969, 1998

36] Formby B. and Wiley T.S. Progesterone Inhibits Growth and Induces Apoptosis in Breast Cancer Cells: Inverse Effect on Expression of p53 and Bcl-2. Ann Clin Lab Sc. 28(6):360-9, 1998

37] Gambell R.D. Use of Progestogens in Post-menopausal Women. Int J Fertil. 34:315-321, 1989

38] Gompel A., Malet C., Spritzer P., La Lardrie J.-P., et al. Progestin Effect on Cell Proliferation and 17â-hydroxysteroid Dehydrogenase Activity in Normal Human Breast Cells in Culture. J Clin Endocrinol Metab 63:1174, 1986

39] Gompel A., Sabourin J.C., Martin A., Yaneva H., et al. Bcl-2 Expression in Normal Endometrium during the Menstrual Cycle. Am J Path. 144:1196-1202, 1994

40] Gozzo et al Xenoestrogens, pollution & health: a critical review.J Pharm Belg 1998 Jul-Aug;53(4):278-86

41] Guo D., et al. Protection by chlorophyllin and indole-3-carbinol against 2-amino-1-methyl-6-phenylimidazo[4,5-b]pyridine (PhIP)-induced DNA adducts and colonic aberrant crypts in the F344 rat. Carcinogenesis. 16(12):2931-2937, 1995

42] Hamnridge, K.M. et al Zinc Nutrtional Staus During Pregnancy: A longitudinal Study Am J Clin Nutr 37, 1983

43] Hankinson S.E. Circulating Concentrations of Insulin-like Growth Factor-I and Risk of Breast Cancer. The Lancet. 351(9113):1393-1396, 1998

44] Hess, F.M. et al Zinc Excretion in Young Women on Low Zinc Intakes and Oral Contraceptives. J Nutr 107 1977

45] Hreshchyshn M.M., et al. Effects of Natural Menopause, Hysterectomy, and Oophorectomy on Lumber Spine and Femoral Neck Bone Densities. Obstet Gynecol. 72:631-638, 1988

44] Hrushesky W.J.M. Breast Cancer, Timing of Surgery, and the Menstrual Cycle: Call for Prospective Trial. J Women's Health. 5:555-566, 1996

45] Hrushesky W.J. Menstrual Cycle Timing of Breast Cancer Resection: Prospective Study is Overdue. J Natl Cancer Inst. 87(2):143-4, 1995

46] Inoh A., Kamiya K., Fujii Y. and Yokoro K. Protective Effect of Progesterone and Tamoxifen in Estrogen-induced Mammary Carcinogenesis in Ovariectomized W/Fu Rats. Jpn J Cancer Res. 76:699-704, 1985

47] Jacobson J.L. and Jacobson S.W. Intellectual Impairment in Children Exposed to Poly-chlorinated Biphenyls in Utero. N Eng J Med. 335:783-789, 1996

48] Jellinck P.H., Michnovicz J.J. and Bradlow H.L. Influence of Indole-3-carbinol on the Hepatic Microsomal Formation of Catechol Estrogens. Steroids. 56(8):446-450, 1991

49] Kandouz M., Siromachkova M., Jacob D., Marquet B.C., et al. Antagonism between Estradiol and Progestin on Bcl-2 Expression in Breast Cancer Cells. Int J Cancer. 68:120-125, 1996

50] Katdare M., et al. Prevention of mammary preoplastic transformation by naturally-occurring tumor inhibitors. Cancer Letters. 111(1-2):141-147, 1997

51] Kirschner M.A. The Role of Hormones in the Etiology of Human Breast Cancer. Cancer. 39(6):2716-2726, 1977

52] Krimsky S. Hormonal Chaos: The Scientific and Social Origins of the Environmental Endocrine Hypothesis. Baltimore, Md.: Johns Hopkins University Press, 2000

53] Lee, J.R. What your doctor may not tell you about premenopause. Warner Books 1999

54] Leis H.P. Endocrine Prophylaxis of Breast Cancer with Cyclic Estrogen and Progesterone. Intern Surg. 45:496-503, 1966

55] Liehr J.G. Catechol Estrogens as Mediators of Estrogen-induced Carcinogenesis. Cancer Res. 35:704, 1994

56] Liehr J.G. Genotoxic Effects of Estrogens. Mutat Res. 238(3):269-276, 1990

57] Liehr J.G. Mechanisms of Metabolic Activation and Inactivation of Catecholestrogens: A Basis of Genotoxicity. Polycyclic Aromatic Compounds. 6:229-239, 1994

58] Liehr J.G., et al. 4-Hydroxylation of Estradiol by Human Uterine Myomerium and Myoma Microsomes: Implications for the Mechanism of Uterine Turmorigenesis. Proc Nat Acad Sci. 92:1229-1233, 1995

59] Limanova Z., et al. Frequent Incidence of Thyropathies in Women with Breast Carcinoma. Vnitr Lek. 44(2):76-82, 1998

60] Lipson S.F. and Ellison P.T. Reference Value for Lutal 'Progesterone' Measured by Salivary Radioimmunoassay. Fertil Steril 61(3): 448-454, 1994

61] Lizotte L The woman with too much copper. Total health 19: 49 19997

62] Llang J., et al. Indole-3-carbinol prevents cervical cancer in human papilloma virus type 16 (HPV16) transgenic mice. Cancer Research. 59:3991-3997, 1999

63] MacLusky N.J., Naftolin F., Krey L.C. and Franks S. The Catechol Estrogens. J Steroid Biochem. 15:111-124, 1981

64] Mahesh V.B., Brann D.W. and Hendry L.G. Diverse Modes of Action of Progesterone and Its Metabolites. J Steroid Biochem Molec Biol., Dept of Cell Biology, Baylor College of Medicine, Houston, Tex. 56:67-77, 1996

65] Malloy V. L., et al. Interaction between a semisynthetic diet and indole-3-carbinol on mammary tumor incidence in Balb/cfC3H mice. Anticancer Research. 17(6D):4333-4337, 1997

66] Matzkin H., et al. Immunohistochemical evidence of the existence and localization of aromatase in human prostatic tissues. Prostate. 21:309-314, 1992

67] Meng Q., et al. Indole-3-carbinol is a negative regulator of estrogen receptor- signaling in human tumor cells. Journal of Nutrition. 130:2927-2931, 2000

68] Mohr P.E., Wang D.Y., Gregory W.M., Richards M.A. and Fentiman I.S. Serum Progesterone and Prognosis in Operable Breast cancer. Brit J Cancer. 73:1552-1555, 1996

69] Moyer D.L., et al. Prevention of Endometrial Hyperplasia by Progesterone during Long Term Estradiol Replacement: Influence of Bleeding Pattern and Secretory Changes. Fertil Steril. 59:992-997, 1993

70] Munday M.R., et al. Correlations between Progesterone, Oestradiol and Aldosterone Levels in the Premenstrual Syndrome. Clin Endocrinol. 14:1-9,1981

72] Muneyvirci-Delale O et al Sex steroid hormones modulate serum ionized magnesium and calcium levels throughout the menstrual cycle in women. Fertil Steril, May; 69(5): 958-62 1998

73] Nagata C., et al. Relations of Insulin Resistance and Serum Concentrations of Estradiol and Sex Hormone-binding Globulin to Potential Breast Cancer Risk Factors. Jpn J Cancer Res. 91(9):948-953, 2000

74] Nolan KR Copper toxicity syndrome J Orthomol Psych 12:270-282 1983

75] O'Brien P.M.S., Selby C. and Symonds E.M. Progesterone, Fluid and Electrolytes in Premenstrual Syndrome. Brit Med J. 1:1161-1163, 1980

76] Osborne M.P., et al. Upregulation of Estradiol C16-alpha-hydroxylation in HumanBreast Tissue: A Potential Biomarker of Breast Cancer Risk. J Nat Cancer Inst. 85(23):1917-1993, 1993

77] Pujol P., Hilsenbeck S.G., Chamness G.C. and Elledge R.M. Rising Levels of Estrogen Receptor in Breast Cancer over 2 Decades. Cancer. 74:1601-1606, 1994

78] Rajapakse et al Defining the impact of weakly estrogenic chemicals on the action of steroidal estrogens.Tox Sci 60(2):296-304 2001

79] Reed M.J. and Purohit A. Breast Cancer and the Role of Cytokines in Regulating Estrogen Synthesis: An Emerging Hypothesis. Endocrine Rev. 18:701-715, 1997

80] Reidel H.H., et al. Ovarian Failure Phenomena after Hysterectomy. J Reprod Med. 31:597-600, 1986

81] Rodriquez C., Calle E.E., Coates R.J., Miracle-McMahill H.L., Thun M.J. and Heath C.W. Estrogen Replacement Therapy and Fatal Ovarian Cancer. Am J Epidemiol. 141:828-834, 1995

82] Rodriguez C., Calle E.E. and Coates R.J., et al. Estrogen Replacement Therapy and Fatal Ovarian Cancer. Am J Epidemiol. 141:828-834, 1995

83] Sabourin J.C., Martin A., Baruch J., Truc J.B., et al. Bcl-2 Expression in Normal Breast Tissue during the Menstrual Cycle. Int J Cancer. 59:1-6, 1994

84] Schairer C., et al. Menopausal Estrogen and Estrogen-Progestin Replacement Therapy and Breast Cancer Risk. JAMA 283:485-491, 2000

85] Shering S.G., et al. Thyroid Disorders and Breast Cancer. Eur J Cancer Prev. 5(6):504-506, 1996

86] Sherwood RA, Rocks BF, et al. Magnesium and the premenstrual syndrome. Ann Clin Bioc 23:667-70 1986

87] Shi-Zhong Bu, De-Ling Yin, Xiu-Hai Ren, Li-Zhen Jiang, et al. Progesterone Induces Apoptosis and Up-regulation of p53 Expression in Human Ovarian Carcinoma Cell Lines. Am Cancer Soc. 1944-1950, 1997

88] Siddle N., et al The effect of Hysterectomy on the Age at Ovarian Failure: Identification of a Subgroup of Women with Premature Loss of Ovarian Function and Literature Review. Fertil Steril. 47:94-100, 1987

89] Smyth P.P. The Thyroid and Breast Cancer: A Significant Association? Ann Med. 29(3):189-191, 1997

90] Stoewsand G. S. Bioactive organosulfur phytochemicals in Brassica oleracea vegetables - a review. Food Chem Toxicol . 33(6):537-543, 1995

91] Stoll B.A. Adiposity as a Risk Determinant for Postmenopausal Breast Cancer. Int J Obes Relat Metab Disord. 24(5): 527-533, 2000

92] Stoll B.A. Dietary Supplements of Dehydroepiandrosterone in Relation to Breast Cancer Risk. Eur J Clin Nutr. 53(10):771-775, 1999

93] Stoll B.A. Western Nutrition and the Insulin Resistance Syndrome: A Link to Breast Cancer. Eur J Clin Nutr. 53(2):83-87, 1999

94] Stone S.C., et al. The Acute Effect of Hysterectomy on Ovarian Function. Am J Obstet Gynecol. 121:193-197, 1975

95] Talamini R. Selected Medical Conditions and Risk of Breast Cancer. Brit J Cancer. 75(11):1699-1703, 1997

96] Vir, S.C. et al Serum and Hair Concentrations of Copper in Pregnancy Am J Clin Nutr 34 1981

97] Watts, D.L. Trace Elements and other Essential Nutrients Writers Block Books 1997

98] Watts, D.L. The Effects of oral contraceptive agents on Nutritional status Am Chiro March 1985

99] Watts, DL Nutritional relationships of copper J Orthomol Med 4:99-108 1989

100] Wattenburg L.W., et al. Inhibition of polycyclic aromatic hydrocarbon-induced neoplasia by naturally occurring indoles. Cancer Research. 38(5):1410-1413, 1978

101] Werbach, M. Nutritional Influences on Illness. Third Line Press. 199

102] Yuan F., et al. Anti-estrogenic activities of indole-3-carbinol in cervical cells: implications for prevention of cervical cancer. Anticancer Research. 19:1673-1680, 1999

# Xenoestrogens

Pesticides (DDT, DDE, 2,4, 5-T, Dieldrin,
endosulfan, Dioxins
methoxychlor, kepone,
toxafene, chloropicrin
lindane, chlordane, artrazine)

Metals    Arsenic Cadmium

Petroleum products
(methyl benzine, toluene,
car fumes, PCB)

Plastics

(PVC, lunch wraps, etc)

Hormones
a. From Doctors
(The Pill &
Hormone Replacement therapy)
b. From Food 1) Poultry industry
2) Antibiotics in animal feed

# Hormone system interactions

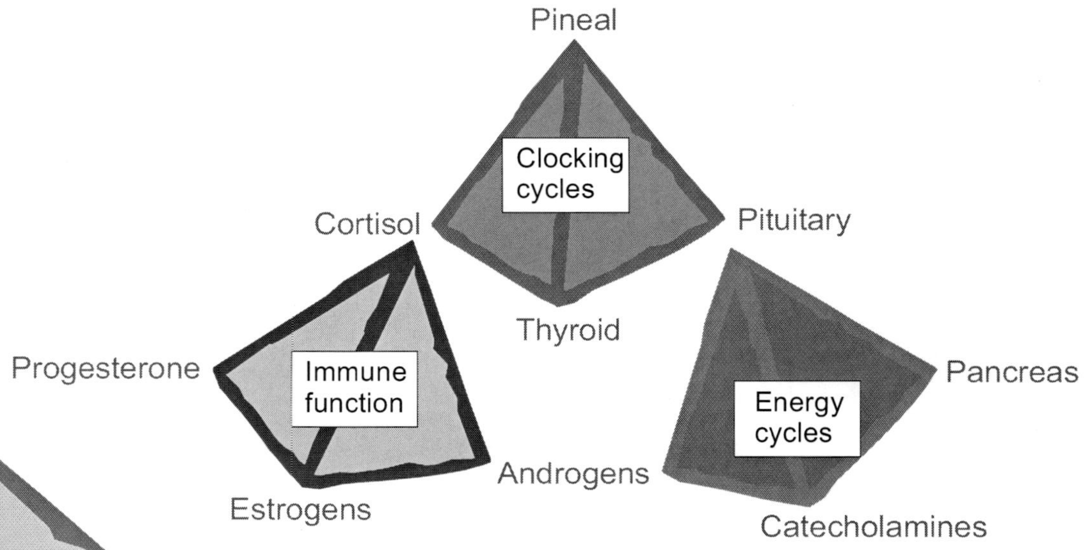

Pineal

Pituitary

Pancreas

Clocking cycles

Energy cycles

Thyroid

Catecholamines

Cortisol

Androgens

Immune function

Estrogens

Progesterone

Normal Copper balance depends on Estrogen: progesterone balance

$$\frac{E}{P}$$

Cu

Zn

Mg

## Mineral systems and balance

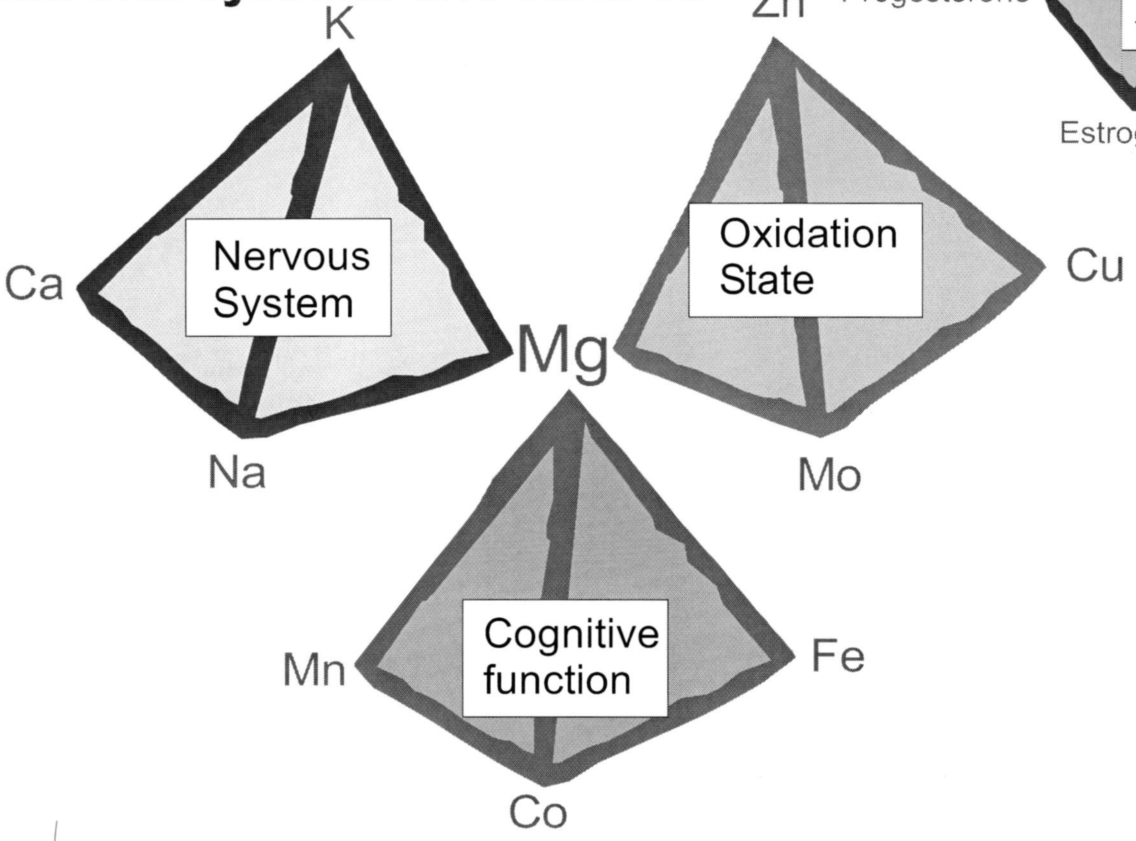

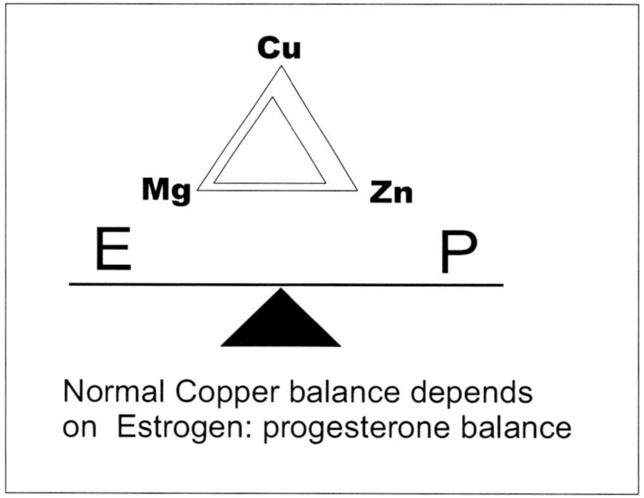

Cu

Zn

Oxidation State

Mo

Mg

Fe

Cognitive function

Co

Mn

K

Nervous System

Na

Ca

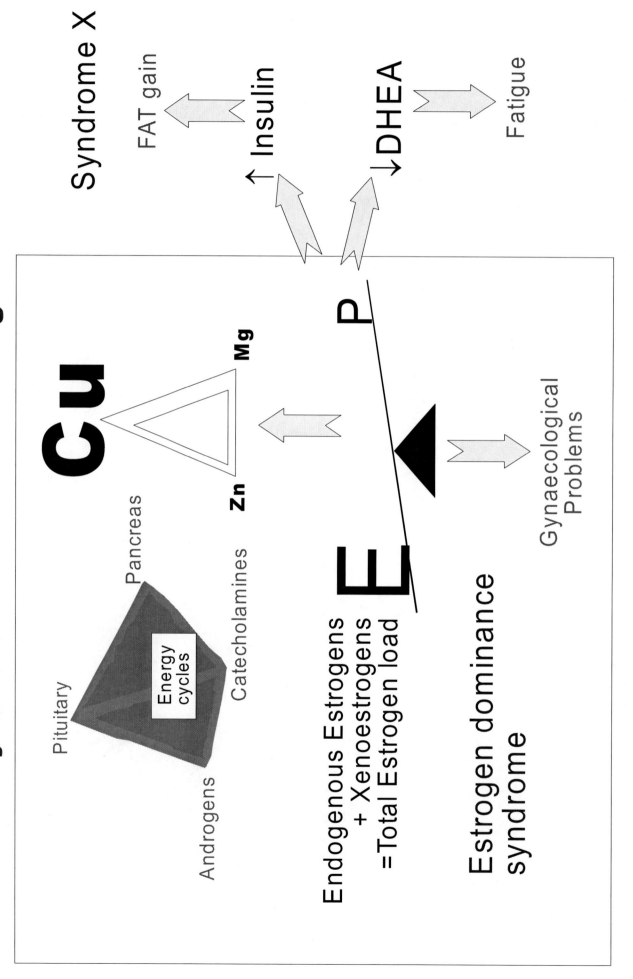

# Syndrome X meets Estrogen dominance

Syndrome X

FAT gain

↑ Insulin

↓DHEA

Fatigue

Cu

Pituitary

Pancreas

Energy cycles

Catecholamines

Androgens

Zn

Mg

P

E

Gynaecological Problems

Endogenous Estrogens
+ Xenoestrogens
=Total Estrogen load

Estrogen dominance syndrome

# Effect on Menstrual cycles and Copper

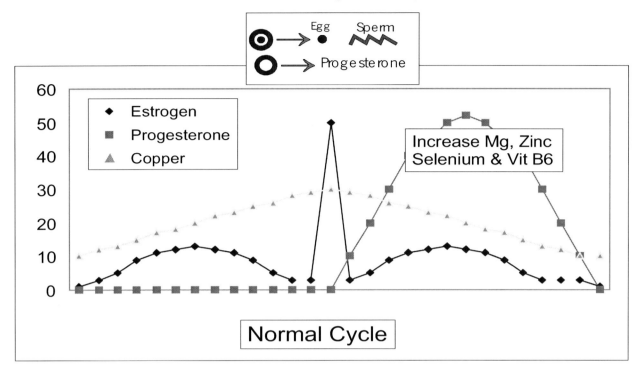

Egg • Sperm

Progesterone

Estrogen
Progesterone
Copper

Increase Mg, Zinc
Selenium & Vit B6

Normal Cycle

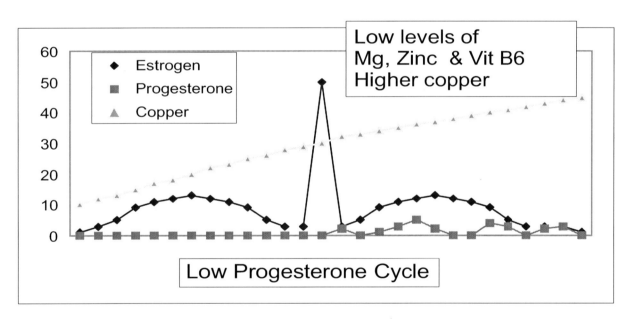

Low levels of
Mg, Zinc & Vit B6
Higher copper

Estrogen
Progesterone
Copper

Low Progesterone Cycle

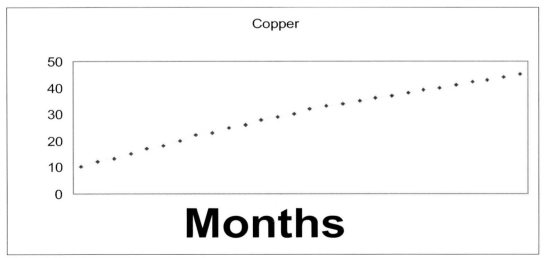

Copper

# Months

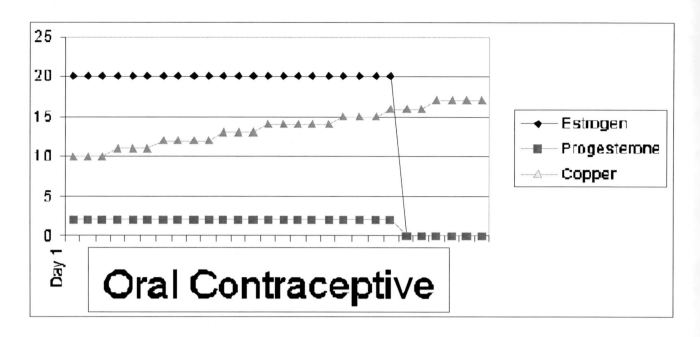

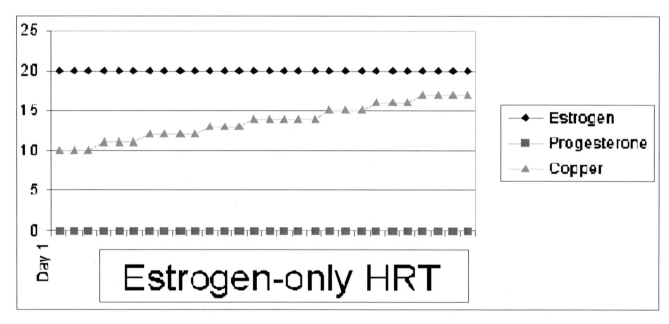

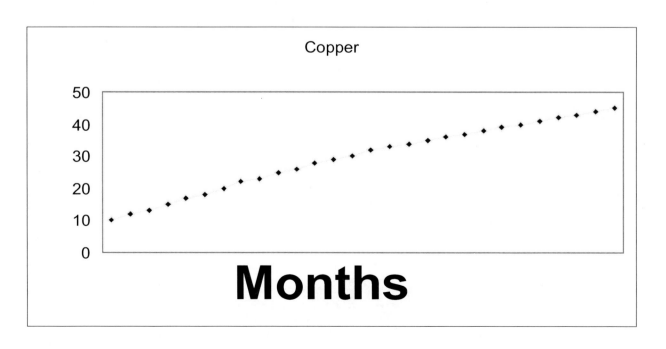

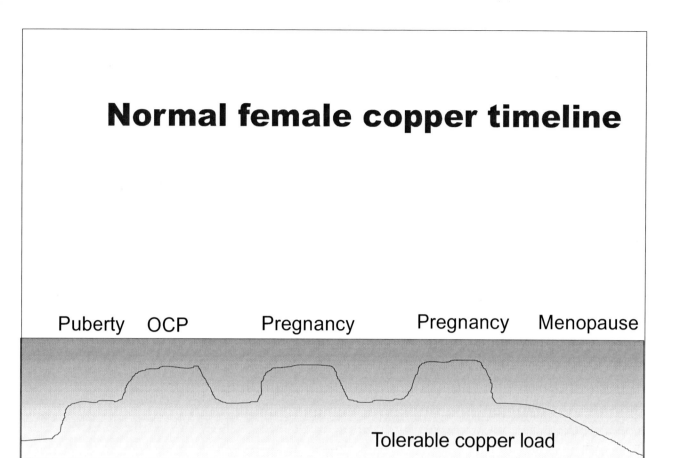

Time in years

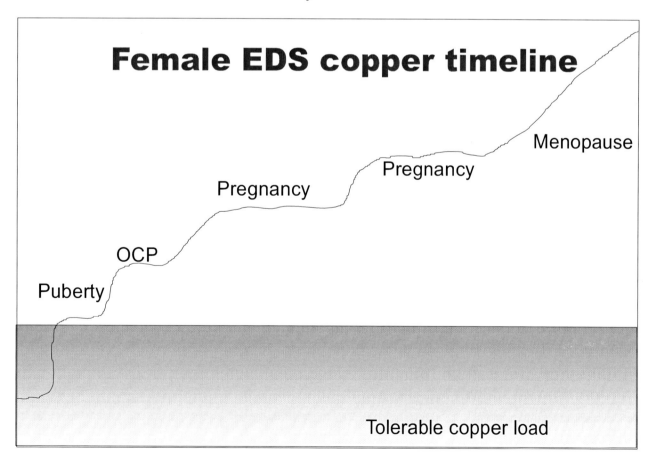

Time in years

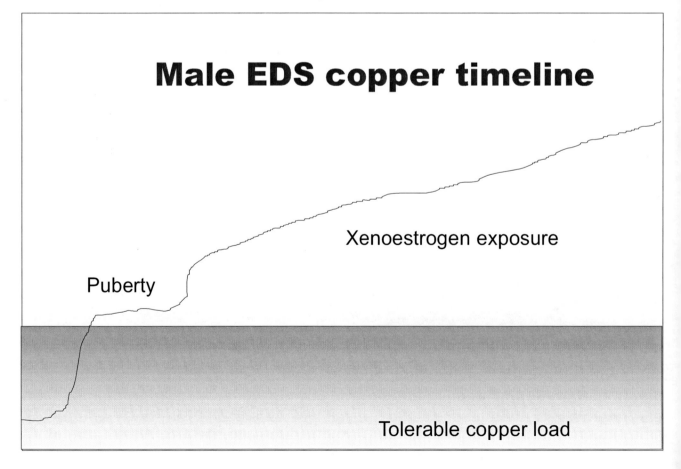

# Normal Male copper timeline

Puberty

Tolerable copper load

Time in years

# Male EDS copper timeline

Xenoestrogen exposure

Puberty

Tolerable copper load

# Some technical stuff: Why the cations are so important

For those who want more nitty gritty about the importance of minerals in biological systems, this section may help to clarify some points. Reductionism leads to Holism and this is why.

**Charged Ions**

| Cations | Anions |
|---|---|
| Positive charge | Negative charge |
| Gives up electrons | Accepts electrons |
| Sodium (Na$^+$) | Chloride (Cl$^-$) |
| Magnesium (Mg$^{++}$) | Sulphate (SO$_4$$^{2-}$) |
| Chromate (Cr$^{++}$) | Phosphate (PO$_4$$^{3-}$) |

When electrons are added or taken away from any atom or molecule, charges are created that have been arbitrarily labeled as positive or negative. If you take away an electron you make the ion more positive. Because the proton (hydrogen ion) is the most basic of ions, it has been given an elctronegativity value of zero. All other ions are either more electronegative or less electronegative.

# Natural production of Hydrogen ion (proton)

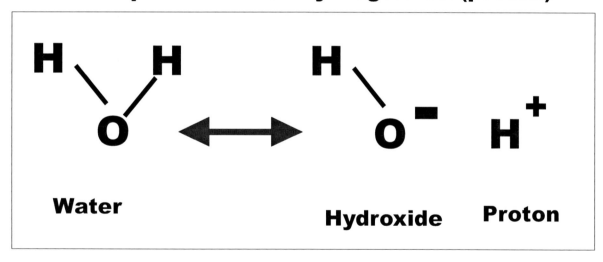

Water ⟷ Hydroxide Proton

Because of the prevalence of water in biological systems (99 out of every 100 molecules), there will always be protons present. These create the pH (acidity level). If water is left to its own devices the pH will be 7 (neutral). Life forms had to deal with this from the very first cell. There are many mechanisms of how this works and most biochemistry textbooks will have a chapter on acid-base balance. So the production of protons (hydrogen ion) is rather different from the other ions we find in abundance. Protons form spontaneously from water.

For metallic ions like sodium, electrons are "taken" away from the metallic atom and this creates a "lack" of an electron, which we arbitrarily say is a positive charge. Some atoms will give more electrons and therefore might have different valences (charge values). Biological examples are copper and iron.

If you look at the graph of elctronegativity from Lithium to Fluoride we notice several points. The cluster of ions around minus 3 includes Potassium, Sodium, Calcium and Magnesium. These form the Nervous system tetrahedron (see Chapter on this). They are relatively easy to deal with and of these magnesium is the most free to roam in cells.

# Metallic Cations

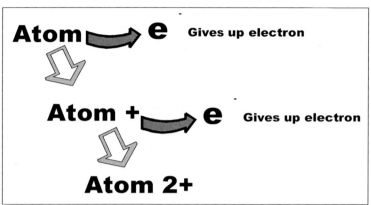

As we "climb" the graph we progressively come across zinc then, then hydrogen then copper. The less electronegative the more pressure there is on the cell to "contain" these metals. We need to store them safely and to mobilize them when they are need. The higher the position on the graph the more "dangerous" the metal. Systems such as Metallothionine, Lipoic acid, Ferritin and Ceruloplasmin help us control such atoms. But environmental toxins mess up the systems. Isn't it interesting how the most elctronegative elements are added to drinking water?

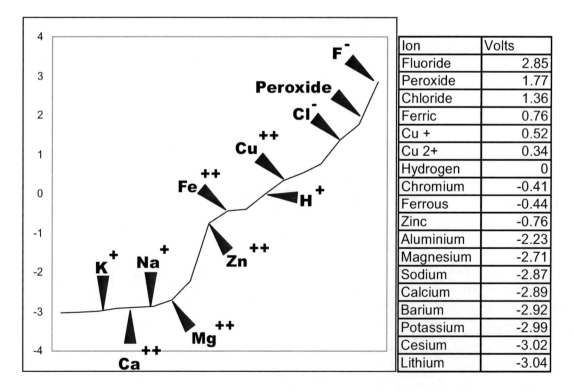

| Ion | Volts |
|---|---|
| Fluoride | 2.85 |
| Peroxide | 1.77 |
| Chloride | 1.36 |
| Ferric | 0.76 |
| Cu + | 0.52 |
| Cu 2+ | 0.34 |
| Hydrogen | 0 |
| Chromium | -0.41 |
| Ferrous | -0.44 |
| Zinc | -0.76 |
| Aluminium | -2.23 |
| Magnesium | -2.71 |
| Sodium | -2.87 |
| Calcium | -2.89 |
| Barium | -2.92 |
| Potassium | -2.99 |
| Cesium | -3.02 |
| Lithium | -3.04 |

Because of the importance of metals to higher life forms, disruption to these nutrients gives rise to very common symptoms, which can be analyzed and interpreted. We know quite a bit about these metals and what happens when they are low or too high. We also know the *reasons* why they vary from normal. The bottom line is that symptoms are caused because a nutrient is either low or being interfered with by another compound. This is Diagnostic Orthomolecular Medicine.

Nutritional Medicine is in a unique position to examine the factors that drive humans from energetic to fatigued. Allopathic medicine is very good at picking up the obvious conditions like anaemia and Heart failure, but not good at restoring wellness.

## Nutritional Medicine

**Fatigued**                                      **Energetic**

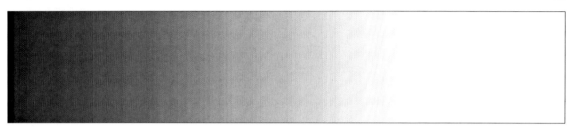

**Anaemia**
**Heart failure**

Reductionists would breakdown the causes of chronic illness into the below mentioned categories, and we will examine why this might be a handy way of understanding why our patients get fatigued. These problems have all been covered elsewhere in this book. Fixing the patient involves understanding *why* these things have happened. I cannot stress enough that any abnormal test is not a diagnosis; it is the beginning of another investigation. Just giving Magnesium or DHEA on the basis of low levels doesn't adhere to the ideology of DOM. Find out *why* these things are low and fix the reason!

# Causes of chronic illness

## Imbalance

## deficiency

| minerals | hormones | immune system |
|----------|----------|---------------|
| minerals | hormones | immune system |

## excess   copper manganese

## toxin   toxic metals chemicals

## digestion/dysbiosis

## Channelopathy

# Energy & Fatigue

## Patterns of fatigue

1. Unrefreshed sleep, daytime sleepiness
2. Fixed "energy coupon" type
3. Postprandial
4. Late afternoon
5. PM crash and second wind
6. Heavy limb type
7. Myalgic type

## Patterns of fatigue

| | Mg | Fe | VitC | Zn | Cr | Se | Copper Xs | Mycoplasma |
|---|---|---|---|---|---|---|---|---|
| 1. Unrefreshed sleep daytime sleepiness | ✓ | ± | | ± | | ± | | |
| 2. Fixed "energy coupon" type | ± | ✓ | ✓ | | | | | |
| 3. Postprandial | ± | | | ✓ | ± | ± | | |
| 4. Late afternoon | | | | ✓ | ✓ | | | |
| 5. PM crash and second wind | | ✓ | ✓ | | | | | |
| 6. Heavy limb type | ✓ | ± | | | | ✓ | | |
| 7. Myalgic type | ✓ | ± | ✓ | | | ✓ | | ✓ |

Fatigue is a very vague symptom and the clinician should try to ascertain what type of fatigue the patient has. A list of subtypes is shown below with a table suggesting some reasons for these. Note the importance of the divalent cations.

# Sleep disorders

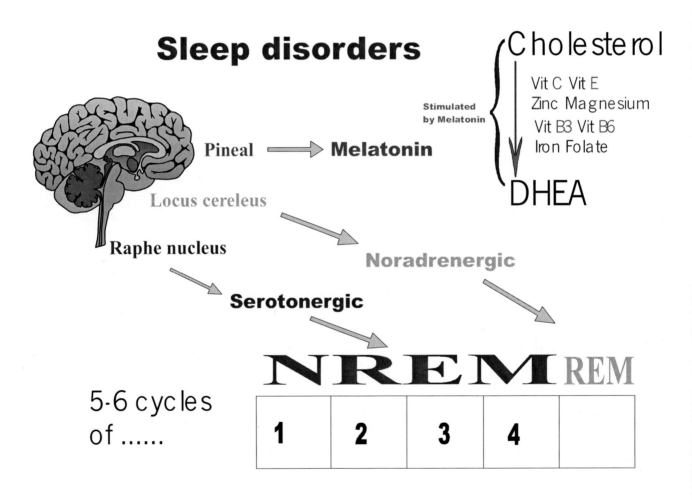

Disruption to the sleep-wake cycle is often overlooked as a cause of fatigue. Most doctors who have worked shifts have completely forgotten that your day is rather different if you didn't sleep well! The process of sleep can be broken down into initiation, perpetuation and termination of sleep. This involves the Melatonin, Serotonin and Noradrenaline.

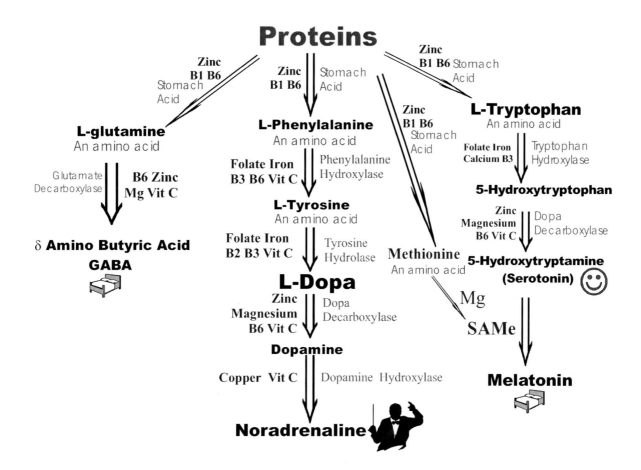

These neurotransmitters must be synthesised from Amino acids, and the brain cells need many cofactors to complete the task. Deficiencies in any one of these may be associated with abnormal sleep pattern and therefor a cause of fatigue.

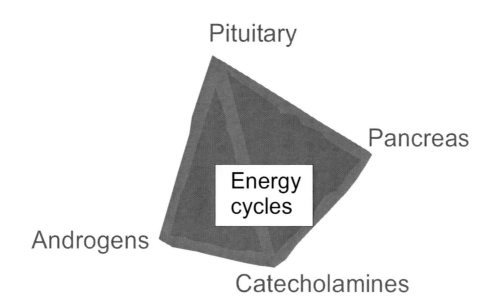

If we examine the balance of hormones that affect energy levels, we can understand that imbalances between these endocrine glands will affect energy. Just giving the obvious hormone does not really fix the problem at all.

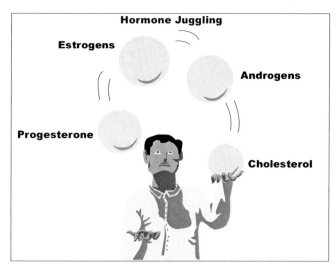

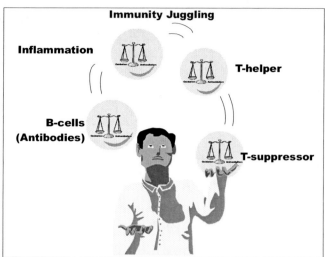

In fact, for the sex hormones, we have seen that the juggling act can be a difficult one for the organs involved, adrenal, gonads, liver, brain, bone etc. Poor juggling can lead to fatigue and most doctors who prescribe "natural hormone therapies" would readily agree.

In addition, the Immune system must juggle many factors as well. In the case of chronic fatigue, we frequently see over- and under-stimulated immune systems. The juggler has messed up.

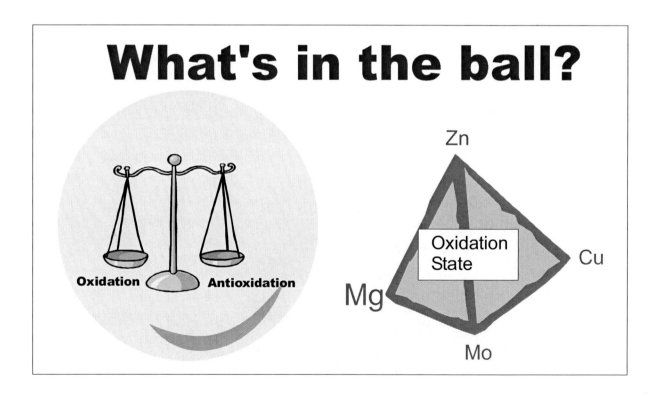

So what's in the ball? It turns out that oxidation state affect each ball in the juggling act. If we breakdown the components of the oxidation balance we find the divalent cations again.

With respect to mineral balance (of the divalnet cations), the delicate cogs that keep balanced will upset by "spanners" such as Xenoestrogens and Heavy metals.

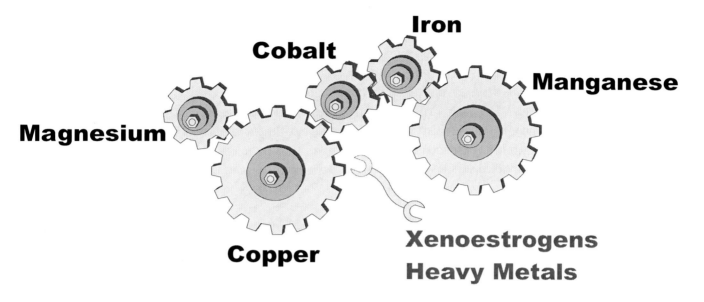

So at the end of the day fatigue may occur for two reasons. The nutrient isn't there or the nutrient is blocked. A good example is mercury. Mercury causes Channelopathies and has a severe effect on the Mitochondria as shown.

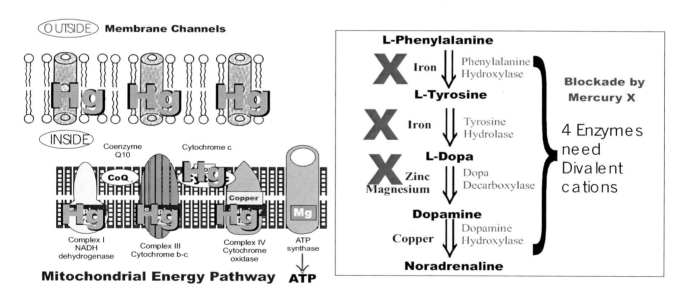

So for a cell that makes noradrenaline, this would block 3 of the 4 enzymes needed to make this compound. This would lead to fatigue, depression and cognitive dysfunction.

So the bottom line is fatigue is generated by the same forces as any other problem.

Essential Fatty Acid (EFA) metabolism has received much attention in recent years. Good oils, bad oils and all the ascribed pathology and wonder cures that go with such writing. Udo Erasmus's book "Fats that heal, Fats that Kill" is one of the best attempts at putting this work into practical terms. Just as John R Lees's book apparent take home message seemed to be "give progesterone for everything", so it seems that the take home message from Erasmus's book was "give Omega-3 EFA's to everyone". Regularly throughout his book he constantly mentions the importance of the supporting nutrients B3, B6, Vitamin C, Zinc and magnesium. In fact, in his second printing he mentions Zinc 43 times! His most poignant statement is " a deficiency of any of the above five (B3, B6, Vitamin C, Zinc or Magnesium) nutrients may mimic the degenerative symptoms of EFA deficiency". If we look at his list of LA/LNA (Linoleic acid and Linolenic Acid) deficiency symptoms and we look at a list of zinc deficiency symptoms, there is a

## Linolenic Acid deficiency symptoms

eczema-like skin eruptions
loss of hair
liver degeneration
behavioral disturbances
kidney degeneration
excessive water loss through the skin
drying up of glands

susceptibility to infections
failure of wound healing
sterility in males
miscarriage in females
arthritis-like conditions
heart and circulatory problems
growth retardation

very strong overlap.

Is Udo Erasmus confused between Zinc and Linolenic acid? On page 50 of his book he says, "LA and LNA substantially shorten the time required for fatigued muscles to recover after exercise. They facilitate the conversion of lactic acid to water and carbon dioxide". The last time I looked at the system that managed Lactic acid I found an enzyme called lactate dehydrogenase, which is a Zinc dependent enzyme. This was part of the Cori Cycle, which

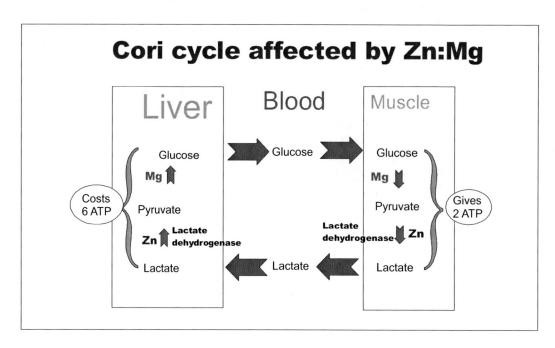

# Carbonic Anhydrase

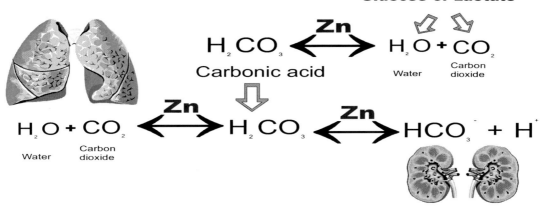

Glucose or Lactate

$$H_2CO_3 \xleftrightarrow{\text{Zn}} H_2O + CO_2$$

Carbonic acid          Water     Carbon dioxide

$$H_2O + CO_2 \xleftrightarrow{\text{Zn}} H_2CO_3 \xleftrightarrow{\text{Zn}} HCO_3^- + H^+$$

Water   Carbon dioxide

sent lactate back to the liver for processing.

If Lactate isn't converted back to glucose by lactate dehydrogenase and gets converted to Water and carbon dioxide instead, then these by-products are sent into the blood stream as Carbonic acid . This is the job of Carbonic acid anhydrase, which is also a zinc dependent enzyme!

To transport water and carbon dioxide out of the body, Carbonic Anhydrase converts them to carbonic acid. The

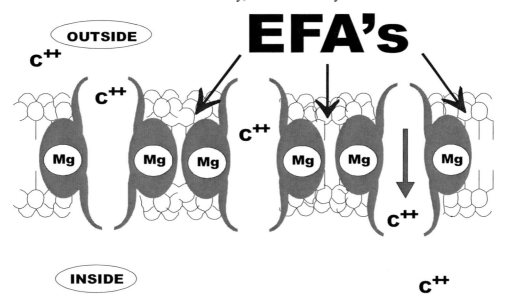

lung converts this back to Carbon dioxide and water and excretes both. The Kidney converts it to bicarbonate and hydrogen ion (proton) and excretes these.

Either way it is Zinc that is the most important divalent cation in this process of lactate metabolism. So why the mix up? There are two possibilities. The first is that these functions were always about EFA's and the Zinc is required for the their correct working in the body. The second is that EFA's affect the transport of zinc into cells. They improve intracellular levels of minerals. Let's look at this possibility. EFA's make up a significant part of the cell wall. Ion transport systems come in various shapes and sizes, but one model is shown below. The outer protein grabs the ion and closes the outer "claws" which drags the ion into the membrane channel. The inner "claw" opens and allows the ion to enter the cell. The process is driven by a Magnesium dependent ATP pumps. The region of the cell membrane next to the "claw" needs to be flexible enough to be "squashed" by the ion channel protein as it opens the outer "claw" and the inner "claw". This flexibility is provided by the EFA's in the membrane. Therefore EFA's influence the transmembrane passage of ions like Zinc. Therefore the observed effects of EFA's could be explained by the improvement in intracellular levels of zinc (or any other ion).

Therefore the connection between EFA's and ions like zinc is established. Cations need EFA's to be transported into cells. Therefore EFA abnormalities will lead to cation deficiencies in cells, which will affect enzyme function.

Pyrroles have been found in excessive amounts in patients with Autism and Schizophrenia. Treatment with Zinc and/ or B6 has resulted in reductions of Pyrroluria over 3-6 months treatment. Authors have also noted the high frequency of dysbiosis and leaky gut in Autism patients (and indeed many patients with chronic illness).

So here we have 3 unconnected observations. Zinc /B6 treatment, probiotics and gut restoration lead to a slow improvement in Pyrroluria (and hopefully symptoms).

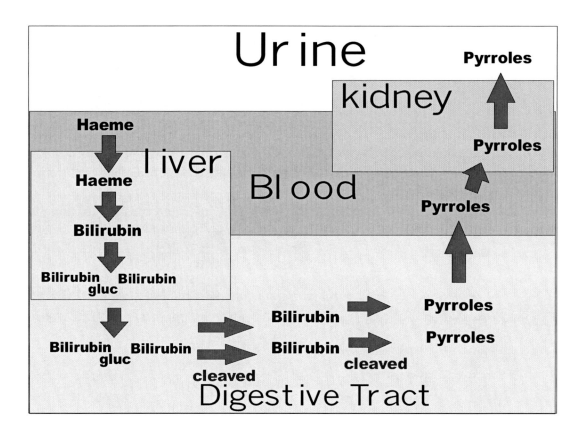

So let us revise the hypothesis again. Haeme returns to the liver for breakdown. Iron is recycled and haeme is converted to bilirubin. Bilirubin is conjugated to Bilirubin glucuronide (a magnesium dependent enzyme) and this is excreted in the bile. This compound is split in the intestine by the enzyme beta-glucuronidase whose activity is inducible to excessive levels. The unusually high levels of bilirubin are affected by the enzymes of gut bacteria resulting in altered fragments of bilirubin, which are pyrrole in chemical structure. In the presence of leaky gut, these compounds are absorbed with higher frequency than normally occurring bilirubin fragments. These absorbed Pyrroles are then excreted by the kidney into the urine.

| Zinc and B6 in digestion | | |
|---|---|---|
| **Role of Zinc in digestion** | **Role of B6 in digestion** | |
| 1] Gustin (produced by parotid) | 1] Hydrochloric acid | |
| 2] Hydrochloric acid | 2] Picolinate production | |
| 3] Carboxypeptidase | 3] Na/K pump in intestinal wall | |
| 4] Aminopeptidase | | |
| 5] Control of intestinal flora | **But activation of B6 requires Zinc and B2** | |

**Why dysbiosis leads to pyrroles**

1] Increased activity of beta-glucuronidase which cleaves Bilirubin glucuronide

2] Unusually high levels are affected by gut bacteria to create bilirubin fragments

3] These fragments are altered to the observed pyrrole compounds

4] Dysbiosis increases the conversions

5] Dysbiosis usually means "leaky gut" which increases the likelihood of pyrroles being absorbed

6] Absorbed pyrroles are excreted in the urine

Let's look at the function of zinc and B6 in digestion. Zinc is the principle cation involved in digestion of food. It supports both upper and lower gut function as listed. Vitamin B6's role is also listed, but B6 cannot be activated without Zinc (and B2). Therefore normal B6 supplements may not work as well as say Pyridoxal-5-phosphate supplements in the presence of zinc deficiency or zinc blockade (say, by Copper, Mercury, Cadmium, Aluminium, Antimony or Lead). Therefore low zinc or zinc blockade will lead to dysbiosis and increased activity of beta-glucuronidase thereby increasing bilirubin fragments (measured as pyrroles). Zinc is required for the digestion of proteins especially gluten (which is 60% glutamine). Any reduction in glutamine will cause a reduction in nourishment to the cells of the intestinal wall. This reduced maintenance and the resultant dysbiosis increases the permeability of a normally "tight" barrier, leading so the so-called "leaky gut syndrome". Therefore dysfunction of the cation Zinc may lead to "leaky gut". The increased permeability will allow more substances (like pyrroles) to be absorbed in the bloodstream.

Therefore if zinc is low or blocked there will be an excess of gut pyrroles and an increased absorption of these. Therefore, Zinc deficiency or Zinc blockade will lead to Pyrroluria. And therefore Cation dysfunction will lead to Pyrroluria

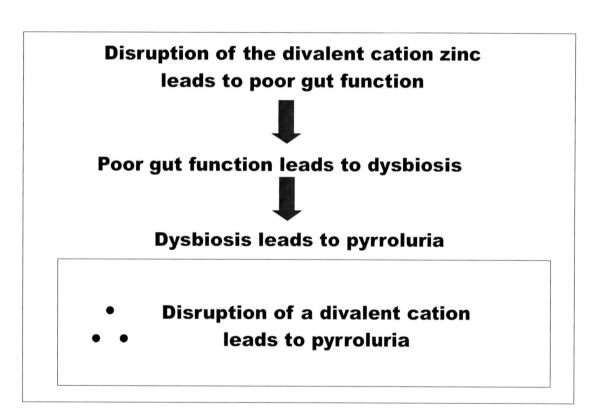

The next 2 pages show how bilirubin cleavage is the start of pyrrole creation. The fragments acted on by gut bacteria just like the "blue diaper syndrome".

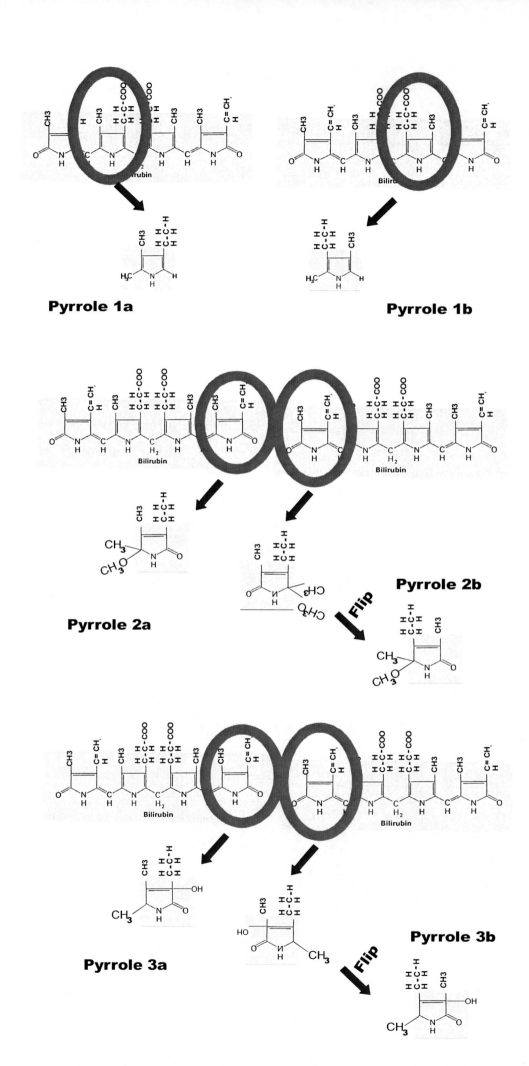

**Pyrrole 1a**

**Pyrrole 1b**

**Pyrrole 2a**

**Pyrrole 2b**

*Flip*

**Pyrrole 3a**

**Pyrrole 3b**

*Flip*

253

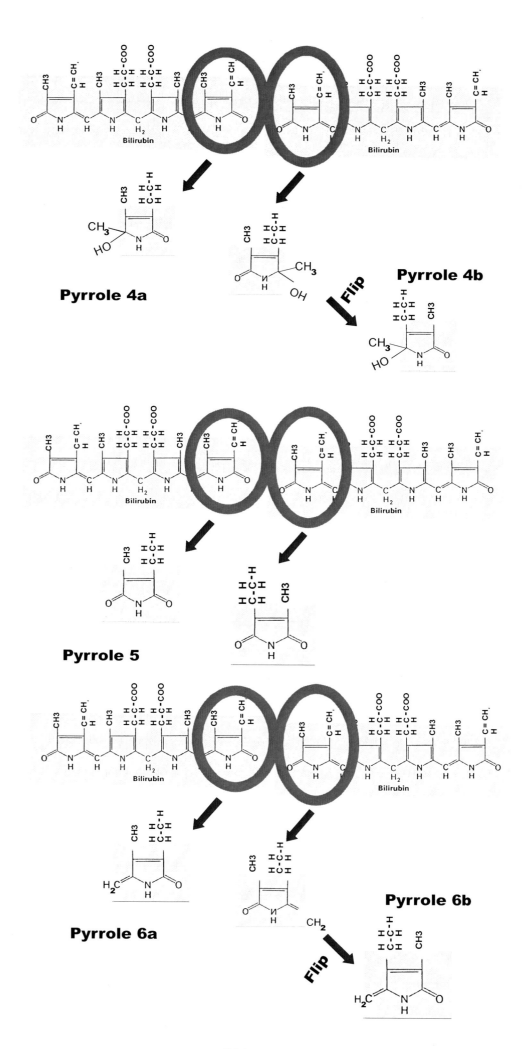

Pyrrole 4a

Flip

Pyrrole 4b

Pyrrole 5

Pyrrole 6a

Flip

Pyrrole 6b

A large proportion of methylation is provided by S-adenosyl-methionine (SAMe), which has become a popular over-the-counter supplement in recent years. SAMe's methylating role is summarised below. The range of functions is impressive. It includes 2 neurotransmitter conversions and providing "methyl tags" for DNA.

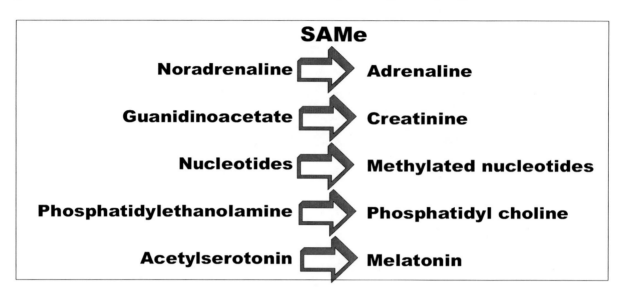

The deviation from normal that one sees can occur for several reasons outlined in the diagram. Low levels are due to supply problems. That is malabsorption of the key nutrients needed to make SAMe or failure of the nutrients to traverse cell membranes to reach their ultimate destination (Channelopathies). High levels are due to toxins (see "Cation dysfunction and Overmethylation").

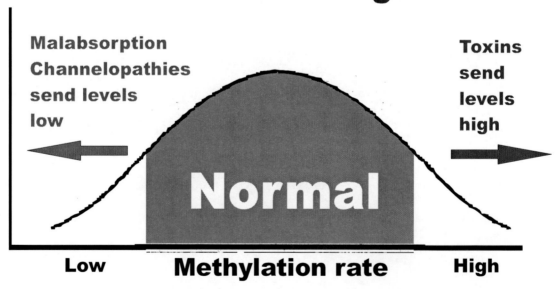

The production of SAMe relies on adequate supplies of the amino acid methionine, magnesium and ATP. Amino acids come from protein breakdown, which requires the initial effect of permanent denaturing by Hydrochloric acid. The analogy is one of making a sculpture from a large log. We start with a chainsaw to roughly carve out the shape before using carving tools. Hydrochloric acid is the chainsaw and pancreatic peptidases are the carving tools. Zinc, Vitamins B1 & B6 are needed for the production of Hydrochloric acid and Zinc is required for the function of Carboxypeptidase and Aminopeptidase. Therefore low levels of zinc in the gut will cause hypochlorhydria and poor protein digestion leading to low levels of amino acids like methionine. The next step involves ATP and magnesium. Magnesium absorption from the intestine also requires stomach acid, and so Zinc depletion will lead to Magnesium deficiency. If we study the major ions involved in ATP production wee see that Magnesium and Iron are major requirements. Iron also needs hydrochloric acid in order to be in the correct form for absorption. Therefore low gut zinc will lead to iron deficiency too. And either low Iron or magnesium will lead to low ATP, which will lead to Undermethylation. Therefore low gut zinc will lead to Undermethylation.

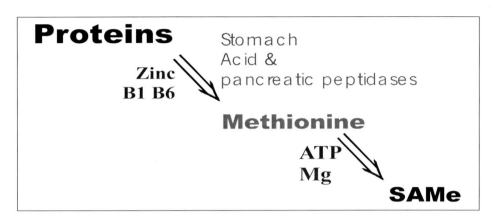

The major sites of ATP production are glycolysis, The Krebs (TCA) cycle and the electron transport chain. Examination of the roles of magnesium and iron show these divalent cations to major contributors to cellular ATP production. Therefore disruption to these divalent cations will cause low ATP levels.

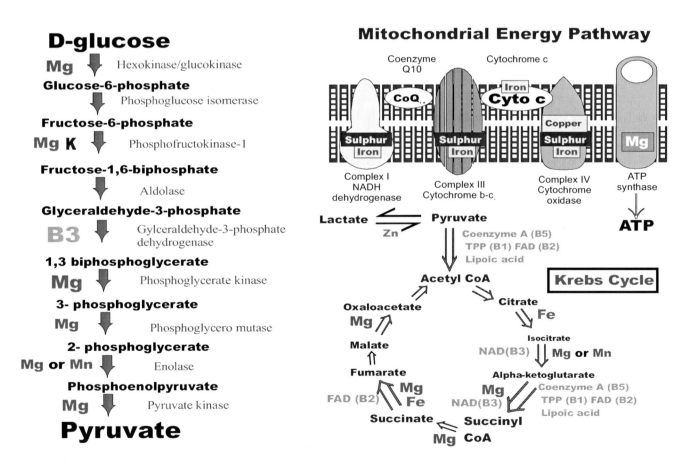

Therefore if divalent cations (like Zinc, Magnesium or Iron) are low or blocked there will be a decrease in SAMe. And therefore Cation dysfunction will lead to Undermethylation.

A large proportion of methylation is provided by S-adenosyl-methionine (SAMe), which has become a popular over-the-counter supplement in recent years. SAMe's methylating role is summarised below. The range of functions is impressive. It includes 2 neurotransmitter conversions and providing "methyl tags" for DNA.

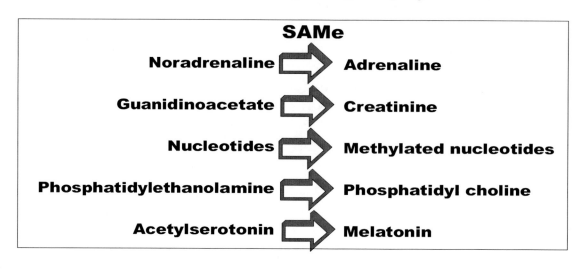

DNA contains segments called transcription units, which code for proteins.

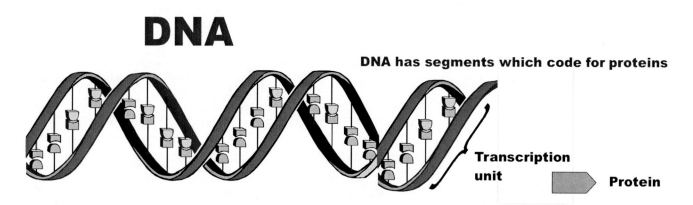

In the recently born science of Epigenetics, it was discovered that gene expression is not just "on or off"; it is more like a volume control. The way to silence (or muffle) gene expression is to attach "methyl tags" to the segment you want to block. In order to provide enough tags, you need to produce enough SAMe to muffle many DNA containing cells. You have to "tool up". The more genes you wish to stifle, the more SAMe you need.

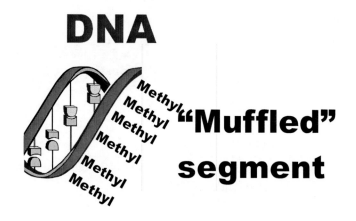

Another source of such DNA is when abnormal DNA replication occurs (or abnormal DNA is inserted into the cell). The Cell has 2 choices to deal with this situation. It can spontaneously abort (apoptosis) or it can tuck the abnormal DNA away somewhere and start again.

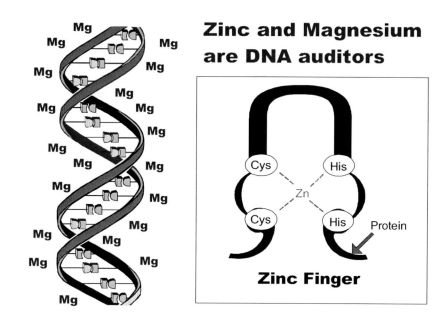

**Zinc and Magnesium are DNA auditors**

**Zinc Finger**

When DNA is copied in preparation for cell division, there is a clever cellular "auditing" system. This provided in the mostly by the minerals Zinc and Magnesium. When these are abundant, they ensure that DNA replication is correct. "We, Zinc and Magnesium herby certify that this is a true copy of the original DNA"; or something similar to that.

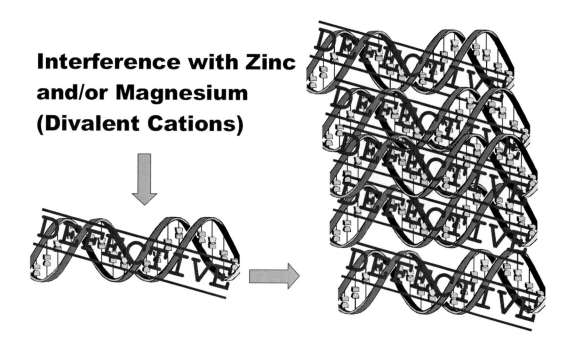

**Interference with Zinc and/or Magnesium (Divalent Cations)**

So we see how low levels (or blockade) of Zinc and/or magnesium will lead to defective DNA synthesis. Other reasons that DNA might be "wrong" for the cell would include chronic intracellular infections like viruses or Mycoplasma's. The cell might try to "silence" this kind of genetic information too, until the organism disables the attempt.

**How to stop Defective DNA being transcribed into proteins?**

Methyl    Methyl   Methyl

Methyl                                    Methyl

Methyl                                    Methyl

**Who provides the Methyl groups?**

# SAMe

Methyl    Methyl    Methyl

If defective DNA is made as a result of low levels or blockade of the divalent cations, then the defective DNA must be silenced until apoptosis can occur. Silencing involves SAMe, which provides the methyl tags.

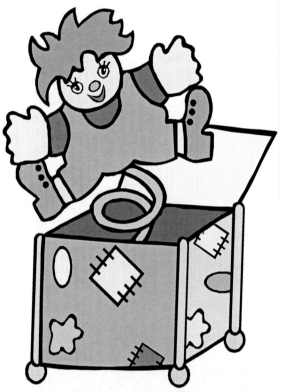

**Bad gene keeps popping up**

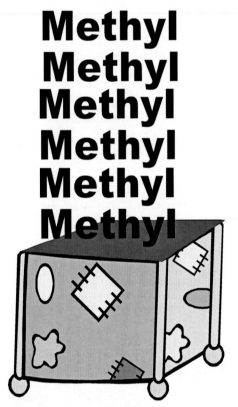

**Methyl**
**Methyl**
**Methyl**
**Methyl**
**Methyl**
**Methyl**

**Methyl "tags" keep gene "volume" low**

This is analogous to having a jack-in-the-box that keeps popping out to scare you. Stack some methyl groups on his lid to keep him under control.

The other choice apart from just silencing the genes is to program the cell to die (apoptosis). Two important requirements for this process are 1] Good ATP levels in the cell and 2] the abundance of Cytochrome C (the mobile cytochrome in the electron transport chain).

The major sites of ATP production are glycolysis, The Krebs (TCA) cycle and the electron transport chain. Examination of the roles of magnesium and iron show these divalent cations to major contributors to cellular ATP production. Therefore disruption to these divalent cations will cause low ATP levels and difficulty in aborting an abnormal cell line. If a cell cannot abort, then it will try to silence any abnormal DNA segments with methyl tags. Therefore in this way low levels or blockade of divalent cations lead to increased methylation.

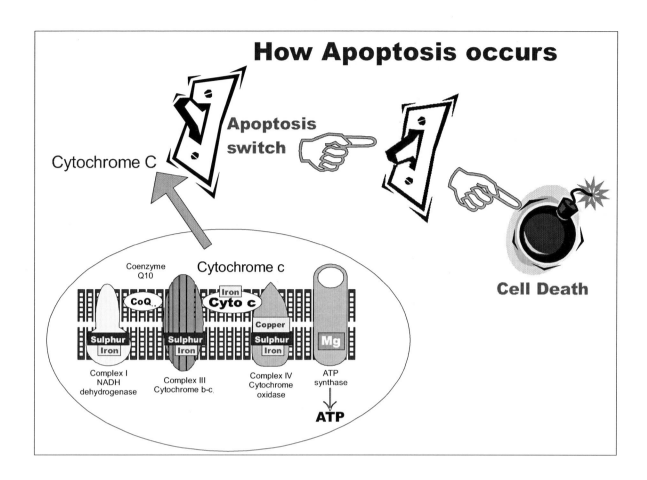

Another mechanism of Apoptosis is the ability of Cytochrome C to leave the Mitochondria and initiate Apoptosis in the cytosol. It is an Iron containing Cytochrome and therefore vulnerable to blockade by Heavy Metals and Copper overload. Again low level (or blockade) of this divalent cation will lead to reduced apoptosis.

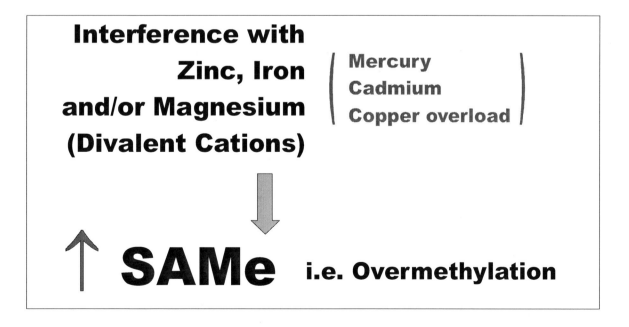

Therefore if divalent cations (like zinc, Magnesium or Iron) are low or blocked there will be an increase in SAMe to deal with the situation. And therefore Cation dysfunction will lead to Overmethylation.

# Current Cytochrome Media Publications
Prices Valid from 1st Februaury 2007

| Product | Type | RRP |
|---|---|---|
| Nutrition: The Good, The Bad & The Politics | Book | $25 |
| Practitioner's Guide to Hair Analysis | Book | $28 |
| Magnesium, Zinc, Iron, Copper etc | Book | $28 |
| Degenerative Diseases of the Brain Book | Book | $28 |
| Brain Foods, Brain Poisons (Autism) | Book | $28 |
| Textbook Of Nutritional Medicine | Book | $75 |
| Whirlwind Tour of Medicine | Audio CD | $25 |
| The Use of Hair Analysis in Chronic Illness | Audio CD | $25 |
| Nutritional Aspects of Arthritis | Audio CD | $25 |
| Nutritional Aspects of Sleep Disorders | Audio CD | $25 |
| Nutritional Aspects of Immunity | Audio CD | $25 |
| Cancer profiling in Nutritional Medicine | Audio CD | $25 |
| Nutritional Aspects of Depression | Audio CD | $25 |
| Nutritional Aspects of Diabetes | Audio CD | $25 |
| Nutritional Aspects of Haemochromatosis | Audio CD | $25 |
| Too Much, Too Young | Audio CD | $25 |
| Introduction to Nutritional Medicine | Audio CD | $25 |
| Brain Foods, Brain Poisons Autism (A) | Audio CD | $25 |
| How to Read A Tissue Mineral Analysis | DVD | $25 |
| Introduction to Nutritional Medicine | DVD | $25 |
| Nutritional Aspects of Arthritis | DVD | $25 |
| Nutritional Aspects of Immunity | DVD | $25 |
| Cancer profiling in Nutritional Medicine | DVD | $25 |
| Nutritional Aspects of Depression | DVD | $25 |
| Nutritional Aspects of Diabetes | DVD | $25 |
| Nutritional Aspects of Haemochromatosis | DVD | $25 |
| Nutritional Aspects of Sleep Disorders | DVD | $25 |
| Brain Foods, Brain Poisons Autism (DVD) | DVD | $25 |
| Degenerative Diseases of the Brain Slide Show | DVD | $25 |
| Oral Chelation Therapies Slide Show | DVD | $25 |

How to find more information.

see www.nutritionreviewservice.com.au

this website will allow you to

1] download an order form to fax

2] order books on-line

3] find a reseller near you

You can also

Ring 08 9342 0471 to order  by credit card

# Suggested Reading List.

1] Edelman, Eva <u>Natural Healing for Schizophrenia and other Common Mental Disorders.</u> Borage Books

2] Ellis, Gregory <u>Autism Body-Brain Connection</u> Targeted Body Systems Publishing

3] Holford, Patrick <u>The Optimum Nutrition Bible</u> Judy Piatkus Ltd

4] Koch Manfred <u>Laugh with Health</u> Renaissance & New Age Creations

5] Lee John R <u>What your Doctor may not tell you about Premenopause</u> Warner Books

6] Lee John R <u>What your doctor may not tell you about breast cancer</u> Warner Books

7] Buist, R <u>The Cholesterol Myth</u> Pan Macmillan Publishers

8] Heinerman, John <u>Nature's Vitamins and Minerals</u> Prentice Hall

9] Aihara, Herman <u>Acid & Alkaline</u> George Ohsawa Macrobiotic Foundation

10] McGilvery <u>Biochemistry A functional Approach</u> Saunders

11] Mark & Marks <u>Basic Medical Biochemistry</u> Williams & Wilkins

12] Osiecki, H <u>The Physician's Handbook of Clinical Nutrition</u> Bioconcepts Publishing

13] Osiecki H <u>The Nutrient Bible</u> Bioconcepts Publishing

14] Osiecki, H <u>Cancer A Nutritional/Biochemical approach</u> Bioconcepts Publishing

15] Pelton et al <u>Drug-Induced Nutrient depletion handbook</u> Lexi-comp Inc

16] Reavley Nicola <u>The New Encyclopaedia of Vitamins, Mineral Supplements and Herbs</u> Bookman Press.

17] Watts, David <u>Trace elements and other essential nutrients</u> Writers Block

18] Zelikoff, J <u>Immunotoxicology of Environmental and Occupational Metals.</u> Taylor & Francis

19] Stringer, G <u>Clinical Issues in Diagnosis of Mercury Toxicity</u> Toowoomba Ed Ctr QLD

20] Williams,R <u>A Physician's Handbook on Orthomolecular Medicine</u> Keats Health Science Books

21] Tabrizian, I <u>Nutritional Medicine Fact & Fiction</u> NRS Publications

22] Tabrizian, I <u>Another dose of Nutritional Medicine</u> NRS Publications

23] Tabrizian, I <u>Practitioner's Guide to reading a TMA</u> NRS Publications

24] Amen, D <u>Healing ADD</u> Berkley Books

25] Medina J <u>What you need to know about Alzheimer'sNew</u> Harbinger Publications

26] Penrose, R <u>Shadows of the Mind</u> Vintage Press

27] Erdmann <u>The Amino Revolution</u> Century Paperbacks

28] Finnin , B <u>Essential Guide to Amino Acids</u> Musashi Publishing

29] Pressman, A <u>The GSH Phenomenon</u> St Martin's Press

30] Passwater, R <u>Trace elements, Hair Analysis and Nutrition</u> Keats Publishing

31] Groff, J et al <u>Advanced Nutrition & Human Metabolism</u> West Publishing

32] Lane, N <u>Oxygen</u> Oxford University Press

33] Mann, J <u>Murder, Magic & Medicine</u> Oxford University Press